SECOND EDITION

CHEMOTHERAPY AND BIOTHERAPY GUIDELINES

AND RECOMMENDATIONS FOR PRACTICE

EDITED BY
Martha Polovich, MN, RN, AOCN®
Julie M. White, RN, BSN, OCN®
Linda O. Kelleher, RN, MS

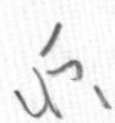

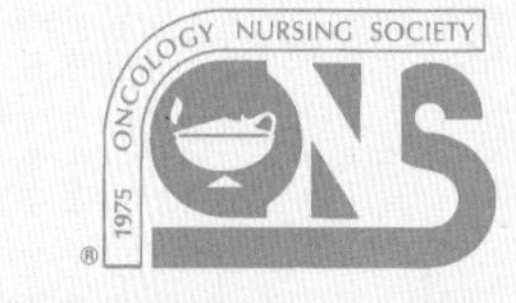

Oncology Nursing Society
Pittsburgh, PA

ONS Publishing Division
Publisher: Leonard Mafrica, MBA, CAE
Director, Commercial Publishing/Technical Editor: Barbara Sigler, RN, MNEd
Production Manager: Lisa M. George, BA
Technical Editor: Judith A. DePalma, PhD, RN
Staff Editor: Lori Wilson, BA
Copy Editor: Amy Nicoletti, BA
Graphic Designer: Dany Sjoen

Chemotherapy and Biotherapy Guidelines and Recommendations for Practice (Second Edition)

First printing, May 2005
Second printing, December 2005
Third printing, September 2006
Fourth printing, June 2007
Fifth printing, December 2007

Library of Congress Control Number: 2005927151

ISBN 1-890504-53-X

Publisher's Note

This manual is published by the Oncology Nursing Society (ONS). ONS neither represents nor guarantees that the practices described herein will, if followed, ensure safe and effective patient care. The recommendations contained in this manual reflect ONS's judgment regarding the state of general knowledge and practice in the field as of the date of publication. The recommendations may not be appropriate for use in all circumstances. Those who use this manual should make their own determinations regarding specific safe and appropriate patient-care practices, taking into account the personnel, equipment, and practices available at the hospital or other facility at which they are located. The editors and publisher cannot be held responsible for any liability incurred as a consequence from the use or application of any of the contents of this manual. Figures and tables are used as examples only. They are not meant to be all-inclusive, nor do they represent endorsement of any particular institution by ONS. Mention of specific products and opinions related to those products do not indicate or imply endorsement by ONS.

ONS publications are originally published in English. Permission has been granted by the ONS Board of Directors for foreign translation. (Individual tables and figures that are reprinted or adapted require additional permission from the original source.) However, because translations from English may not always be accurate or precise, ONS disclaims any responsibility for inaccuracies in words or meaning that may occur as a result of the translation. Readers relying on precise information should check the original English version.

Printed in the United States of America

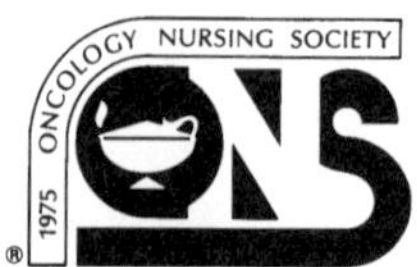

Oncology Nursing Society
Integrity • Innovation • Stewardship • Advocacy • Excellence • Inclusiveness

Contributors

Editors

Martha Polovich, MN, RN, AOCN®
Oncology Clinical Nurse Specialist
Southern Regional Medical Center
Riverdale, Georgia
Fundamentals of Administration: Safe Handling; Mucositis

Julie M. White, RN, BSN, OCN®
Supervisor of Nursing Care
Cancer Care Associates – South Tulsa
Tulsa, Oklahoma
Anorexia; Constipation; Nursing Management of Biotherapy Side Effects

Linda O. Kelleher, RN, MS
Consultant, Oncology Clinical Specialist
Pensacola, Florida
Introduction; Cancer Therapy Goals and Response; Principles of Chemotherapy

Authors

Lois A. Almadrones, RN, MS, FNP, MPA
Clinical Nurse Specialist
Gynecologic Oncology Outpatient
Memorial Sloan-Kettering Cancer Center
New York, New York
Neurotoxicity

Nancy Bowles, RN, BSN, OCN®, CRNI
Director of Clinical Operations
Norton Healthcare, Louisville Oncology
Louisville, Kentucky
Administration of IV Cytotoxic Agents

Theresa Clark, RN
Patient Educator
Patient and Family Education
Cancer Treatment Centers of America
Tulsa, Oklahoma
Care of the Patient Receiving Cancer Therapy

Cindy Jo Horrell, CRNP, MS, AOCN®
Oncology Nurse Practitioner
The Regional Cancer Center
Erie, Pennsylvania
Hepatotoxicity; Pancreatitis

Anne M. Ireland, RN, MSN, AOCN®
Oncology Consultant
Fletcher Allen Health Care
Burlington, Vermont
Alopecia; Alterations in Sexuality and Reproductive Function

Alice S. Kerber, MN, RN, AOCN®
Clinical Nurse Specialist
St. Joseph's Hospital
Atlanta, Georgia
Ethical Issues Related to Cancer Therapy; Legal Issues Related to Cancer Therapy

Kristine B. LeFebvre, MSN, RN, AOCN®
Education Associate
Oncology Nursing Society
Pittsburgh, Pennsylvania
Clinical Practicum; Anorexia; Cutaneous Toxicity; Ocular Toxicity

Eileen Duffey Lind, MSN, RN, CPNP, CPON®
Pediatric Oncology Nurse Practitioner
Dana-Farber Cancer Institute
Boston, Massachusetts
Secondary Malignancies; Post-Treatment Care

Rebecca Long, MSN, RN, OCN®
Consultant – Owner
LONGin' for Quality Health Care
Ephrata, Washington
Cardiac Toxicity; Pulmonary Toxicity

Paula M. Muehlbauer, RN, MSN, OCN®
Clinical Nurse Specialist
Surgical Oncology and Immunotherapy
Clinical Center Nursing Department
National Institutes of Health
Bethesda, Maryland
Principles of Biotherapy

MiKaela Olsen, RN, MS, OCN®
Oncology and Bone Marrow Transplant Clinical Nurse Specialist
Sidney Kimmel Comprehensive Cancer Center at The Johns Hopkins Hospital
Baltimore, Maryland
Gastrointestinal and Mucosal Side Effects

Maureen H. Quick, RN, MS, OCN®
Oncology Nurse Educator/Consultant
Bloomington, Minnesota
Fatigue

Elizabeth Randall, BSN, RN, BC
Unit Educator
St. Jude Children's Hospital
Memphis, Tennessee
Secondary Malignancies; Post-Treatment Care

Stephanie Shields, PharmD
Oncology Clinical Pharmacist
Southern Regional Medical Center
Riverdale, Georgia
Characteristics of Cytotoxic Agents

Tracy Skripac, RN, CNS, MSN, AOCN®, CHPN
Independent Pain and Oncology Nurse Consultant
Canfield, Ohio
Administration of Oral Cytotoxic Agents; Hemorrhagic Cystitis; Nephrotoxicity

Michael Steinberg, BA, BS, PharmD, BCOP
Clinical Pharmacy Specialist in Oncology
Assistant Professor of Pharmacy Practice
Massachusetts College of Pharmacy
Worcester, Massachusetts
Characteristics of Biologic Agents

Wendy Stiver, RN, BSN, MA, OCN®
Instructor/Oncology Care Coordinator
Methodist Hospital of Southern California
Arcadia, California
Pretreatment; Treatment

Cynthia L. Teeple, APRN, BC, MSN, AOCN®
Oncology Nurse Practitioner
Oncology Practice of Abraham Mittelman, MD
Cancer Institute
White Plains, New York
Myelosuppression: Anemia and Thrombocytopenia

Shirley A. Triest-Robertson, RN, PhD, AOCNS
Oncology Clinical Nurse Specialist
St. Vincent Regional Cancer Center
Green Bay, Wisconsin
Treatment Schedule

Jennifer S. Webster, MN, MPH, RN, AOCN®
Clinical Nurse Specialist/Nurse Practitioner
Georgia Cancer Specialists
Atlanta, Georgia
Cancer Therapy Goals and Response; Immediate Complications of Cytotoxic Therapy

Barbara J. Wilson, MS, RN, OCN®, AOCN®, CS
Clinical Nurse Specialist
Oncology Services
WellStar Health System
Marietta, Georgia
Myelosuppression: Introduction and Neutropenia

Field Reviewers

Janice Beschorner, RN, MS, AOCN®
Clinical Nurse Specialist
University of Chicago Hospitals
Chicago, Illinois

Eileen M. Glynn-Tucker, RN, MS, AOCN®
Oncology Clinical Nurse Specialist
Green Oaks, Illinois

Jeanne Held-Warmkessel, MSN, RN, AOCN®, APRN-BC
Clinical Nurse Specialist
Fox Chase Cancer Center
Philadelphia, Pennsylvania

Angela Klimaszewski, MSN, RN
Nurse Consultant
ADK Communications
Canton, New York

Elizabeth Randall, BSN, RN, BC
Unit Educator
St. Jude Children's Hospital
Memphis, Tennessee

Jean Rosiak, RN, BSN, OCN®
Medical Consultant
Milwaukee, Wisconsin

Gail M. Sulski, RN, MS, FNP, AOCN®
Blood and Marrow Transplant Nurse Practitioner
City of Hope/Samaritan Bone Marrow Transplantation Program
Banner Good Samaritan Regional Medical Center
Phoenix, Arizona

Cindy von Hohenleiten, RN, MN
Oncology Clinical Specialist
Amgen Inc.
Suwanee, Georgia

Jan Watkins, RN, MS, OCN®
Oncology Program Coordinator
Liberty Hospital
Liberty, Missouri

Table of Contents

Preface

This edition of the Oncology Nursing Society (ONS) *Chemotherapy and Biotherapy Guidelines and Recommendations for Practice* (2005) is built on the strengths of the previous editions of *Cancer Chemotherapy Guidelines and Recommendations for Practice* (1984, 1988, 1992, 1996, 1999), *Biotherapy: Recommendations for Nursing Course Content and Clinical Practicum* (1995), and *Chemotherapy and Biotherapy Guidelines and Recommendations for Practice* (2001). In addition, the editors and authors have participated in the ONS Chemotherapy and Biotherapy Course and are knowledgeable about both the educational aspects of the course and the clinical aspects of chemotherapy and biotherapy administration and patient care.

The editors of the new edition have responded to suggestions made by users of previous editions and course participants. Based on these suggestions, the content has been reorganized to make it easier to follow, evidence has been cited to provide support for statements of practice, and lists of acronyms and generic/brand-name equivalents are included in the front of the manual for easy reference. The manual also features a comprehensive index to facilitate location of specific content.

The *Guidelines* are again presented in an outline format, which nurses have said they find easy to use. New tables and figures have been added, and previous tables have been updated to provide key information to supplement the text. Information on newly approved drugs (available at the time of publication) also has been included to keep nurses apprised of the latest developments in drug therapy. This manual used evidence where possible. As with other ONS publications, *Chemotherapy and Biotherapy Guidelines and Recommendations for Practice* uses the levels of evidence from strongest to weakest (that is, research-based to non–research-based).

ONS gratefully acknowledges the authors and editors who have participated in previous editions of this manual as well as the editors and authors of the material presented in this edition. The content has undergone an extensive peer review by both outside reviewers and chemotherapy trainers updating the content for the Chemotherapy and Biotherapy Course. Thanks to all who have participated in the development of this publication.

Abbreviations Used in This Manual

ABVD—doxorubicin, bleomycin, vinblastine, dacarbazine

ADCC—antibody-dependent cellular cytotoxicity

ADLs—activities of daily living

ADP—adenosine diphosphate

AHRQ—Agency for Healthcare Research and Quality

ALARA—as low as reasonably achievable

ALL—acute lymphocytic leukemia

AML—acute myelogenous leukemia

ANC—absolute neutrophil count

APC—antigen-presenting cells

ASCO—American Society of Clinical Oncology

ASHP—American Society of Health-System Pharmacists

AST—aspartate aminotransferase

AUC—area under the plasma concentration versus time curve

bFGF—basic fibroblast growth factor

BMT—bone marrow transplant

BSA—body surface area

BSC—biological safety cabinet

BUN—blood urea nitrogen

CBC—complete blood count

CDC—Centers for Disease Control and Prevention

CFU-GM—colony-forming unit–granulocyte macrophage

CHF—congestive heart failure

CIN—chemotherapy-induced neutropenia

CINV—chemotherapy-induced nausea and vomiting

CML—chronic myelogenous leukemia

CN—cranial nerve

CNS—central nervous system

COG—Children's Oncology Group

COPD—chronic obstructive pulmonary disease

CPR—cardiopulmonary resuscitation

CR—complete response

CSF—colony-stimulating factor

CT—computed tomography

CTEP—Cancer Therapy Evaluation Program

CTZ—chemoreceptor trigger zone

CVC—central venous catheter

D5W—5% dextrose in water

DES—diethylstilbestrol diphosphate

DHHS—Department of Health and Human Services

DIC—disseminated intravascular coagulation

DMSO—dimethyl sulfoxide

DNA—deoxyribonucleic acid

DSMB—Data Safety Monitoring Board

EAB—Ethical Advisory Board

ECG—electrocardiogram

ECOG—Eastern Cooperative Oncology Group

EGFR—epidermal growth factor receptor

EPO—erythropoietin

FDA—U.S. Food and Drug Administration

5-FU—5-fluorouracil

$5HT_3$—5-hydroxytryptamine-3

FSH—follicle-stimulating hormone

G-CSF—granulocyte–colony-stimulating factor

GFR—glomerular filtration rate

GI—gastrointestinal

GM-CSF—granulocyte macrophage–colony-stimulating factor

GVHD—graft-versus-host disease

HCT—hematocrit

HEPA—high-efficiency particulate air

Hgb—hemoglobin

HIV—human immunodeficiency virus

HRT—hormone replacement therapy

IARC—International Agency for Research on Cancer

IgG—immunoglobulin G

IL—interleukin

IM—intramuscular

IND—investigational new drug

INS—Intravenous Nurses Society

IRB—Institutional Review Board

IT—intrathecal

IV—intravenous

JCAHO—Joint Commission on Accreditation of Healthcare Organizations

LAK—lymphokine-activated killers

LFT—liver function test

LH—luteinizing hormone

LOC—level of consciousness

MASCC—Multinational Association for Supportive Care in Cancer

MHC—major histocompatibility complex

MOPP—mechlorethamine, vincristine, procarbazine, prednisone

MRI—magnetic resonance imaging

MSDS—material safety data sheet

MUGA—multiple-gated acquisition

MVPP—mechlorethamine, vinblastine, procarbazine, prednisone

NCCN—National Comprehensive Cancer Network

NCI—National Cancer Institute

NF-κB—Nuclear factor-κB

NG—nasogastric

NIH—National Institutes of Health

NIOSH—National Institute for Occupational Safety and Health

NK—natural killer

NPO—nothing by mouth

NRC—U.S. Nuclear Regulatory Commission

NS—normal saline

NSAID—nonsteroidal anti-inflammatory drug

OHRP—Office for Human Research Protections

OSHA—Occupational Safety and Health Administration

PBPC—peripheral blood progenitor cells

PD—progressive disease

PEG—percutaneous endoscopic gastrostomy

PICC—peripherally inserted central catheter

po—oral

PPE—personal protective equipment

PR—partial response

psi—pounds per square inch

PT—prothrombin time

PTT—partial thromboplastin time

RBC—red blood cell

rHu—recombinant human

RIT—radioimmunotherapy

RNA—ribonucleic acid

RSO—radiation safety officer

SIADH—syndrome of inappropriate antidiuretic hormone

SQ—subcutaneous

SSRI—selective serotonin reuptake inhibitor

TC—cytotoxic T cells

TH—helper T cells

TLS—tumor lysis syndrome

TM—memory T cells

TNF—tumor necrosis factor

TPN—total parenteral nutrition

TS—suppressor T cells

VA—vestibular apparatus

VAD—vascular access device

VC—vomiting center

VEGF—vascular endothelial growth factor

VP—ventricular peritoneal

WBC—white blood cell

WHO—World Health Organization

Generic Medications and Brand-Name Equivalents

This list is not comprehensive; more than one company may manufacture or market a product by the same name. Although every effort was made to ensure the accuracy of this information at press time, product and company information change frequently; therefore, the publishers and contributors disclaim responsibility for the accuracy of this list. Before using this information, verify it to ensure that it is up-to-date. Cited trademark status pertains to the United States only. Not all products listed are available in the United States. This list is not an assertion of trademark ownership or an endorsement of any product.

Aldesleukin (IL-2, Proleukin®, Chiron Corp., Emeryville, CA)

Alemtuzumab (anti-CD52, Campath®, Genzyme Corp., Cambridge, MA)

Altretamine (Hexalen®, MGI Pharma, Bloomington, MN)

Anastrozole (Arimidex®, AstraZeneca, Wilmington, DE)

Aprepitant (Emend®, Merck & Co., Inc., Whitehouse Station, NJ)

Arcitumomab (CEA-Scan®, Immunomedics, Inc., Morris Plains, NJ)

Arsenic trioxide (Trisenox®, Cell Therapeutics, Inc., Seattle, WA)

Asparaginase (E. coli asparaginase, Elspar®, Merck & Co., Inc., Whitehouse Station, NJ)

Attapulgite, activated (Kaopectate®, Pfizer Inc., New York, NY)

Azacitidine (Vidaza®, Pharmion Corp., Boulder, CO)

Bevacizumab (anti-VEGF, Avastin®, Genentech, Inc., South San Francisco, CA)

Bicalutamide (Casodex®, AstraZeneca, Wilmington, DE)

Bismuth subsalicylate (Pepto-Bismol®, Procter & Gamble, Cincinnati, OH; Kaopectate®, Pfizer Inc., New York, NY)

Bleomycin sulfate (Blenoxane®, Bristol-Myers Squibb, Princeton, NJ)

Bortezomib (Velcade®, Millennium Pharmaceuticals, Inc., Cambridge, MA)

Busulfan (Myleran®, GlaxoSmithKline, Research Triangle Park, NC)

Calcium polycarbophil (FiberCon®, Wyeth Consumer Healthcare, Madison, NJ; Equalactin®, Numark Laboratories, Edison, NJ)

Capecitabine (Xeloda®, Hoffmann-La Roche Inc., Nutley, NJ)

Carboplatin (Paraplatin®, Bristol-Myers Squibb, Princeton, NJ)

Carmustine (BiCNU®, Bristol-Myers Squibb, Princeton, NJ)

Cetuximab (Erbitux™, ImClone Systems, New York, NY, and Bristol-Myers Squibb, Princeton, NJ)

Chlorambucil (Leukeran®, GlaxoSmithKline, Research Triangle Park, NC)

Cisplatin (Platinol®, Bristol-Myers Squibb, Princeton, NJ)

Cladribine (Leustatin®, Ortho Biotech, Bridgewater, NJ)

Clofarabine (Clolar™, Genzyme Corp., Cambridge, MA)

Cyclophosphamide (Cytoxan®, Bristol-Myers Squibb, Princeton, NJ)

Cytarabine (cytosine arabinoside; ARA-C; Cytosar-U®, Sicor, Inc., Irvine, CA)

Cytarabine liposomal (DepoCyt®, SkyePharma, New York, NY)

Dacarbazine (DTIC-Dome®, Bayer Pharmaceuticals, West Haven, CT)

Dactinomycin (actinomycin-D, Cosmegen®, Merck & Co., Inc., Whitehouse Station, NJ)

Darbepoetin alfa (Aranesp®, Amgen Inc., Thousand Oaks, CA)

Daunorubicin (Cerubidine®, Bedford Laboratories, Bedford, OH)

Daunorubicin liposomal (DaunoXome®, Gilead, Foster City, CA)

Denileukin diftitox (Ontak®, Ligand Pharmaceuticals, San Diego, CA)

Dexamethasone (Decadron®, Merck & Co., Inc., Whitehouse Station, NJ)

Diphenoxylate hydrochloride and atropine sulfate (Lomotil®, Pfizer Inc., New York, NY)

Docetaxel (Taxotere®, Aventis Pharmaceuticals Inc., Bridgewater, NJ)

Dolasetron mesylate (Anzemet®, Aventis Pharmaceuticals Inc., Bridgewater, NJ)

Doxorubicin (Adriamycin®, Bedford Laboratories, Bedford, OH)

Doxorubicin liposomal (Doxil®, Ortho Biotech, Bridgewater, NJ)

Dronabinol (Marinol®, Solvay Pharmaceuticals, Marietta, GA)

Epirubicin (Ellence®, Pfizer Inc., New York, NY)

Erlotinib (Tarceva™, Genentech, Inc., South San Francisco, CA)

Erythropoietin (epoetin alfa; Procrit®, Ortho Biotech, Bridgewater, NJ; Epogen®, Amgen Inc., Thousand Oaks, CA)

Estradiol (Estrace®, Bristol-Myers Squibb, Princeton, NJ)

Estramustine (Emcyt®, Pfizer Inc., New York, NY)

Estrogens, esterified (Menest®, Monarch Pharmaceuticals, Inc., Bristol, TN)

Etoposide (VP-16; Etopophos®, Bristol-Myers Squibb, Princeton, NJ; VePesid®, Bristol-Myers Squibb, Princeton, NJ)

Exemestane (Aromasin®, Pfizer Inc., New York, NY)

Filgrastim (Neupogen®, Amgen Inc., Thousand Oaks, CA)

Floxuridine (FUDR™, Mayne Pharma, Paramus, NJ)

Fludarabine (Fludara®, Berlex Laboratories, Inc., Richmond, CA)

Fluorouracil (5-fluorouracil; 5-FU; Adrucil®, Sicor, Inc., Irvine, CA)

Flutamide (Eulexin®, Schering Corp., Kenilworth, NJ)

Fulvestrant (Faslodex®, AstraZeneca, Wilmington, DE)

Gefitinib (Iressa®, AstraZeneca, Wilmington, DE)

Gemcitabine (Gemzar®, Eli Lilly & Co., Indianapolis, IN)

Gemtuzumab ozogamicin (anti-CD33, Mylotarg®, Wyeth, Madison, NJ)

Goserelin (Zoladex®, AstraZeneca, Wilmington, DE)

Granisetron (Kytril®, Roche Pharmaceuticals, Nutley, NJ)

Generic Medications and Brand-Name Equivalents *(Continued)*

Haloperidol (Haldol®, Ortho-McNeil Pharmaceutical, Inc., Raritan, NJ)

Hydroxyurea (Hydrea®, Bristol-Myers Squibb, Princeton, NJ; Mylocel®, MGI Pharma, Inc., Bloomington, MN)

Ibritumomab tiuxetan (Zevalin®, Biogen Idec, Cambridge, MA)

Idarubicin (Idamycin PFS®, Pfizer Inc., New York, NY)

Ifosfamide (Ifex®, Bristol-Myers Squibb, Princeton, NJ)

Imatinib mesylate (Gleevec®, Novartis Pharmaceuticals Corp., East Hanover, NJ)

Interferon alfa-2a (Roferon-A®, Hoffmann-La Roche Inc., Nutley, NJ)

Interferon alfa-2B (Intron A®, Schering Corp., Kenilworth, NJ)

Interferon gamma (IFN-γ; Actimmune®, InterMune, Inc., Brisbane, CA)

Irinotecan (Camptosar®, Pfizer Inc., New York, NY)

Lepirudin (Refludan®, Berlex Laboratories, Richmond, CA)

Letrozole (Femara®, Novartis Pharmaceuticals Corp., East Hanover, NJ)

Leukocyte interleukin injection (Multikine®, CEL-SCI Corp., Vienna, VA)

Leuprolide (Lupron®, TAP Pharmaceutical Products, Inc., Lake Forest, IL)

Levamisole (Ergamisol®, Janssen Pharmaceutica, Titusville, NJ)

Lomustine (CeeNu®, Bristol-Myers Squibb, Princeton, NJ)

Loperamide (Imodium® AD, McNeil Consumer & Specialty Pharmaceuticals, Ft. Washington, PA; Kaopectate® II, Pfizer Inc., New York, NY; Maalox® Antidiarrheal, Novartis Consumer Health, Parsippany, NJ)

Lorazepam (Ativan®, Biovail Corp., Mississauga, Ontario, Canada)

Mechlorethamine hydrochloride (nitrogen mustard; Mustargen®, Merck & Co., Inc., Whitehouse Station, NJ)

Melphalan (Alkeran®, GlaxoSmithKline, Research Triangle Park, NC)

Mercaptopurine (6-MP; Purinethol®, Teva Pharmaceuticals, North Wales, PA)

Methotrexate (MTX; generic, multiple manufacturers)

Metoclopramide (Reglan®, Baxter Healthcare Corp., Deerfield, IL)

Mitomycin (Mutamycin®, Bristol-Myers Squibb, Princeton, NJ)

Mitotane (Lysodren®, Bristol-Myers Squibb, Princeton, NJ)

Mitoxantrone (Novantrone®, Serono, Inc., Rockland, MA)

Octreotide (Sandostatin®, Novartis Pharmaceuticals Corp., East Hanover, NJ)

Ondansetron (Zofran®, GlaxoSmithKline, Research Triangle Park, NC)

Oprelvekin (IL-11, Neumega®, Wyeth, Madison, NJ)

Oxaliplatin (Eloxatin™, Sanofi-Synthelabo Inc., New York, NY)

Paclitaxel (Taxol®, Bristol-Myers Squibb, Princeton, NJ)

Paclitaxel protein-bound particles for injectable suspension, albumin-bound (Abraxane™, American Pharmaceutical Partners, Inc., Schaumburg, IL)

Palifermin (Kepivance™, Amgen Inc., Thousand Oaks, CA)

Palonosetron (Aloxi®, MGI Pharma, Inc., Bloomington, MN)

Pegaspargase (PEG-L-asparaginase, Oncaspar®, Enzon Pharmaceuticals, Bridgewater, NJ)

Pegfilgrastim (Neulasta®, Amgen Inc., Thousand Oaks, CA)

Pemetrexed (Alimta®, Eli Lilly & Co., Indianapolis, IN)

Pentostatin (Nipent®, SuperGen, Dublin, CA)

Personal lubricants (Astroglide®, Bio-Film, Inc., Vista, CA; Replens®, Lil' Drug Store Products, Inc., Cedar Rapids, IA; K-Y® jelly, McNeil-PPC, Skillman, NJ)

Polyoxyl castor oil (Cremophor® EL, BASF, Florham Park, NJ)

Procarbazine (Matulane®, Sigma-Tau Pharmaceuticals, Gaithersburg, MD)

Prochlorperazine (Compazine®, GlaxoSmithKline, Research Triangle Park, NC)

Raltitrexed (Tomudex®, AstraZeneca, Wilmington, DE)

Rasburicase (Fasturtec®/Elitek®, Sanofi Synthelabo, New York, NY)

Rituximab (anti-CD20, Rituxan®, Genentech, Inc., South San Francisco, CA, and Biogen Idec, Cambridge, MA)

Sargramostim (Leukine®, Berlex Laboratories, Richmond, CA)

Streptozocin (Zanosar®, Sicor, Inc., Irvine, CA)

Tamoxifen (Nolvadex®, AstraZeneca, Wilmington, DE)

Temozolomide (Temodar®, Schering Corp., Kenilworth, NJ)

Teniposide (VM-26, Vumon®, Bristol-Myers Squibb, Princeton, NJ)

Thalidomide (Thalomid®, Celgene Corp., Summit, NJ)

Thioguanine (6-thioguanine, 6-TG, GlaxoSmithKline, Research Triangle Park, NC)

Thiotepa (generic, multiple manufacturers)

Topotecan (Hycamtin®, GlaxoSmithKline, Research Triangle Park, NC)

Toremifene citrate (Fareston®, Orion Pharma, Espoo, Finland)

Tositumomab and iodine I-131 tositumomab (Bexxar®, Corixa Corp., Seattle, WA)

Trastuzumab (anti-HER2/neu, Herceptin®, Genentech, Inc., South San Francisco, CA)

Trimetrexate (Neutrexin®, MedImmune, Inc., Gaithersburg, MD)

Uracil and tegafur (UFT®, Bristol-Myers Squibb, Princeton, NJ)

Valrubicin (Valstar®, Anthra Pharmaceuticals, Princeton, NJ)

Vinblastine (generic, multiple manufacturers)

Vincristine (generic, multiple manufacturers)

Vindesine (Eldisine® [in Canada], Eli Lilly & Co., Indianapolis, IN)

Vinorelbine (Navelbine®, GlaxoSmithKline, Research Triangle Park, NC)

I. Introduction

A. Definition of cancer

1. Cancer historically has been described as a large group of malignant diseases with some or all of the following characteristics (Gribbon & Loescher, 2000; Volker, 2005).
   a) Abnormal cell proliferation caused by a series of cellular and/or genetic alterations or translocations
   b) Lack of controlled growth and division that leads to the formation of tumors and to invasion of tissues that are proximate to tumor cells
   c) Ability to spread (metastasize) to distant site(s) and establish secondary tumors
2. With the discovery of new information about molecular and cellular activity, the current thinking is that cancer may be only a few diseases (Loescher & Whitesell, 2003) that result from faulty or abnormal genetic expression caused by changes that have occurred in DNA.
   a) The transcription of DNA into a single strand of messenger RNA may be changed.
   b) When abnormal messenger RNA exists, the synthesis of amino acids will be changed; thus, the protein structure will be abnormal, as well.
3. Normal cells may undergo the changes as outlined by Loescher and Whitesell (2003) because of
   a) Spontaneous transformation: In this case, there is no suspected causative agent identified, but the cell characteristics become those typical of cancer cells.
   b) Exposure to chemical or physical carcinogens or biologic agents such as viruses: Environmental factors have been extensively studied without definitive causation attributed in most cases. Exposure to substances such as benzenes, radiation, and some chemotherapeutic agents has been implicated in the development of cancers (International Agency for Research on Cancer, 2000; U.S. Department of Health and Human Services [DHHS], 2002).
   c) Genetic alterations: Mutations are permanent changes in DNA sequencing of the base pairs, resulting in a cell with malignant properties. Some mutations are of no concern, but those that give rise to a clone of malignant cells form tumors (Giarelli, Jacobs, & Jenkins, 2002; Loescher & Whitesell, 2003).
4. Figure 1 provides a summary of selected characteristics of tumor cells. The properties of transformed cells are changes in the cytology, cell membrane, and growth and development.

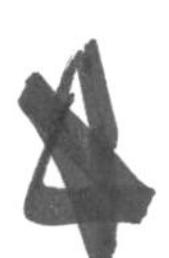

5. Grading and differentiation: Differentiation is based on how closely tumor cells resemble normal cells in their structure and maturity. It is the process of cells developing and becoming fully mature and fully functional. Cells are obtained by biopsy or surgical removal for examination by a cytopathologist. Cancer cells tend to appear different from those of the surrounding tissue. A tumor's level of differentiation can vary over time, and cells with several grades of differentiation may exist within a single tumor. The higher the grade, the more aggressive the tumor (Greene et al., 2002; Griffin-Brown, 2000).
   a) GX—grade cannot be assessed
   b) G1—well differentiated (resembles the parent cell)
   c) G2—moderately differentiated
   d) G3—poorly differentiated (bears little resemblance to the parent cell)
   e) G4—undifferentiated (impossible to tell which cell is the parent)
6. Staging: The purpose of staging is to determine the extent of disease. Staging criteria are unique for each type of cancer.
   a) In general, evaluating stage for solid tumors includes assessing the involvement of three factors.
      (1) T—tumor (local involvement, invasion): The primary tumor is measured to document its size and to determine the depth of invasion of the tumor.
      (2) N—nodes (nodal involvement): Lymph nodes in the area of the primary tumor are examined for the evidence of disease spread. Their size, number, and location are documented.
      (3) M—metastasis (metastatic involvement): Studies are done to determine if the primary tumor has metastasized to distant location(s) (Greene et al., 2002).

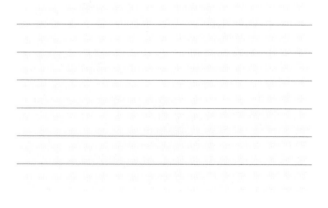

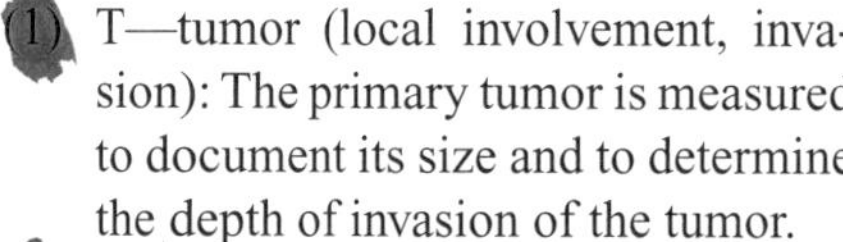

Figure 1. Clonal Evolution in Cancer

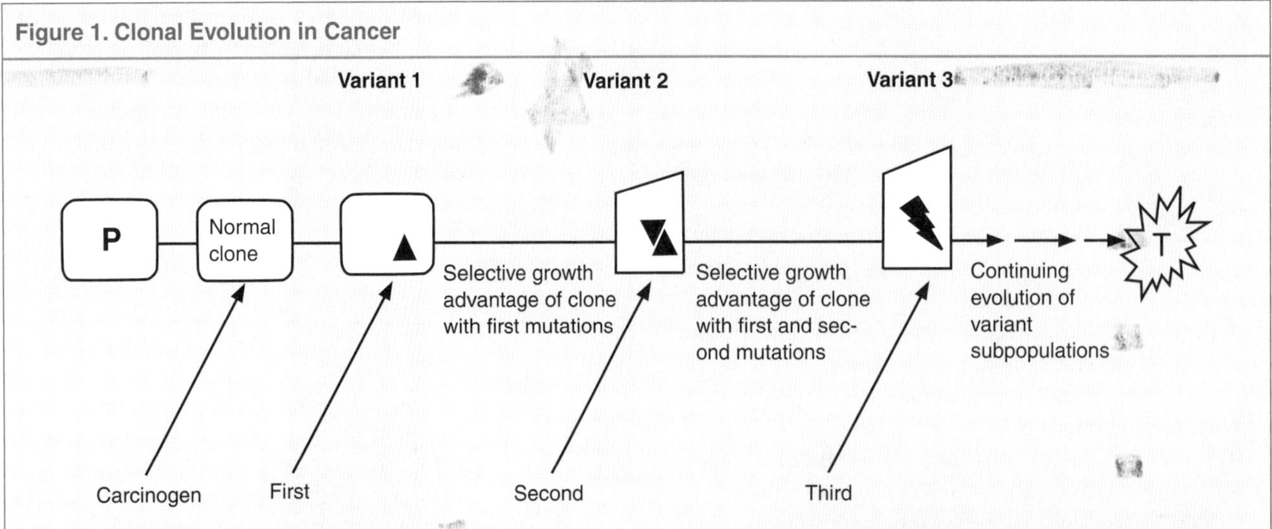

Specific genetic alterations in evolving tumors may range from gene mutations to major chromosomal aberrations (genetic instability). This figure illustrates a carcinogen-induced genetic change in a progenitor normal cell P, which produces a cell with selective growth advantage allowing clonal expansion to begin. In this case, gene mutations produce variant cells. Because they are at a disadvantage metabolically or immunologically, most variant cells are nonviable. If one variant has a selective advantage, its progeny becomes the predominant subpopulation until another variant appears. The sequential selection of variant subpopulations in each tumor (T) differs because of genetic instability, which positively or negatively affects cell proliferation.

Note. From "Biology of Cancer" (p. 18), by J. Gribbon and L.J. Loescher in C.H. Yarbro, M.H. Frogge, M. Goodman, and S.L. Groenwald (Eds.), *Cancer Nursing: Principles and Practice* (5th ed.), 2000, Sudbury, MA: Jones and Bartlett. Copyright 2000 by Jones and Bartlett. Reprinted with permission.

b) Hematologic malignancies are not staged in this manner. Lymphomas, leukemias, and multiple myeloma are recognized as systemic diseases as opposed to solid tumors.

c) Not all pediatric tumors are staged according to these criteria. See Foley, Fochtman, Baggott, and Kelly (2001) for pediatric staging criteria.

7. Depending upon the clinical presentation, laboratory values, and suspected malignancy, specimens obtained may be submitted for cytogenetics, assays for cell surface markers, and other studies.

B. Treatment modalities: A variety of modalities are used to treat cancer. Treatment may include one or more of the following interventions.

1. Surgery (Frogge & Cunning, 2000; Szopa, 2005)
   - *a)* Is a precise local treatment
   - *b)* May remove all of the primary tumor or a portion of it
   - *c)* May be the method of obtaining specimens for cytopathology
   - *d)* May be the only treatment a patient requires
   - *e)* May be preceded or followed by other modalities
   - *f)* May be utilized in the palliative setting to alleviate or lessen symptoms that are intolerable
2. Radiation therapy (Hilderley, 2000; Witt, 2005)
   - *a)* Like surgery, is also local treatment in that a beam is directed at precise target
   - *b)* May follow surgery to prevent recurrence of the primary tumor
   - *c)* Is more effective in some diseases than others
   - *d)* Is sometimes utilized after chemotherapy because radiation can permanently damage bone marrow, making it impossible to give chemotherapy in the doses needed for curative therapy
   - *e)* Often given in combination with chemotherapy (chemoradiation)
3. Chemotherapy/hormonal therapies (Temple & Poniatowski, 2005; Tortorice, 2000)
   - *a)* Are systemic therapies, rather than local treatments, as drugs are distributed throughout the body by the blood stream
   - *b)* May be used as single drugs or more commonly in combination with other drugs
   - *c)* Are limited by toxic effects on normal tissues

d) May have a tumoricidal effect in hormone-sensitive tumors because of reduction or blockage of the source of the hormone or receptor site where hormone is active

4. Biotherapy/targeted agents (Gale, 2005)
   a) Are systemic treatments, like chemotherapeutics and hormonal therapies
   b) May modify the patient's own immune defenses
   c) May be so specific as to target a single receptor on the surface of tumor cells
   d) May require a paradigm shift in nursing's assessment and management of side effects and toxicities
   e) May be combined with other treatment modalities
   f) May promote tumor regression
   g) May stimulate hematopoiesis

C. The drug development process: Although there is a sense of urgency to develop new and better therapies, public protection is of paramount importance. Steps to develop new anticancer agents are complex as well as time- and resource-consuming. The National Cancer Institute (NCI), a division of the National Institutes of Health (NIH) and the U.S. government, examines thousands of chemicals yearly to discover new agents for testing. Only a small percentage are selected for preclinical testing, and even fewer are tested in phase I clinical trials.

1. Development of new cytotoxic and other therapeutic agents (see Table 1)
   a) Preclinical studies: Laboratory research utilizing animal models often is conducted collaboratively between NCI and pharmaceutical companies. The NCI Cancer Therapy and Evaluation Program (CTEP) will seek pharmaceutical sponsorship early once an agent is discovered because NCI does not market new agents. Pharmaceutical companies may seek CTEP codevelopment (Berg, 2000; Wong & Westendorp, 2000).
   b) Preclinical studies do not involve human subjects. Studies comprise a four-step process involving lab analysis and animal subjects (Giacalone, 1997; Wong & Westendorp, 2000).
      (1) Researchers undertake empirical or rational research to develop a new agent or a derivative of an existing agent that is more effective, has fewer side effects, or is less toxic than existing agents.
      (2) The new agent is tested in vitro in various tumor cell lines. If the agent is effective, researchers undertake in vivo testing using mice or other research animals.
      (3) The agent is tested for stability and solubility and dose.
      (4) Researchers perform studies involving animals to predict the initial dose that will be used in human studies.

2. Clinical trials involving humans: The purpose of a clinical trial is to study a new agent or

Table 1. History of Cancer Therapy

Period	Events
Pre 20th Century	• 1500s: Heavy metals are used systemically to treat cancers; however, their effectiveness is limited and their toxicity is great (Burchenal, 1977). • 1890s: William Coley, MD, develops and explores the use of Coley's tonics, the first nonspecific immunostimulants used to treat cancer.
World War I	• Sulfur-mustard gas is used for chemical warfare; servicemen who are exposed to nitrogen mustard experience bone marrow and lymphoid suppression (Gilman, 1963; Gilman & Philips, 1946).
World War II	• Congress passes National Cancer Institute (NCI) Act in 1937. • Alkylating agents are recognized for their antineoplastic effect (Gilman & Philips). • Thioguanine and mercaptopurine are developed (Guy & Ingram, 1996). • 1946: NCI-identified cancer research areas include biology, chemotherapy, epidemiology, and pathology. • 1948: Divisions within NCI and external institutions are identified to conduct research (Zubrod, 1984). • Folic acid antagonists are found to be effective against childhood acute leukemia (Farber et al., 1948). • Antitumor antibiotics are discovered.
1950s	• 1955: National Chemotherapy Program, developed with congressional funding, is founded to develop and test new chemotherapy drugs. • 1957: Interferon is discovered. • The Children's Cancer Group, the first cooperative group dedicated to finding effective treatments for pediatric cancer, is formed.

(Continued on next page)

Table 1. History of Cancer Therapy *(Continued)*

Period	Events
1960s–1970s	• Development of platinum compounds begins. • Multidrug therapy improves remission rate without severe toxicity; MOPP (Mustargen, Oncovin, procarbazine, prednisone), the first combination chemotherapy, is used and found to be curative against Hodgkin disease (Scofield et al., 1991). • Clinical trials of Bacillus Calmette-Guérin and *Corynebacterium parvum*, nonspecific immunostimulants, begin. • Chemotherapy is used with surgery and radiation as cancer treatment. • Development of hybridoma technology begins. • NCI starts its Biological Response Modifier Program.
1970s	• The National Cancer Act of 1971 provides funding for cancer research; director is appointed by and reports to the president of the United States. • Doxorubicin phase I trials begin. • Adjuvant chemotherapy begins to be a common cancer treatment (Bonadonna et al., 1985; Fisher et al., 1986).
1980s	• Community Clinical Oncology Programs are developed in 1983 to contribute to NCI chemotherapy clinical trials. • Use of multimodal therapies increases (Eilber et al., 1984; Marcial et al., 1988). • Focus turns to symptom management to alleviate dose-limiting toxicities related to neutropenia, nausea and vomiting, and cardiotoxicity. • Clinical trials for dexrazoxane (ICRF-187) as a cardioprotectant begin (Speyer et al., 1988). • New chemotherapeutic agents are available. • Researchers begin to investigate recombinant DNA technology. • Trials of monoclonal antibodies and cytokines begin. • Effector cells (lymphokine-activated killer cells and tumor-infiltrating lymphocytes) are grown ex vivo. • 1986: U.S. Food and Drug Administration (FDA) approves interferon alfa. • 1989: FDA approves erythropoietin.
1990s	• New classifications of drugs (e.g., taxanes) are developed. • In clinical trials, paclitaxel is found to be effective against ovarian and breast cancers (Rowinsky et al., 1992). • FDA approves G-CSF and GM-CSF, interleukin-2, interleukin 11, rituximab, trastuzumab, and denileukin diftitox. • Clinical trials of gene therapy and antiangiogenic agents begin. • FDA approves filgrastim for use in bone marrow transplantation and chemotherapy-induced neutropenia, severe chronic neutropenia, and peripheral blood stem cell transplantation. • FDA approves ondansetron for prevention of chemotherapy-induced nausea and vomiting; other 5-hydroxytryptamine-3 ($5HT_3$) receptor antagonists are in clinical trials (Perez, 1995). • As a result of improved symptom management, dose intensity becomes a focus. • FDA approves new analogs (e.g., vinorelbine) (Abeloff, 1995). • Researchers focus on the sequencing of agents (Bonadonna et al., 1995). • The genetic basis of cancers becomes an important factor in cancer risk research (e.g., BRCA1 for breast cancer, renal cell cancer) (Gnarra et al., 1995; Hoskins et al., 1995; Miki et al., 1994). • Aromatase inhibitors are approved for breast cancer treatment. This approval marks a step forward for hormonal therapy.
2000s	• The Children's Oncology Group, a cooperative group combining the efforts of several groups, is formed to further the advancement of cancer treatment for children. • Scientists complete a working draft of the human genome. • FDA approves gemtuzumab ozogamicin. • FDA approves imatinib mesylate, the first molecularly targeted anticancer drug, for use against chronic myelogenous leukemia. • FDA approves approved porfimer sodium injection photodynamic therapy for the treatment of high-grade dysplasia associated with Barrett's esophagus. • Trials involving tumor necrosis factors, angiogenesis inhibitors, and monoclonal antibodies continue.

G–CSF—granulocyte–colony-stimulating factor; GM–CSF—granulocyte macrophage–colony-stimulating factor

combination of agents by involving human volunteers in a scientific experiment. Researchers seek to evaluate the safety, effectiveness, and toxicities of a new drug or drug combinations in humans. Clinical trials are vital to improved patient care. They have played an important role in the reduction of cancer morbidity and mortality (Kosta & Gullatte, 2001).

a) Policies and entities relevant to the protection of human research subjects: In addition to strict federal regulation, multiple regulatory groups oversee the participation of individuals in research.

(1) Regulations are set forth in the Code of Federal Regulations, *Protection of Human Subjects,* 45 CFR 46 (DHHS, 2003).

(2) Institutional Review Boards (IRBs)

(3) Ethical Advisory Boards (EABs)

(4) Data Safety Monitoring Boards (DSMBs)

(5) Office for Human Research Protections (OHRP), within the United States

(6) DHHS

(7) U.S. National Commission for the Protection of Human Subjects of Biomedical and Behavioral Research (Berg, 2000)

b) Drug approval process

(1) If the trial involves a new agent, the U.S. Food and Drug Administration (FDA) approves the agent as an investigational new drug (IND).

(2) Researcher protocols are designed within the academic environment, through NCI, by pharmaceutical companies, or by cooperative research groups.

(3) Table 2 presents an overview of the phases of a clinical trial (Breslin, 2000). Funding may originate from public or private sources.

)A approves the new drug for rcial use when studies docu- ; efficacy and safety.

ig is marketed commercially.

(6) Postmarketing studies are conducted to define new uses for approved drugs, as well as for unexpected toxicities.

c) Pediatric involvement in clinical trials

(1) More than 90% of pediatric patients with cancer (in contrast to only 2%–3% of adult patients) receive treatment at centers affiliated with a multi-institution collaborative research group, such as the Children's Oncology Group (COG). Of patients younger than 15 years old, 50%–60% are enrolled in clinical trials. Of adolescents (15–19 years), 10% are enrolled in clinical trials, as are 2% of young adults (20–30 years). One goal of the COG is to increase the number of young patients participating in clinical trials, especially the number of adolescents and young adults (Bleyer, 2000).

(2) In general, new drugs are tested in adults before researchers undertake studies involving children. In clinical trials with children, the first dose of the agent being studied is usually 80% of the maximum tolerated adult dose.

(3) Because a child's size and metabolism differ significantly from those of an adult, drug data derived from adults may not apply to children. See Smyth and Weindling (1999) for a discussion of protocols that limit the risks of transient hypoxemia and infection and otherwise take into account the uniqueness of the pediatric population.

Trials

Phase	Primary Goals	Characteristics
I	• Establish maximum tolerated dose and dosing schedule • Evaluate toxicity • Determine pharmacokinetics	• Relapsed/refractory disease • Small number of patients • Dose-escalating cohorts • Variety of tumor types • Pharmacokinetic studies
II	• Determine antitumor activity • Evaluate toxicity	• Groups of patients with same tumors • Measurable disease to assess response rates
	• Establish efficacy by assessing survival, time to progression • Obtain quality-of-life data	• Randomization between experimental treatment and standard treatment and/or control group • Large numbers of patients
IV	• Expand "off-label" use • Further assess toxicity data	• Postmarketing trials of commercially available drugs

Note. From "History and Background" (p. 5), by S. Breslin in A.D. Klimaszewski, J.A. Aikin, M.A. Bacon, S.A. DiStasio, H.E. Ehrenberger, and B.A. Ford (Eds.), *Manual for Clinical Trials Nursing,* 2000, Pittsburgh, PA: Oncology Nursing Society. Copyright 2000 by the Oncology Nursing Society. Reprinted with permission.

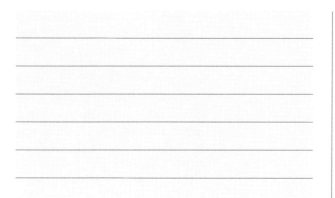

(4) In phase IV studies, dosages may be changed or combinations of approved agents altered in an attempt to maintain or improve cure rate while increasing quality of life and decreasing the late effects of treatment. Incorporating phase IV trials into studies involving children is less common (Gattuso, 2004).

d) Nurses' roles regarding clinical trials: Nurses may

(1) Help patients find clinical trials. A helpful resource in this regard is the NIH's Clinical Trials Web site (http://clinicaltrials.gov/), which lists clinical trials and provides education about clinical trials for the consumer.

(2) Support prospective participants as individuals decide whether to enroll. When a patient is considering participation in a clinical trial, he or she may be facing many stressors in addition to the enrollment decision. Possible stressors include a new diagnosis of cancer or disease progression. Nurses can ease stress and help with decision making by

(a) Ensuring that the patient and/or family understands the purpose of participation in the clinical trial.

(b) Providing educational materials as required. Make certain that all materials presented to patients and families are developmentally appropriate and that content is accurate.

(3) Ensure informed consent if the patient decides to participate: The institution's IRB will review/revise the consent document for format and appropriateness of reading level for the patient and family. A signed consent to participate does not take the place of providing study participants with ongoing information after enrollment. U.S. regulations about informed consent are set forth in the Code of Federal Regulations 45 CFR 46 (DHHS, 2003). This document is the result of a 1995 working group from NCI, the Office of Protection from Research Risks, and the FDA (Klimaszewski, Anderson, & Good, 2000).

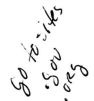

(a) A consent document must (Klimaszewski et al., 2000)

i) State the purposes, duration, and procedures involved in participation.

ii) Describe foreseeable risks and/or benefits of participation.

iii) Disclose treatment alternatives or courses of therapy, if any, that could be advantageous for the patient.

iv) Include a statement describing the extent of confidentiality the study will afford and how confidentiality is protected.

v) State whether compensation is provided.

vi) Include the name of a contact person who can answer questions about the study and the participant's rights.

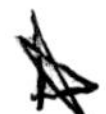

vii) State that participation is voluntary and may be revoked at any time by the patient.

(b) A nurse should ensure that the parents of pediatric patients understand the concepts of assent and dissent as they relate to a child's participation in research. Assent is a child's affirmative agreement to participate in research. Allowing the right to assent honors a child's autonomy to the extent that he or she has developed the capacity to make informed choices (Baylis, Downie, & Kenny, 1999). Dissent is a child's active refusal to participate in research.

i) Both the National Commission for the Protection of Human Subjects of Biomedical and Behavioral Research and the American Academy of Pediatrics Committee on Bioethics recommend honoring a child's dissent; the position taken by DHHS is not as clear-cut. DHHS recommends that dissent be handled on a case-by-case basis and leaves the final determination to the relevant IRB (Broome, 1999). DHHS recommends that the IRB consider the child's age, psychological state, and maturity level and ensure that all explanations are clear, concise, and age-appropriate (Baylis et al., 1999; Broome, 1999).

ii) In regard to pediatric research, parents provide informed consent. Obviously, difficulties arise when parents give consent but the child dissents and vice versa.

(4) Work with trial participants as appropriate. Make certain that all participation by nursing is within the scope of practice guidelines for the state where the patient is receiving care (Frank-Stromborg & Christensen, 2001).

(5) Have a variety of additional responsibilities depending upon the phase of the clinical trial (Aikin, 2000).

(a) Verify that the patient or parent has given informed consent.

(b) Clarify technical explanations of procedures and treatments.

(c) Document pretreatment assessment data (Frank-Stromborg & Christensen, 2001).

(d) Have emergency medications and equipment available as appropriate.

(e) Instruct the patient to report changes or symptoms experienced during and after drug administration.

(f) Administer the drug(s) according to the protocol.

(g) Assess and evaluate drug reactions. Use NCI Common Terminology Criteria for Adverse Events (available online at http://ctep.info.nih.gov/reporting/ctc.html) to document individual toxicities and identify trends in the study population.

(h) Follow up with telephone calls to assess the patient for delayed or chronic side effects as appropriate.

References

Abeloff, M. (1995). Vinorelbine (Navelbine) in the treatment of breast cancer: A summary. *Seminars in Oncology, 22*(Suppl. 5), 1–4.

Aikin, J.L. (2000). Nursing roles in clinical trials. In A.D. Klimaszewski, J.L. Aikin, M.A. Bacon, S.A. DiStasio, H.E. Ehrenberger, & B.A. Ford (Eds.), *Manual for clinical trials nursing* (pp. 273–276). Pittsburgh, PA: Oncology Nursing Society.

Baylis, F., Downie, J., & Kenny, N. (1999). Children and decision making in health research. *IRB: A Review of Human Subjects Research, 21*(4), 5–10.

Berg, D.T. (2000). Sponsoring agencies: Industry. In A.D. Klimaszewski, J.L. Aikin, M.A. Bacon, S.A. DiStasio, H.E. Ehrenberger, & B.A. Ford (Eds.), *Manual for clinical trials nursing* (pp. 33–35). Pittsburgh, PA: Oncology Nursing Society.

Bleyer, A. (2000). COG to lead the adolescent and young adult initiative. *Children's Oncology News, 1*(1), 8.

Bonadonna, G., Valagussa, P., Rossi, A., Brambilla, C., Zambetti, M., & Veronesi, U. (1985). Ten-year experience with CMF-based adjuvant chemotherapy in resectable breast cancer. *Breast Cancer Research and Treatment, 5,* 95–115.

Bonadonna, G., Zambetti, M., & Valagussa, P. (1995). Sequential or alternating doxorubicin and CMF regimens in breast cancer with more than three positive nodes: Ten-year results. *JAMA, 273,* 542–547.

Breslin, S. (2000). History and background. In A.D. Klimaszewski, J.L. Aikin, M.A. Bacon, S.A. DiStasio, H.E. Ehrenberger, & B.A. Ford (Eds.), *Manual for clinical trials nursing* (pp. 3–6). Pittsburgh, PA: Oncology Nursing Society.

Broome, M.E. (1999). Consent (assent) for research with pediatric patients. *Seminars in Oncology Nursing, 15,* 96–103.

Burchenal, J.H. (1977). The historical development of cancer chemotherapy. *Seminars in Oncology, 4,* 135–148.

Eilber, F.R., Morton, D.L., Eckhardt, J., Grant, T., & Weisenburger, T. (1984). Limb salvage for skeletal and soft tissue sarcomas. *Cancer, 53,* 2579–2584.

Farber, S., Diamond, L.K., Mercer, R.D., Sylvester, R.F., & Wolff, J.A. (1948). Temporary remissions in acute leukemia in children produced by folic acid antagonist, 4-aminopteroly-glutamic acid (aminopterin). *New England Journal of Medicine, 238,* 787–793.

Fisher, B., Fisher, E., & Redmond, C. (1986). Ten-year results from the NSABP clinical trial evaluating the use of L-phenylalanine mustard (L-PAM) in the management of primary breast cancer. *Journal of Clinical Oncology, 4,* 929–941.

Foley, G., Fochtman, D., Baggott, C., & Kelly, K.P. (2001). *Nursing care of children and adolescents with cancer* (3rd ed.). Philadelphia: Saunders.

Frank-Stromborg, M., & Christensen, J. (2001). Legal issues in chemotherapy administration. In M.M. Gullatte (Ed.), *Clinical guide to antineoplastic therapy: A chemotherapy handbook* (pp. 281–295). Pittsburgh, PA: Oncology Nursing Society.

Frogge, M.H., & Cunning, S.M. (2000). Surgical therapy. In C.H. Yarbro, M.H. Frogge, M. Goodman, & S.L. Groenwald (Eds.), *Cancer nursing: Principles and practice* (5th ed., pp. 272–283). Sudbury, MA: Jones and Bartlett.

Gale, D.M. (2005). Nursing implications of biotherapy and molecular targeted therapy. In J.K. Itano & K.N. Taoka (Eds.), *Core curriculum for oncology nursing* (4th ed., pp. 763–784). St. Louis, MO: Elsevier.

Gattuso, J.S. (2004). Clinical trials. In N.E. Kline (Ed.), *Essentials of pediatric oncology nursing: A core curriculum* (2nd ed., pp. 80–81). Glenview, IL: Association of Pediatric Oncology Nurses.

Giacalone, S.B. (1997). Cancer clinical trials. In S.E. Otto (Ed.), *Oncology nursing* (3rd ed., pp. 641–665). St. Louis, MO: Mosby.

Giarelli, E., Jacobs, L.A., & Jenkins, J. (2002). Cancer prevention, screening, and early detection: Human genetics. In K. Jennings-Dozier & S. Mahon (Eds.), *Cancer prevention, detection, and control: A nursing perspective* (pp. 99–141). Pittsburgh, PA: Oncology Nursing Society.

Gilman, A. (1963). The initial clinical trial of nitrogen mustard. *American Journal of Surgery, 105,* 574–578.

Gilman, A., & Philips, F.J. (1946). The biological actions of therapeutic applications of b-chloroethyl amines and sulfides. *Science, 103,* 409–415.

Gnarra, J., Lerman, M., Zbar, B., & Linehan, W.M. (1995). Genetics of renal-cell carcinoma and evidence for a critical role for von Hippel-Lindau in renal tumorigenesis. *Seminars in Oncology, 22,* 3–8.

Greene, F.L., Page, D.L., Fleming, I.D., Fritz, A., Balch, C.M., Haller, D.G., et al. (Eds.). (2002). *AJCC cancer staging manual* (6th ed.). New York: Springer

Gribbon, J., & Loescher, L.J. (2000). Cancer biology. In C.H. Yarbro, M.H. Frogge, M. Goodman, & S.L. Groenwald (Eds.), *Cancer nursing: Principles and practice* (5th ed., pp. 18–34). Sudbury, MA: Jones and Bartlett.

Griffin-Brown, J. (2000). Diagnostic evaluation, classification, and staging. In C.H. Yarbro, M.H. Frogge, M. Goodman, & S.L. Groenwald (Eds.), *Cancer nursing: Principles and practice* (5th ed., pp. 214–239). Sudbury, MA: Jones and Bartlett.

Guy, J.L., & Ingram, B.A. (1996). Medical oncology—The agents. In R. McCorkle, M. Grant, M. Frank-Stromborg, & S.B. Baird (Eds.), *Cancer nursing: A comprehensive textbook* (2nd ed., pp. 359–394). Philadelphia: Saunders.

Hilderley, L.J. (2000). Principles of radiation therapy. In C.H. Yarbro, M.H. Frogge, M. Goodman, & S.L. Groenwald (Eds.), *Cancer nursing: Principles and practice* (5th ed., pp. 286–299). Sudbury, MA: Jones and Bartlett.

Hoskins, K., Stopfer, J., Calzone, K., Merajver, S., Rebbeck, T., Garber, J., et al. (1995). Assessment and counseling for women with a family history of breast cancer. *JAMA, 273,* 577–585.

International Agency for Research on Cancer. (2000, June). *IARC monographs on the evaluation of carcinogenic risks to humans ionizing radiation, part 2: Some internally deposited radionuclides* (Vol. 78, pp. 14–21). Retrieved August 28, 2004, from http://www-cie.iarc.fr/htdocs/announcements/vol78.htm

Klimaszewski, A.D., Anderson, S., & Good, M. (2000). Informed consent. In A.D. Klimaszewski, J.L. Aikin, M.A. Bacon, S.A. DiStasio, H.E. Ehrenberger, & B.A. Ford (Eds.), *Manual for clinical trials nursing* (pp. 213–219). Pittsburgh, PA: Oncology Nursing Society.

Kosta, J.A., & Gullatte, M.M. (2001). Clinical trials. In M.M. Gullatte (Ed.), *Clinical guide to antineoplastic therapy: A chemotherapy handbook* (pp. 321–327). Pittsburgh, PA: Oncology Nursing Society.

Loescher, L.J., & Whitesell, L. (2003). The biology of cancer. In A.S. Tranin, A. Masny, & J. Jenkins (Eds.), *Genetics in oncology practice: Cancer risk assessment* (pp. 23–56). Pittsburgh, PA: Oncology Nursing Society.

Marcial, V.A., Pajak, T.F., Kramer, S., Davis, L.W., Steta, J., Laramore, G.E., et al. (1988). Radiation Therapy Oncology Group (RTOG) studies in head and neck cancer. *Seminars in Oncology, 15,* 39–60.

Miki, Y., Swensen, J., Shattuck-Eidens, D., Futreal, P.A., Harshman, K., Tavtigian, S., et al. (1994). A strong candidate for the breast and ovarian cancer susceptibility gene BRCA1. *Science, 266,* 66–71.

Perez, E. (1995). Review of the preclinical pharmacology and comparative efficacy of 5-hydroxytryptamine-3 receptor antagonists for chemotherapy-induced emesis. *Journal of Clinical Oncology, 13,* 1036–1043.

Rowinsky, E., Onetto, N., Canetta, R., & Arbuck, S. (1992). Taxol: The first of the taxanes, an important new class of antitumor agents. *Seminars in Oncology, 19,* 646–662.

Smyth, R.L., & Weindling, A.M. (1999). Research in children: Ethical and scientific aspects. *Lancet, 354*(Suppl. 11), 21–24.

Speyer, J., Green, M., Dramer, E., Rey, M., Sanger, J., Ward, C., et al. (1988). Protective effect of the bispiperazinedione ICRF-187 against doxorubicin-induced cardiac toxicity in women with advanced breast cancer. *New England Journal of Medicine, 319,* 745–752.

Szopa, T.J. (2005). Nursing implications of surgical treatment. In J.K. Itano & K.N. Taoka (Eds.), *Core curriculum for oncology nursing* (4th ed., pp. 736–747). St. Louis, MO: Elsevier.

Temple, S.V., & Poniatowski, B.C. (2005). Nursing implications of antineoplastic therapy. In J.K. Itano & K.N. Taoka (Eds.), *Core curriculum for oncology nursing* (4th ed., pp. 785–801). St. Louis, MO: Elsevier.

Tortorice, P.V. (2000). Chemotherapy: Principles of therapy. In C.H. Yarbro, M.H. Frogge, M. Goodman, & S.L. Groenwald (Eds.), *Cancer nursing: Principles and practice* (5th ed., pp. 352–384). Sudbury, MA: Jones and Bartlett.

U.S. Department of Health and Human Services. (2002). *Report on carcinogens* (10th ed.). Washington, DC: Author.

U.S. Department of Health and Human Services. (2003, October). *Code of federal regulations* (Title 45, Vol. 1, Part 46). Washington, DC: U.S. Government Printing Office. Retrieved November 27, 2004, from http://frwebgate4.access.gpo.gov/cgi-bin/waisgate.cgi?WAISdocID=91939125304+51+0+0&WAISaction=retrieve

Volker, D.L. (2005). Biology of cancer and carcinogenesis. In J.K. Itano & K.N. Taoka (Eds.), *Core curriculum for oncology nursing* (4th ed., pp. 443–464). St. Louis: MO: Elsevier.

Witt, M.E. (2005). Nursing implications of radiation therapy. In J.K. Itano & K.N. Taoka (Eds.), *Core curriculum for oncology nursing* (4th ed., pp. 748–762). St. Louis, MO: Elsevier.

Wong, S.F., & Westendorp, J. (2000). Investigational agents and procurement of research study drugs. In A.D. Klimaszewski, J.L. Aikin, M.A. Bacon, S.A. DiStasio, H.E. Ehrenberger, & B.A. Ford (Eds.), *Manual for clinical trials nursing* (pp. 93–98). Pittsburgh, PA: Oncology Nursing Society.

Zubrod, C.G. (1984). Origins and development of chemotherapy research at the National Cancer Institute. *Cancer Treatment Reports, 68,* 9–19.

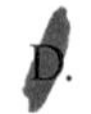

D. Ethical issues related to cancer therapy

1. Healthcare realities that present potential ethical issues
   - *a)* Technologic advances: Advances in technology may allow healthcare professionals to sustain the patient's life longer than ever before. However, this ability may not always be employed for the "right" reasons. Life-sustaining measures may be employed because the healthcare professional
     - (1) Did not discuss the wishes of the patient before a crisis developed
     - (2) Was reluctant to or did not communicate medical treatment options with a grief-stricken family
     - (3) Feared legal liability
     - (4) Followed traditional treatment protocol, which emphasizes treatment

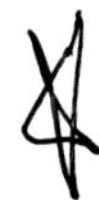

rather than supportive care measures (Marsee, 1994; Pence, 2004; Sheridan, 2000).

b) Changing healthcare environment: Cutbacks in nursing personnel, reallocation of resources, consolidation, and corporatization have resulted in growing administrative dominance over clinical practice (Agency for Healthcare Research and Quality [AHRQ], 2000; Benoliel, 1993; Institute of Medicine, 2004).

c) Increasing numbers of uninsured and insufficiently insured individuals: Children and the working poor are most affected by lack of coverage (Hoffman, Schoen, Rowland, & Davis, 2001; McCabe, 1993), and some people with insurance are unable to obtain reimbursement for certain treatments, such as bone marrow transplant (BMT) (Barr et al., 1996).

d) Increases in a culturally diverse populace: This presents a range of issues, including cultural and communication challenges (Balsa, Seiler, McGuire, & Bloche, 2003).

e) Use of unproven cancer treatments: Increasing use of unproven treatments, either in conjunction with or as a substitute for conventional treatment, is the result of many factors, including the unpredictable nature of individual response to cancer and its treatment, the need for control, belief in individual rights and determination, and cultural and spiritual beliefs (Fletcher, 1992).

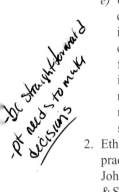

2. Ethical issues that oncology nurses face in daily practice (Cassells, Jenkins, Lea, Calzone, & Johnson, 2003; Ersek, Scanlon, Glass, Ferrell, & Steeves, 1995; Ferrell & Rivera, 1995; Glass, 1994; Gruber, 1998) relate to
   - *a)* End-of-life decisions
   - *b)* Informed consent
   - *c)* Patient autonomy
   - *d)* The right to refuse treatment
   - *e)* Undertreatment of pain
   - *f)* The healthcare environment and reform
   - *g)* Access to care
   - *h)* Confidentiality
   - *i)* Scientific integrity
   - *j)* Nurse-physician conflicts
   - *k)* Physician-family conflicts
   - *l)* Participation in clinical research.

3. The Joint Commission on Accreditation of Healthcare Organizations (JCAHO, 2003) requires that a nurse be able to request an ethics consultation within the clinical institution to assist in evaluating the decision-making capacity of an individual as well as to assist with problem resolution.

4. The characteristics of ethical decisions: Ethical decisions maximize the following (Monagle, 1998).
   - *a)* Autonomy: Independent decision making by an individual in accordance with his or her own best interest
   - *b)* Nonmaleficence: The duty to do no harm
   - *c)* Beneficence: The duty to act in the best interest of the involved person
   - *d)* Justice: Equitable distribution of available resources
   - *e)* Veracity: Truth telling
   - *f)* Fidelity: Faithfulness to promises made
   - *g)* Advocacy: Support given to others to assist in their decision-making ability

E. Legal issues related to cancer therapy: Adhering to national, state, and institutional standards is a fundamental responsibility of all nurses.

1. The acts and standards guiding nursing practice (Frank-Stromborg & Chamorro, 1996)
   - *a)* Nurse practice acts: State laws that define nursing performance in fundamental terms for each state
   - *b)* Oncology Nursing Society *Statement on the Scope and Standards of Oncology Nursing Practice* (Brant & Wickham, 2004) describes the minimum standard of care to which a patient with cancer is entitled.
   - *c)* *Infusion Nursing Standards of Practice* (Infusion Nurses Society, 2000) describes the current standard of nursing practice for IV therapy.
   - *d)* Institution-specific standards may be set forth in
     - (1) Standards of practice
     - (2) Nursing policy and procedure manuals
     - (3) Job descriptions.

2. Common legal issues
   - *a)* Medication errors: A nurse is the final checkpoint in the medication-administration process; therefore, legal issues regarding medication errors frequently affect nurses.
     - (1) Prevalence

(a) In the Institute of Medicine's report (Kohn, Corrigan, & Donaldson, 2000), 3.7% of inpatients experienced an adverse event related to a medication error.
(b) Preventable adverse drug events caused one out of five injuries or deaths to patients in hospitals (AHRQ, 2000).
(c) Sixty-three percent of the oncology nurses that participated in a 1999 study by Schulmeister reported chemotherapy errors in their institutions.

(2) Risks associated with the administration of cytotoxic agents (Birner, 2003; Fischer, Alfano, Knobf, Donovan, & Beaulieu, 1996; Schulmeister, 1997)
(a) Toxicity
(b) Low margin for dosing error (Use of high-dose ablative therapy leaves practically no margin for error.)
(c) Widely varying dosages and administration schedules (Doses and schedules may be patient-specific.)
(d) Doses often are modified based on the patient's clinical status.

(3) Types of chemotherapy medication errors (Schulmeister, 1999)
(a) Administration of the wrong dose (under- or overdosing)
(b) Schedule and timing errors
(c) Use of the wrong drug
(d) Infusion rate errors
(e) Omission of drugs or hydration
(f) Improper drug preparation
(g) Route errors (e.g., intrathecal [IT] versus IV)
(h) Administration to the wrong patient

(4) Factors contributing to medication errors in chemotherapy (Schulmeister, 1999): Most medical errors are system-related and not attributable to individual negligence or misconduct (AHRQ, 2000).

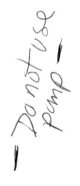

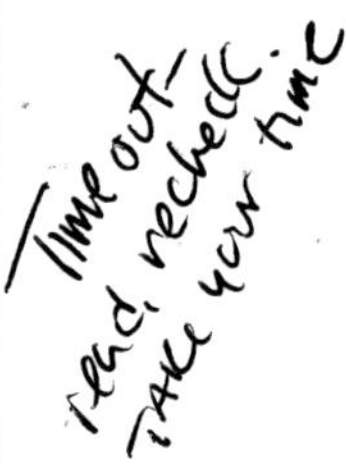

(a) Stress
(b) Understaffing
(c) Lack of experience administering chemotherapy
(d) Unclear or ambiguous chemotherapy orders
(e) Lack of experience administering the specific chemotherapy drug with which the error occurred
(f) Fatigue
(g) Illegible handwriting
(h) Inaccessibility of information about chemotherapy drugs
(i) Chemotherapy drug packaging or vial difficult to read or understand

(5) Strategies for preventing medication errors have been described by Floriddia (2000) and the American Society of Health-System Pharmacists (ASHP, 2002), which include the following.
(a) Verify all pertinent clinical patient information, including patient's height, weight, laboratory results, and body surface area (BSA).
(b) Ensure that up-to-date drug information and other resources are readily available to clinicians.
(c) Institutional policy should not permit verbal orders for chemotherapy.
(d) Use preprinted, standardized forms or computer-generated forms to order cytotoxic drugs when possible.
(e) Avoid the use of abbreviations, acronyms, coined names, and other ambiguous methods of communicating drug information.
(f) Provide ongoing education to patients about their medications, and encourage them to ask questions and seek clarification before their drugs are administered.
(g) Ensure adherence to institutional policies and procedures.
(h) Verify all chemotherapy doses and dosing calculation (see section V, Treatment Schedule). Institution should develop a systematic method of dose verification.
(i) Review orders in an environment with minimal distractions.
(j) Ensure that only experienced oncology nurses who are competent

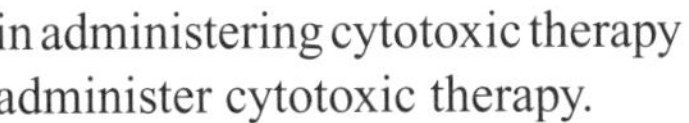

in administering cytotoxic therapy administer cytotoxic therapy.

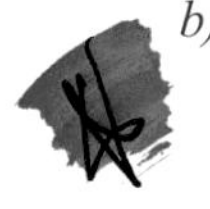

b) Documentation issues (Gialanella, 2004; Schulmeister, 1993): The duty to keep accurate records is one of the nurse's most fundamental legal responsibilities. The patient's medical record is scrutinized in the event of litigious action and is believed to reflect the care rendered (i.e., "If it wasn't charted, it wasn't done").

(1) Common documentation errors include
- *(a)* Omitting observations of significance.
- *(b)* Failing to document the patient's response to an intervention.
- *(c)* Failing to document patient teaching.

(2) Documentation should include the following direct and indirect nursing actions.
- *(a)* Telephone conversations, particularly those in which the nurse gives the patient instructions or advice
- *(b)* Pertinent conversations with the patient, family, or other caregivers
- *(c)* Interagency referrals
- *(d)* Cytotoxic drug administration: See Appendices 1 and 2.
- *(e)* The record should include
  - i) Patient's name
  - ii) Date and time of therapy
  - iii) Drug name, dose, route of administration, and infusion duration
  - iv) Volume and type of fluids administered
  - v) Assessment of the site before and after infusion
  - vi) Information about infusion device (e.g., vein selection, needle size, type of device, infusion pump)
  - vii) Verification of blood return before, during, and after IV therapy
- *(f)* Patient assessment and evaluation of the patient response to and tolerance of treatment
- *(g)* Patient and family education related to drugs received, toxicities, toxicity management, and follow-up care
- *(h)* Post-treatment or discharge instructions

c) Issues related to informed consent: The patient must give an informed consent for treatment, enrollment in a clinical trial, or participation in nursing research (Baylis, 1999; Berry, Dodd, Hinds, & Ferrell, 1996).

(1) Informed consent implies the right of the patient to refuse or discontinue treatment at any time.

(2) Nurses must assure patients that ongoing support and care will be provided if they decline or discontinue treatment connected with the trial or research.

(3) Nurses and physicians have complementary roles in the informed consent process.

(4) Elements of the informed consent process include competence, disclosure, understanding, voluntariness, and consent (Beauchamp & Childress, 1994; Monagle, 1998).

References

Agency for Healthcare Research and Quality. (2000). *Translating research into practice: Reducing errors in health care* (AHRQ Publication No. 00-PO58). Rockville, MD: Author. Retrieved August 27, 2004, from http://www.ahrq.gov/research/errors.htm

American Society of Health-System Pharmacists. (2002). ASHP guidelines on preventing medication errors with antineoplastic agents. *American Journal of Health-System Pharmacists, 59,* 1648–1668.

Balsa, A., Seiler, N., McGuire, T., & Bloche, M. (2003). Clinical uncertainty and healthcare disparities. *American Journal of Law and Medicine, 29*(2–3), 203–219.

Barr, R., Furlong, W., Henwood, J., Feeny, D., Wegener, J., Walker, I., et al. (1996). Economic evaluation of allogeneic bone marrow transplantation: A rudimentary model to generate estimates for the timely formulation of clinical policy. *Journal of Clinical Oncology, 14,* 1413–1420.

Baylis, F., Downie, J., & Kenny, N. (1999). Children and decision making in health research. *IRB: A Review of Human Subjects Research, 21*(4), 5–10.

Beauchamp, T.L., & Childress, J.F. (1994). *Principles of biomedical ethics* (4th ed.). New York: Oxford University Press.

Benoliel, J.Q. (1993). The moral context of oncology nursing. *Oncology Nursing Forum, 20*(Suppl.10), 5–12.

Berry, D.L., Dodd, M.J., Hinds, P.S., & Ferrell, B.R. (1996). Informed consent: Process and clinical issues. *Oncology Nursing Forum, 23,* 507–512.

Birner, A. (2003). Safe administration of chemotherapy. *Clinical Journal of Oncology Nursing, 7,* 158–162.

Brant, J.M., & Wickham, R.S. (Eds.). (2004). *Statement on the scope and standards of oncology nursing practice.* Pittsburgh, PA: Oncology Nursing Society.

Cassells, J.M., Jenkins, J., Lea, D.H., Calzone, K., & Johnson, E. (2003). An ethical assessment framework for addressing global genetic issues in clinical practice. *Oncology Nursing Forum, 30,* 383–390.

Ersek, M., Scanlon, C., Glass, E., Ferrell, B.R., & Steeves, R. (1995). Priority ethical issues in oncology nursing: Current approaches and future directions. *Oncology Nursing Forum, 22,* 803–807.

Ferrell, B.R., & Rivera, L.M. (1995). Ethical decision making in oncology: A case study approach. *Cancer Practice, 3,* 94–99.

Fischer, D., Alfano, S., Knobf, M., Donovan, C., & Beaulieu, N. (1996). Improving the cancer chemotherapy use process. *Journal of Clinical Oncology, 14,* 3148–3155.

Fletcher, D.M. (1992). Unconventional cancer treatments: Professional, legal, and ethical issues. *Oncology Nursing Forum, 19,* 1351–1354.

Floriddia, D.G. (2000). *Management of medical errors.* Paper presented at the American Pharmaceutical Association Annual Meeting, Washington, DC. Retrieved August 24, 2004, from http://www.medscape.com/viewarticle/419163?src=search

Frank-Stromborg, M., & Chamorro, T. (1996). Legal responsibilities of the nurse. In R. McCorkle, M. Grant, M. Frank-Stromborg, & S.B. Baird (Eds.), *Cancer nursing: A comprehensive textbook* (2nd ed., pp. 1388–1408). Philadelphia: Saunders.

Gialanella, K. (2004). Documentation. *Advance for Nurses, 6*(14), 17–19.

Glass, E. (1994, December). Coordinator's message: Ethics SIG survey results. *Ethics Special Interest Group Newsletter, 5*(2), 1, 4.

Gruber, A. (1998). Social systems and professional responsibility. In J. Monagle & D. Thomasma (Eds.), *Health care ethics: Critical issues for the 21st century* (pp. 392–397). Gaithersburg, MD: Aspen.

Hoffman, C., Schoen, C., Rowland, D., & Davis, L. (2001). Gaps in health care coverage in working age Americans and the consequences. *Journal of Health Care for the Poor and Underserved, 12,* 272–289.

Infusion Nurses Society. (2000). Infusion nursing standards of practice. *Journal of Intravenous Nursing, 23*(Suppl. 6).

Institute of Medicine. (2004). *Keeping patients safe: Transforming the work environment of nurses.* Washington, DC: National Academies Press.

Joint Commission on Accreditation of Healthcare Organizations. (2003). *Comprehensive accreditation manual for hospitals.* Oakbrook Terrace, IL: Author.

Kohn, L.T., Corrigan, J.M., & Donaldson, M.S. (Eds.). (2000). *To err is human: Building a safer health system.* Washington, DC: National Academies Press.

Marsee, V. (1994). Ethical dilemmas in the delivery of intensive care to critically ill oncology patients. *Seminars in Oncology Nursing, 10,* 156–164.

McCabe, M.S. (1993). The ethical context of healthcare reform. *Oncology Nursing Forum, 20*(Suppl. 10), 35–43.

Monagle, J. (1998). Ethically responsible creativity-friendship of an understanding heart: A cognitively affective model for bioethical decision-making. In J. Monagle & D. Thomasma (Eds.), *Health care ethics: Critical issues for the 21st century* (pp. 566–577). Gaithersburg, MD: Aspen.

Pence, G.E. (2004). *Classic cases in medical ethics* (4th ed.).New York: McGraw-Hill Higher Education.

Schulmeister, L. (1993). Documentation issues in oncology nursing. *Current Issues in Cancer Nursing Practice Updates, 1*(9), 1–8.

Schulmeister, L. (1997). Preventing chemotherapy dose and schedule errors. *Clinical Journal of Oncology Nursing, 1,* 79–85.

Schulmeister, L. (1999). Chemotherapy medication errors: Description, severity and contributing factors. *Oncology Nursing Forum, 26,* 1033–1042.

Sheridan, C. (2000). Ethical dimensions in cancer care. In B. Nevidjon & K. Sowers (Eds.), *A nurse's guide to cancer care* (pp. 469–478). Philadelphia: Lippincott Williams & Wilkins.

note - drug in solution
time started - duration infused
site assessed - portacath - picc, which lumen - blood return
Before + After administration
response to therapy
teachings - instructions

II. Cancer Therapy Goals and Response

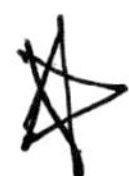

A. Goals of cancer therapy

1. Cure
   - *a)* The desired outcome for all patients, but one that is not always achievable
   - *b)* *Cure* refers to the prolonged absence of detectable disease.
2. Control
   - *a)* An extension of life when cure is unrealistic
   - *b)* Preventing the growth of cancer cells without complete elimination of the disease
3. Palliation
   - *a)* Comfort when supposed cure or control of the disease is impossible
   - *b)* Reduction of side effects and symptoms, including pain (Bender, 1998; Ellison & Chevlen, 2002)
4. Adjuvant therapy: Therapy following the primary treatment modality, such as surgery or radiation. The goal of adjuvant therapy is to target minimal disease or micrometastases for patients at high risk for recurrence (Otto, 2001; Perry, Anderson, & Donehower, 2000).
5. Neoadjuvant therapy: The use of chemotherapy prior to surgery or another treatment modality. Goal is to shrink the primary tumor to improve surgical removal and/or decrease the likelihood of micrometastases (Otto, 2001; Perry et al., 2000).
6. Chemoprevention: Use of selected pharmaceutical agents to prevent cancer in high-risk individuals (e.g., administration of tamoxifen to women whose personal health history indicates they are at a statistically increased risk for developing breast cancer) (Loescher & Reid, 2000; Sporn & Lippman, 2003)
7. Myeloablation: Obliteration of bone marrow in preparation for peripheral blood stem cell or bone marrow transplantation

B. Factors affecting response to treatment

1. Tumor burden: The inverse relationship between the number of tumor cells and response implies that the smaller the tumor, the higher the rate of response (Evans & Bitran, 2001).
2. Rate of tumor growth: Tumor *doubling time* (time for the tumor to double in mass) and *growth fraction* (proportion of proliferating cells in relation to the total number of tumor cells) are important factors affecting response. Chemotherapeutic agents are most active against rapidly growing tumors (Evans & Bitran, 2001; Otto, 2001).
3. Combination versus single-agent therapy (Burris, 2001; Haskell, 2001; Langhorne & Barton-Burke, 2001): Tumor cell populations are heterogeneous; therefore, a combination of agents with different mechanisms of action is able to increase the proportion of cells killed at any one time.
   - *a)* Combination chemotherapy reduces the possibility of drug resistance by using drugs that have different mechanisms of action.
   - *b)* Agents selected for use in combination chemotherapy have a proven efficacy as single agents and have minimally overlapping end organ toxicity.
   - *c)* Combination chemotherapy may use the principle of drug synergy to maximize the effects of another drug. Synergy is affected by the rate of tumor cell proliferation, as well as by whether the drugs are administered sequentially or simultaneously (e.g., leucovorin potentiates the cytotoxicity of 5-fluorouracil [5-FU]) (Brown & Humble, 2001).
4. Dose or dose intensity (dose over total time of delivery) of chemotherapy
   - *a)* Bonadonna, Valagussa, Moliterni, Zambetti, and Brambilla (1995) reported a significant survival benefit for patients with early-stage breast cancer who received ≥ 85% of the standard chemotherapy dose.
   - *b)* Current research efforts are directed toward reducing the amount of time between standard doses of chemotherapy to increase dose density (Citron et al., 2003; Pfreundschuh et al., 2004). By reducing the time between chemotherapy cycles, tumor regrowth may be diminished.
   - *c)* Nurses should be aware that dose reduction or delay resulting from chemotherapy side effects, scheduling conflicts, or any other reason may have a negative impact on patient survival. Proactive management of symptoms and educating patients on the importance of maintaining the prescribed dosing schedule is paramount.
5. Hormone receptor status: Tumors that grow more rapidly in the presence of a certain

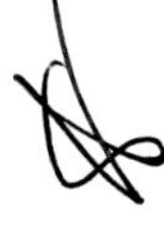

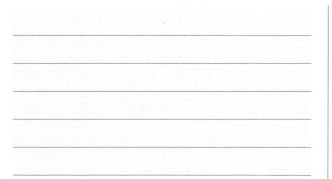

hormone may be suppressed with the administration of an antihormonal agent. This factor has become increasingly important in cancer therapy.

6. Drug resistance: Tumor cells may be inherently resistant to antineoplastic agents or develop resistance after exposure to these drugs. Single-agent or multidrug resistance may occur.
   - *a)* Cells may temporarily be less responsive, because of changes in environment or stimuli, or have permanent resistance (Goldie, 2001).
   - *b)* Preventing drug resistance is one of the primary justifications for combination chemotherapy.
   - *c)* Overcoming established resistance is a focus of current research (Burris, 2001; Kwitkowski & Daub, 2004; Langhorne & Barton-Burke, 2001; Tortorice, 2000). The presence of a multidrug resistant gene is being explored, with current efforts directed to the *p53* gene. Loss of *p53* function has been implicated in the reduced effectiveness of a variety of chemotherapeutic agents (Kwitkowski & Daub).

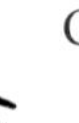

C. Measuring response
1. Measuring tumor response
   - *a)* A tumor is assessed through surgical examination, physical examination, imaging studies, and/or serum tumor markers at the time of diagnosis. Response to treatment administered is determined through comparative measurements of this information. Those tests that provided information upon which to base treatment decisions are repeated.
   - *b)* Tumor response has historically been classified according to the following categories (Perry et al., 2000).
     - (1) *Complete response* (CR): Absence of all signs and symptoms of cancer for at least one month using objective criteria (e.g., quantitative bidimensional tumor measurement)
     - (2) *Partial response* (PR): At least a 50% reduction of measurable tumor mass for one month without development of new tumors
     - (3) *Stable disease* (SD): A reduction in tumor mass of less than 50% or less than a 25% increase in tumor growth
     - (4) *Progressive disease* (PD): Growth of 25% or more or development of new tumors
     - (5) *Relapse:* After CR, a new tumor appears or the original tumor reappears. Or, with PR, a new tumor appears or the original tumor increases in size.
   - *c)* Response Evaluation Criteria in Solid Tumors (RECIST) guidelines: The new guidelines were developed in 1999 by an international task force. These guidelines were presented to scientists and then submitted to NCI for official publication (Therasse et al., 2000). Although not widely used at present, this system continues to gain favor and should facilitate communication between researchers and clinicians.
     - (1) The World Health Organization (WHO) (Therasse et al., 2000) recognizes that new technologies (e.g., computed tomography [CT] scans, magnetic resonance imaging [MRI]) have led to confusion regarding three-dimensional measurement of disease. As a result, the reported response criteria vary among research groups.
     - (2) RECIST guidelines include the following (Therasse et al., 2000).
       - *(a)* Response to a clinical trial is used to decide if an agent or regimen demonstrated results that are promising enough to warrant further testing (prospective end point).
       - *(b)* In further trials, tumor response provides an estimate of benefit for a specific group of patients.
       - *(c)* Response to treatment guides the clinician and patient about continuing with the same therapy.
       - *(d)* If distinctions are not explicit, tumor response can be missed, ignored, or inappropriately evaluated. This may cause incorrect results or conclusions.
       - *(e)* At baseline, tumors must be measurable in at least one dimension

(using metrics) by calipers or a ruler. Baseline measurements must be within four weeks of initiating therapy. (Nonmeasurable lesions include bone lesions, ascites, pleural or pericardial effusions, leptomeningeal disease, and inflammatory breast cancer.)

(f) The same method and technique used at baseline must be used to evaluate response for reporting and follow-up.

(g) If the primary end point is response to treatment, the patient must have at least one measurable lesion at baseline. If only one measurable lesion is present, it must be confirmed by cytology or histology.

(h) Measurable lesions, up to 5 per organ or 10 in total, are identified as "target" lesions. Those selected are the longest in diameter and also suitable for follow-up measurement. The sum of the longest diameter for each lesion is calculated and reported as the baseline sum longest diameter. This sum is used as the reference to compare response. All other non–target lesions are measured and recorded if possible. Their presence or absence can be noted for follow-up but is not included in the response evaluation.

(3) Using RECIST criteria

(a) CR is the disappearance of all target lesions.

(b) PR is a 30% reduction in the sum of the longest diameter of target lesions as compared to the baseline.

(c) PD is a 20% increase in the longest diameter compared to the smallest sum recorded since treatment was initiated.

(d) Follow-up should be protocol-specified. Every other cycle (6–8 weeks) is reasonable for follow-up. Patients who discontinue therapy because of deterioration of their health condition without evidence of PD are identified as "symptomatically deteriorated." At the conclusion of treatment, follow-up will depend upon the goal of the study. If time is the primary end point of the study, measurements must be compared to the baseline. The duration of overall response is measured from when the measurement criteria were met for CR or PR until the first date a recurrence or PD was measured. The duration of stable disease is the time from initiation of therapy until the criteria are met for PD.

(4) Reporting using RECIST results: All patients in the study must be assessed at the end of the study. Patients are assigned to one of the following categories.

(a) CR

(b) PR

(c) Stable disease

(d) PD

(e) Early death from disease

(f) Early death from toxicity

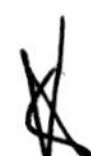

2. Measuring patient response

a) Response according to performance status scales. After tumor type, patient activity level or performance status is the most important factor to consider when determining appropriate treatment (Ellison & Chevlen, 2002). See Table 3, which compares three different performance status scales.

(1) Eastern Cooperative Oncology Group (ECOG) and Zubrod scales: Evaluate adult performance on 0–5 scales; a higher score indicates poorer performance (Oken et al., 1982).

(2) Karnofsky Performance Status scale: Evaluates adult performance in terms of percentage; a lower score indicates poorer performance (Karnofsky & Burchenal, 1949).

(3) Lansky: Evaluates the performance of children ages 10 and younger (Manne et al., 1996)

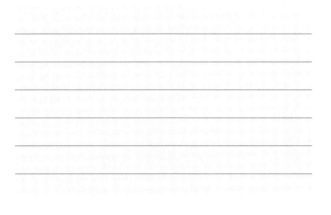

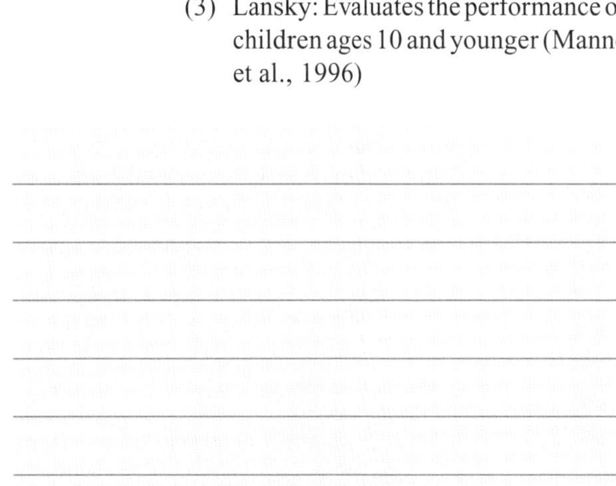

Table 3. Performance Status Scales/Scores[a]

ECOG (Zubrod)		Karnofsky		Lansky[b]	
Score	**Description**	**Score**	**Description**	**Score**	**Description**
0	Fully active, able to carry on all pre-disease performance without restriction	100	Normal, no complaints, no evidence of disease.	100	Fully active, normal
		90	Able to carry on normal activity; minor signs or symptoms of disease.	90	Minor restrictions in physically strenuous activity.
1	Restricted in physically strenuous activity but ambulatory and able to carry out work of a light or sedentary nature, e.g., light housework, office work.	80	Normal activity with effort; some signs or symptoms of disease.	80	Active, but tires more quickly.
		70	Cares for self, unable to carry on normal activity or do active work.	70	Both greater restriction of and less time spent in play activity.
2	Ambulatory and capable of all self care but unable to carry out any work activities. Up and about more than 50% of waking hours.	60	Requires occasional assistance, but is able to care for most of his/her needs.	60	Up and around, but minimal active play; keeps busy with quieter activities.
		50	Requires considerable assistance and frequent medical care.	50	Gets dressed, but lies around much of the day; no active play; able to participate in all quiet play and activities.
3	Capable of only limited self care, confined to bed or chair more than 50% of waking hours	40	Disabled, requires special care and assistance.	40	Mostly in bed, participates in quiet activities.
		30	Severely disabled, hospitalization indicated. Death not imminent.	30	In bed; needs assistance even for quiet play.
4	Completely disabled. Cannot carry on any self care. Totally confined to bed or chair.	20	Very sick, hospitalization indicated. Death not imminent.	20	Often sleeping; play entirely limited to very passive activities.
		10	Moribund, fatal processes progressing rapidly.	10	No play; does not get out of bed.

[a] Karnofsky and Lansky performance scores are intended to be multiples of 10.
[b] The conversion of the Lansky to ECOG scales is intended for NCI reporting purposes only.

Note. From *Oncology Nursing Essentials* (p. 105), by M.P. Lynch, 2002, New York: Professional Publishing Group. Copyright 2002 by Professional Publishing Group. Reprinted with permission.

b) Subjective patient response: Evaluation is based on the patient's perception of changes in symptoms, activity level, quality of life, and other factors. These factors may reflect the effect of treatment even if objective parameters do not demonstrate change (Ellison & Chevlen, 2002).

References

Bender, C. (1998). Implications of antineoplastic therapy for nursing. In J.K. Itano & K.N. Taoka (Eds.), *Core curriculum for oncology nursing* (3rd ed., pp. 641–656). Philadelphia: Saunders.

Bonadonna, G., Valagussa, P., Moliterni, A., Zambetti, M., & Brambilla, C. (1995). Adjuvant cyclophosphamide, methotrexate, and fluorouracil in node-positive breast cancer: The results of 20 years of follow-up. *New England Journal of Medicine, 332,* 901–906.

Brown, D., & Humble, A. (2001). Cellular mechanisms of chemotherapy. In M.M. Gullatte (Ed.), *Clinical guide to antineoplastic therapy: A chemotherapy handbook* (pp. 1–11). Pittsburgh, PA: Oncology Nursing Society.

Burris, H.A. (2001). Combination chemotherapy. In M.C. Perry (Ed.), *The chemotherapy source book* (3rd ed., pp. 69–73). Philadelphia: Lippincott Williams & Wilkins.

Citron, M.L., Berry, D.A., Cirrincione, C., Hudis, C., Winer, E.P., Gradishar, W.J., et al. (2003). Randomized trial of dose-dense versus conventionally scheduled and sequential versus concurrent combination chemotherapy as postoperative adjuvant treatment of node-positive primary breast cancer: First report of Intergroup Trial C9741/Cancer and Leukemia Group B Trial 9741. *Journal of Clinical Oncology, 21,* 1431–1439.

Ellison, N.M., & Chevlen, E.M. (2002). Palliative chemotherapy. In A. Berger, R. Portenoy, & D. Weissman (Eds.), *Principles and practice of palliative care and supportive oncology* (2nd ed., pp. 698–709). Philadelphia: Lippincott Williams & Wilkins.

Evans, A.M., & Bitran, J.D. (2001). Adjuvant chemotherapy. In M.C. Perry (Ed.), *The chemotherapy source book* (3rd ed., pp. 48–69). Philadelphia: Lippincott Williams & Wilkins.

Goldie, J.H. (2001). Drug resistance. In M.C. Perry (Ed.), *The chemotherapy source book* (3rd ed., pp. 37–48). Philadelphia: Lippincott Williams & Wilkins.

Haskell, C.M. (2001). Principles of cancer chemotherapy. In C. Haskell (Ed.), *Cancer treatment* (5th ed., pp. 62–86). Philadelphia: Saunders.

Karnofsky, D.A., & Burchenal, J.H. (1949). The clinical evaluation of chemotherapeutic agents in cancer. In C. MacLeod (Ed.), *Evaluation of chemotherapeutic agents* (pp. 191–205). New York: Columbia University Press.

Kwitkowski, V., & Daub, J. (2004). Clinical applicaitons of genetics in sporadic cancers. *Seminars in Oncology Nursing, 20,* 155–163.

Langhorne, M., & Barton-Burke, M. (2001). Chemotherapy administration: General principles for nursing practice. In M. Barton-Burke, G. Wilkes, & K. Ingwersen (Eds.), *Cancer chemotherapy: A nursing process approach* (3rd ed., pp. 608–643). Sudbury, MA: Jones and Bartlett.

Loescher, L.J., & Reid, M.E. (2000). Dynamics of cancer prevention. In C.H. Yarbro, M.H. Frogge, M. Goodman, & S.L. Groenwald (Eds.), *Cancer nursing: Principles and practice* (5th ed., pp. 135–149). Sudbury, MA: Jones and Bartlett.

Manne, S., Miller, D., Meyers, P., Wollner, N., Steinherz, P., & Redd, W.H. (1996). Depressive symptoms among parents of newly diagnosed children with cancer: A 6-month follow-up study. *Children's Health Care, 25,* 191–209.

Oken, M.M., Creech, R.H., Tormey, D.C., Horton, J., Davis, T.E., McFadden, E.T., et al. (1982). Toxicity and response criteria of the Eastern Cooperative Oncology Group. *American Journal of Clinical Oncology, 5,* 649–655.

Otto, S.E. (2001). Chemotherapy. In S. Otto (Ed.), *Oncology nursing* (4th ed., pp. 638–671). St. Louis, MO: Mosby.

Perry, M.C., Anderson, S.M., & Donehower, R.C. (2000). Chemotherapy. In M. Abeloff, J. Armitage, A. Lichter, & J. Niederhuber (Eds.), *Clinical oncology* (2nd ed., pp. 378–422). Philadelphia: Churchill Livingstone.

Pfreundschuh, M., Truemper, L., Kloess, M., Schmits, R., Feller, A.C., Ruebe, C., et al. (2004). 2-weekly or 3-weekly CHOP chemotherapy with or without etoposide for the treatment of elderly patients with aggressive lymphomas: Results of the NHL-B2 trial of the DSHNHL. *Blood, 104,* 634–641.

Sporn, M.B., & Lippman, S.M. (2003). Chemoprevention of cancer. In D. Kufe, R. Pollack, R. Weichselbaum, R. Bast, T. Ganster, J. Holland, et al. (Eds.), *Cancer medicine* (6th ed., pp. 413–422). Hamilton, Ontario, Canada: BC Decker.

Therasse, P., Arbuck, S.G., Eisenhauer, E.A., Wanders, J., Kaplan, R.S., Rubenstein, L., et al. (2000). New guidelines to evaluate the response to treatment in solid tumors. *Journal of the National Cancer Institute, 92,* 205–214.

Tortorice, P.V. (2000). Chemotherapy: Principles of therapy. In C.H. Yarbro, M.H. Frogge, M. Goodman, & S.L. Groenwald (Eds.), *Cancer nursing: Principles and practice* (5th ed., pp. 352–384). Sudbury, MA: Jones and Bartlett.

be careful about how you talk to pts -
be proactive about things
↑ temp
constipation diarrhea
call office
- follow up calls

III. Principles of Chemotherapy

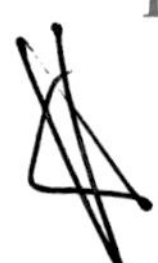

A. Life cycle of cells (Brown & Humble, 2001; Otto, 2001; Vermeulen, Van Bockstaele, & Berneman, 2003): The cell life cycle is a five-stage reproductive process occurring in both normal and malignant cells (see Figure 2).

1. **Gap 0 (G0),** resting phase: Cells are temporarily out of the cycle and not actively proliferating, while all other cellular activities are occurring. Cells continue in this phase until there is a stimulus to enter the active cell cycle, leading to cell division. Because they are not dividing, cells in G0 phase are considered protected from exposure to many chemotherapeutic agents.
2. **Gap 1 (G1),** postmitotic phase: Cells begin an active phase of reproduction. Proteins and RNA are synthesized during this time.
3. **Synthesis (S):** DNA is synthesized.
4. **Gap 2 (G2),** premitotic (or postsynthetic) phase: Further protein synthesis occurs. Preparation for mitotic spindles is occurring. The cell is now prepared to actively divide.
5. **Mitosis (M):** Cell division occurs. Timewise, this is the shortest phase of the cell life cycle. At the conclusion of mitosis, two daughter cells have been formed. They either reenter the life cycle to again reproduce or begin to perform the activities of the tissue they are designed to be (G0).

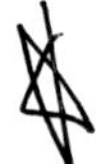

B. Chemotherapeutic agents: Drugs are classified according to pharmacologic action or their effect on cell reproduction (i.e., the cell life cycle as described above). See Table 4.

1. **Cell-cycle– or phase-specific drugs** exert effect within a specific phase of the cell cycle

Figure 2. Cell Life Cycle

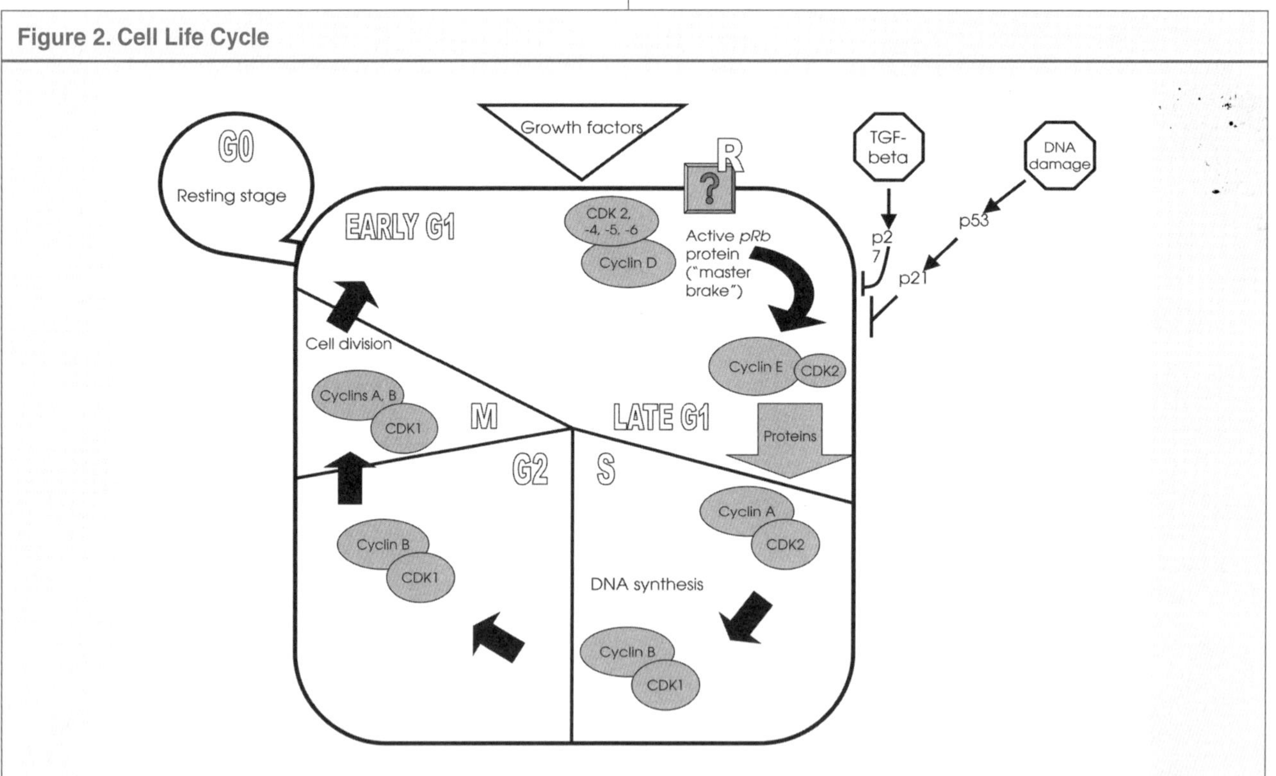

The cell cycle consists of four active stages (G1, S, G2, M) that are controlled by proteins called cyclins. The cyclins (D, E, A, B) activate upon forming complexes with enzymes called cyclin-dependent kinases (CDKs). Upon activation, the cyclin-CDK complexes allow the cell to progress through each specific cell-cycle stage. Present throughout the cell cycle, the cyclin-CDK complexes serve as checkpoints, or monitors, of the cell cycle. Inhibitory proteins—such as p21, p27, and p53—prevent progression through the cell cycle if DNA damage is present or if the nutrients or oxygen necessary to support cellular proliferation is in short supply. Inhibitory proteins, in turn, are regulated by inhibitory growth factors and *TGFB.* Cyclin-CDK complexes and pRb ("the master brake") tightly regulate the R (restriction) point. Once past R, the cell cycle "turns on," and progression through the cell cycle is inevitable. The stability of the inhibitory proteins and cyclin-CDK complexes are altered in cancer. Normal cell-cycle controls are absent and uncontrolled cellular proliferation prevails.

Note. From "Biology of Cancer" (p. 26), by J. Gibbon and L. Loescher in C.H. Yarbro, M.H. Frogge, M. Goodman, and S.L. Groenwald (Eds.), *Cancer Nursing: Principles and Practice* (5th ed.), 2000, Sudbury, MA: Jones and Bartlett. Copyright 2000 by Jones and Bartlett, www.jbpub.com. Adapted with permission.

(Brown & Humble, 2001; Chu & DeVita, 2001; Hande, 1999).

a) These drugs have the greatest tumor-cell kill when given in divided but frequent doses, or as a continuous infusion with a short cycle time. This will allow the maximum number of cells to be exposed to the drug at the specific time in their life cycle where they are vulnerable to the drug.

b) Classifications include antimetabolites, plant alkaloids (camptothecins, epipodophyllotoxins, taxanes, and vinca alkaloids), and miscellaneous agents.

2. **Cell-cycle– or phase-nonspecific drugs** exert effect in all phases of the cell cycle, including the G0 resting phase (Brown & Humble, 2001; Chu & DeVita, 2001; Hande, 1999).

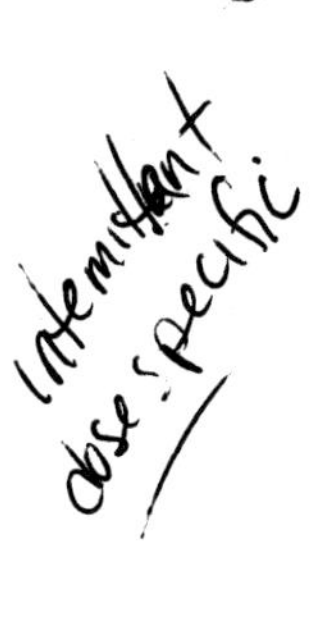

a) Cell-cycle–nonspecific drugs also are effective in treating tumors with more slowly dividing cells.

b) If the cancer is sensitive to the agent used, the drug is incorporated into the cell. The cell kill may not be instantaneous but may occur when the cell attempts to divide. The destruction of tumor cells will be directly proportional to the amount of the drug administered. These drugs are given intermittently, allowing the individual to recover from dose-limiting toxicities before the drug is repeated. The most frequent of the dose-limiting toxicities is the suppression of the bone marrow.

c) Classifications include alkylating agents, antitumor antibiotics, hormonal therapies, and nitrosoureas.

References

Ascherman, J.A., Knowles, S.L., & Atkiss, K. (2000). Docetaxel (Taxotere) extravasation: A report of five cases with treatment recommendations. *Annals of Plastic Surgery, 45,* 438–441.

Brown, D., & Humble, A. (2001). Cellular mechanisms of chemotherapy. In M.M. Gullatte (Ed.), *Clinical guide to antineoplastic therapy: A chemotherapy handbook* (pp. 1–11). Pittsburgh, PA: Oncology Nursing Society.

Camp, M.J., Gullatte, M.M., Gilmore, J.W., & Hutcherson, D.A. (2001). Antineoplastic agents. In M.M. Gullatte (Ed.), *Clinical guide to antineoplastic therapy: A chemotherapy handbook* (pp. 71–279). Pittsburgh, PA: Oncology Nursing Society.

Chu, E. (2003). *Physician's cancer chemotherapy drug manual.* Sudbury, MA: Jones and Bartlett.

Chu, E., & DeVita, V.T. (2001). Principles of cancer management: Chemotherapy. In V.T. DeVita, S. Hellman, & S.A. Rosenberg (Eds.), *Cancer: Principles and practice of oncology* (6th ed., pp. 300–301). Philadelphia: Lippincott Williams & Wilkins.

Cleri, L.B. (2002). *Oncology pocket guide to chemotherapy* (5th ed.). Philadelphia: Elsevier.

Hande, K. (1999). Principles and pharmacology of chemotherapy. In G.R. Lee, J. Foerster, J. Lukens, F. Paraskevas, J.P. Greer, & G.M. Rodgers (Eds.), *Wintrobe's clinical hematology* (10th ed., pp. 2091–2092). Philadelphia: Lippincott Williams & Wilkins.

Otto, S.E. (2001). Chemotherapy. In S.E. Otto (Ed.), *Oncology nursing* (4th ed., pp. 638–671). St. Louis, MO: Mosby.

Pui, C.H., Ribeiro, R.C., Hancock, M.L., Rivera, G.K., Evans, W.E., Riamondi, S.C., et al. (1991). Acute myeloid leukemia in children treated with epipodophyllotoxins for acute lymphoblastic leukemia. *New England Journal of Medicine, 12,* 1682–1687.

Solimando, D.A. (2003). *Drug information handbook for oncology* (3rd ed.). Hudson, OH: Lexi-Comp.

Vermeulen, K., Van Bockstaele, D.R., & Berneman, Z.N. (2003). The cell cycle: A review of regulation, deregulation, and therapeutic targets in cancer. *Cell Proliferation, 36*(3), 131–149.

Weiss, R.B. (2001). Hypersensitivity reactions. In M.C. Perry (Ed.), *The chemotherapy source book* (3rd ed., pp. 436–452). Philadelphia: Lippincott Williams & Wilkins.

Table 4. Characteristics of Cytotoxic Agents

Classification	Mechanism of Action	Medication Name(s)	Route of Administration	Indications	Side Effects	Nursing Considerations
Alkylating agent	Breaks DNA helix strand, thereby interfering with DNA replication	Altretamine (Hexalen®)	po	Ovarian cancer	Nausea, vomiting, myelosuppression, neurotoxicity, hypersensitivity, skin rash, elevation of LFTs, flu-like syndrome, abdominal cramps, diarrhea	Monitor for neurologic toxicity.
		Busulfan (Myleran®)	IV, po	CML, BMT preparation	Myelosuppression, hyperuricemia, hyperpigmentation, alopecia, gynecomastia, sperm or ovarian suppression, seizures, mucositis, pulmonary fibrosis. At high doses, nausea and vomiting.	Monitor blood count closely. If the leukocyte count is < 15,000/mm³, discontinue the drug. Administer seizure prophylaxis. Instruct patients to take on an empty stomach to decrease risk of nausea and vomiting.
		Carboplatin (Paraplatin®)	IV	Ovarian, testicular, head and neck, cervical, bladder, and lung cancers; brain tumors; BMT	Thrombocytopenia, neutropenia, (myelosuppression is more pronounced with renal impairment), nausea, vomiting, hypersensitivity reaction; renal toxicity and hepatic toxicity are uncommon.	Carboplatin exhibits much less renal toxicity than does cisplatin, so rigorous hydration is unnecessary. Monitor blood counts closely, and reduce the dose per protocol.
		Chlorambucil (Leukeran®)	po	CLL, Hodgkin disease, non-Hodgkin lymphoma	Myelosuppression, ovarian or sperm suppression, nausea, vomiting, secondary malignancy, hyperuricemia, pulmonary fibrosis, seizure (increase risk in children with nephrotic syndrome)	Toxicity may increase if the patient has used barbiturates. Contraindicated in patients with seizure history and within one month of radiation and/or cytotoxic therapy.
		Cisplatin (Platinol®)	IV	Ovarian, testicular, bladder, cervical, breast, lung, prostate, and head and neck cancers; multiple myeloma; Hodgkin disease; non-Hodgkin lymphoma; leukemias; Wilms' tumor; brain tumors	Severe nephrotoxicity, nausea, vomiting, myelosuppression, ototoxicity, neurotoxicity, hyperuricemia, hypersensitivity reaction, hypomagnesemia, peripheral neuropathy	Cisplatin has vesicant potential if > 20 ml of concentrated solutions 0.5 mg/ml is extravasated. If less, cisplatin is an irritant. Hold the drug if the patient's serum creatinine is > 1.5 mg/dl; otherwise, irreversible renal tubular damage may occur. Amifostine may be used as a renal protectant. Rigorous hydration is necessary to prevent nephrotoxicity. Use mannitol to achieve osmotic diuresis. Obtain a baseline audiogram.

(Continued on next page)

Table 4. Characteristics of Cytotoxic Agents *(Continued)*

Classification	Mechanism of Action	Medication Name(s)	Route of Administration	Indications	Side Effects	Nursing Considerations
Alkylating agent *(cont.)*		Cyclophosphamide (Cytoxan®)	Intrapleural, IV, po	Breast and ovarian cancers, multiple myeloma, leukemias, lymphoma, neuroblastoma, retinoblastoma	Hemorrhagic cystitis, vomiting, myelosuppression, nausea, alopecia, secondary malignancy, testicular or ovarian failure; with high-dose therapy, syndrome of inappropriate antidiuretic hormone High dose: acute cardiomyopathy	Give the dose, whether IV or po, early in the day. Ensure adequate hydration. If the dose is po, have patients drink plenty of fluids. Have patients empty their bladder frequently to prevent hemorrhagic cystitis. Pelvic irradiation potentiates hemorrhagic cystitis. When used with radiation therapy, potential for radiation recall exists with subsequent doses of cyclophosphamide.
		Dacarbazine (DTIC®)	IV	Malignant melanoma, soft-tissue sarcoma, Hodgkin disease, neuroblastoma	Neutropenia, thrombocytopenia (with nadir at 2–3 weeks or more), severe nausea and vomiting for up to 12 hours, anorexia, alopecia, rash, flu-like syndrome, hypotension, hypersensitivity reaction (uncommon), photosensitivity, hepatic dysfunction	Dacarbazine is an irritant. Administer by infusion over 30–60 minutes. Can cause severe pain and burning at the injection site and along the course of the vein. To reduce these effects, increase the diluent, reduce the infusion rate, and apply cold compresses to the needle insertion site and along the vein. Protect solution from light (pink solution indicates decomposition). Flu-like syndrome may occur up to seven days after drug administration; treat symptoms. Reduce doses for patients with poor renal function.
		Ifosfamide (Ifex®)	IV	Lung, testicular, and head and neck cancers; non-Hodgkin lymphoma; sarcomas	Hemorrhagic cystitis, nausea, alopecia, vomiting, myelosuppression, neurotoxicity	Administer the drug over 30 minutes or more. To prevent hemorrhagic cystitis, always administer ifosfamide with mesna. Mesna may be given orally, as a bolus dose, continuous infusion, or mixed in the bag with the ifosfamide. Mesna dose should be 60%–100% of the ifosfamide dose (based on weight). Refer to package insert for specific dosing recommendations.
		Mechlorethamine (nitrogen mustard, Mustargen®)	IV	Hodgkin disease, non-Hodgkin lymphoma, CLL, CML, mycosis fungoides	Severe nausea, vomiting, alopecia, myelosuppression, pain or phlebitis at IV site, chills, fever, testicular or ovarian failure	Drug is a vesicant. Administer the agent over several minutes, through the side arm of a free-flowing IV. Flush with 125–150 ml NS. If extravasation occurs, the antidote is sodium thiosulfate. Use mechlorethamine as soon after preparation as possible (15–30 minutes); it is extremely unstable. Do not mix mechlorethamine with any other drug.

(Continued on next page)

Table 4. Characteristics of Cytotoxic Agents *(Continued)*

Classification	Mechanism of Action	Medication Name(s)	Route of Administration	Indications	Side Effects	Nursing Considerations
Alkylating agent *(cont.)*		Melphalan (Alkeran®)	IV, po	Multiple myeloma; ovarian, testicular and breast cancers; melanoma, sarcoma, certain types of brain tumors, BMT	Myelosuppression, nausea, vomiting, mucositis, hypersensitivity reaction	Melphalan IV is an irritant. Myelosuppression may be delayed and last four to six weeks, so monitor blood counts carefully. Hold or reduce dose per institutional protocol. Instruct patients to take on an empty stomach.
		Oxaliplatin (Eloxatin®)	IV	Metastatic colorectal cancer	Neurotoxicity, nausea, vomiting, diarrhea, myelosuppression	Consider a dose reduction in patients with renal dysfunction. Monitor for acute, reversible effects and persistent neurotoxicity. For three to four days, patients should avoid consuming cold drinks and foods and breathing cold air (cover mouth with scarf). Do not prepare or infuse in sodium chloride or other chloride-containing solutions. 5% dextrose solution is recommended.
		Temozolomide (Temodar®)	po	Treatment of adult patients with refractory anaplastic astrocytoma who have experienced disease progression on nitrosoureas and procarbazine	Myelosuppression, nausea, vomiting, headache, fatigue, photosensitivity	Warn patient to avoid sun exposure for several days after therapy.
		Thiotepa (Thioplex®)	IV, SQ, IM, IT, intravesical, ophthalmic, intratumoral	Bladder, breast, and ovarian cancers; Hodgkin disease; lymphoma; brain tumors; BMT	Myelosuppression, ovarian or sperm suppression, nausea, vomiting, pain at infusion site, rash, fever, skin burn, mucositis, hemorrhagic cystitis	Thiotepa is primarily excreted in the urine; monitor renal function carefully. Take skin care measures when using high-dose therapy.
Antimetabolite	Azacitidine is believed to cause hypomethylation of DNA and direct cytotoxicity on abnormal hematopoietic cells in the bone marrow. Abnormal cells, including cancer cells, no longer respond to normal growth control mechanisms. The cytotoxic effects of azacitidine cause the death of these cells, whereas nonproliferating cells are relatively insensitive to the medication.	Azacitidine (Vidaza®)	SQ	Indicated for the treatment of patients with specific subtypes of myelodysplastic syndrome	Bone marrow suppression (including neutropenia, thrombocytopenia, and anemia), nausea, vomiting, diarrhea, fatigue, fever, erythema at injection site, elevated serum creatinine, renal failure, hypokalemia, renal tubular acidosis, hepatic coma	Gently roll syringe between palms to mix medication immediately prior to administration. Divide doses > 4 ml into two syringes and inject into two separate sites. Rotate sites for administration among thigh, abdomen, and upper arm. Administer new injections at least one inch from old site. Avoid sites that are tender, bruised, red, or hard. Monitor CBC and liver and renal function during therapy. Drug is contraindicated in patients with hypersensitivity to azacitidine or mannitol and those with advanced malignant hepatic tumors. Medication has been shown to have teratogenic effects. Female patients should avoid becoming pregnant while taking this medication. Male patients should be advised not to father a child while receiving therapy.

(Continued on next page)

Table 4. Characteristics of Cytotoxic Agents *(Continued)*

Classification	Mechanism of Action	Medication Name(s)	Route of Administration	Indications	Side Effects	Nursing Considerations
Antimetabolites (*cont.*)	Acts in S phase; inhibits enzyme production for DNA synthesis, leading to strand breaks or premature chain termination	Capecitabine (Xeloda®)	po	Breast cancer, metastatic colon cancer	Diarrhea, hand-foot syndrome, mucositis, nausea, vomiting, anemia, increased bilirubin	Patient education regarding reporting toxicity and dose reduction is critical. Contraindicated in patients with known hypersensitivity to 5-FU. Monitor patients on warfarin closely.
		Cladribine (Leustatin®)	IV	Hairy cell leukemia, non-Hodgkin lymphoma	Myelosuppression, fever, nausea, vomiting, neurotoxicity, hypersensitivity reaction, tumor lysis syndrome	Allopurinol and IV hydration are recommended for patients with high tumor burden to prevent tumor lysis syndrome. Use with caution in patients with liver and renal dysfunction.
	A purine nucleoside antimetabolite that inhibits DNA repair by incorporation into the DNA chain during the repair process.	Clofarabine (Clolar™)	IV	Treatment of patients 1–21 years old with relapsed or refractory acute lymphoblastic leukemia after at least two prior regimens	Nausea, vomiting, diarrhea, bone marrow suppression (including anemia, leukopenia, thrombocytopenia, neutropenia, and febrile neutropenia), infection, hepatobiliary toxicity, renal toxicity; rare cases of systemic inflammatory response syndrome/ capillary leak syndrome and cardiac toxicity, including tachycardia, pericardial effusion, and left ventricular systolic dysfunction, infection	Continuous IV fluid administration during the five days of chemotherapy administration is encouraged to reduce the risk of tumor lysis syndrome and other adverse effects. Use of prophylactic steroids may help to prevent systemic inflammatory response syndrome and capillary leak syndrome. Allopurinol should be given if hyperuricemia is expected. Monitor respiratory status and blood pressure during infusion. Monitor renal and hepatic function during the days of administration. Monitor hematologic status closely following treatment.
		Cytarabine (cytosine arabinoside, ARA-C, Cytosar-U®)	IV, SQ, IT, IM	ALL, AML, CML, Hodgkin and non-Hodgkin lymphoma, CNS leukemia	Myelosuppression, nausea, vomiting, anorexia, fever, mucositis, diarrhea, hepatic dysfunction, pruritus, localized pain and/ or thrombophlebitis at IV site; photophobia (treat with dexamethasone ophthalmic drops) High dose: cerebellar toxicity, keratitis	Determine if the ordered dose is a standard dose or a high dose; administer the agent according to institutional guidelines. For IT administration: Use preservative-free saline. Allopurinol and IV hydration are recommended for newly diagnosed patients with AML or patients with high tumor burden to prevent tumor lysis syndrome.

(Continued on next page)

Table 4. Characteristics of Cytotoxic Agents *(Continued)*

Classification	Mechanism of Action	Medication Name(s)	Route of Administration	Indications	Side Effects	Nursing Considerations
Antimetabolite *(cont.)*		Cytarabine liposomal (DepoCyt®)	IT only	Lymphomatous meningitis	High dose: mucositis, diarrhea	Not used in pediatrics Administer IT only. Patients should lie flat for one hour after lumbar puncture. Monitor closely for immediate toxic reactions.
		Floxuridine (FUDR®)	Intra-arterial, IV	Adenocarcinoma of GI tract with metastasis to liver, gallbladder, or bile duct	Myelosuppression, nausea, vomiting, diarrhea, mucositis, alopecia, photosensitivity, darkening of the veins, abdominal pain, gastritis, enteritis, hepatotoxicity, hand-foot syndrome	Not used in pediatrics Recommendations about dose reduction apply to patients with compromised liver function. Adjust dose per institutional protocol and monitor patient's hepatic function carefully.
		Fludarabine (Fludara®)	IV	CLL, low-grade lymphoma, BMT	Myelosuppression, nausea, vomiting, diarrhea, rash, neurotoxicity, interstitial pneumonitis	Administer this drug as a 30-minute infusion. Fludarabine has been used experimentally as a continuous infusion. Monitor pulmonary function tests. Allopurinol and IV hydration are recommended for newly diagnosed patients with CLL or patients with high tumor burden to prevent tumor lysis syndrome.
		Fluorouracil (5-fluorouracil, 5-FU, Adrucil®)	IV, topical	Colorectal, breast, liver, ovarian, pancreatic, stomach, esophageal, and head and neck cancers	Myelosuppression, nausea, anorexia, vomiting, diarrhea, mucositis, alopecia, photosensitivity, darkening of the veins, dry skin; cardiac toxicity is rare.	Ensure that patient takes year-round photosensitivity precautions; encourage sunscreen use if patient must be exposed. Leucovorin often is given concurrently. Use ice chips in the mouth 10–15 minutes pre- and post-IV bolus to reduce mucositis.
		Gemcitabine (Gemzar®)	IV	Pancreatic, breast, ovarian, and bladder cancers; small cell and non-small cell lung cancer, in conjunction with carboplatin, paclitaxel, or cisplatin	Myelosuppression (especially anemia), nausea, vomiting, fever, flu-like symptoms, rash	Not used in pediatrics Use with NS only. Infuse over 30 minutes; infusion longer than 60 minutes or more than weekly can increase toxicity. Myelosuppression is a dose-limiting toxicity.
		Mercaptopurine (6-MP, Purinethol®)	po, IV (not available in the United States)	ALL, AML, CML, non-Hodgkin lymphoma	Myelosuppression, mucositis, nausea, hyperuricemia	Reduce oral dose by 75% when used concurrently with allopurinol. Patient should take drug on an empty stomach, one hour before meals or two hours after meals.

(Continued on next page)

Table 4. Characteristics of Cytotoxic Agents *(Continued)*

Classification	Mechanism of Action	Medication Name(s)	Route of Administration	Indications	Side Effects	Nursing Considerations
Antimetabolite (*cont.*)		Methotrexate (MTX)	IM, IV, IT, po	Hodgkin disease; lymphoma; leukemias; CNS metastasis; lung, breast, and head and neck cancers; gestational trophoblastic tumor; osteogenic sarcoma; rheumatoid arthritis	Mucositis, nausea, myelosuppression, oral or GI ulceration, renal toxicity, photosensitivity, liver toxicity, neurotoxicity associated with high-dose therapy	High doses must be followed by leucovorin and vigorous hydration. Follow dosing schedule carefully. Monitor serum methotrexate levels until 0.1 mmol. Instruct patient on strict mouth care. Patient must take photosensitivity precautions. Ensure that the patient avoids taking multivitamins with folic acid.
	Disrupts folate-dependent metabolic processes essential for cell replication	Pemetrexed (Alimta®)	IV	Given in combination with cisplatin for the treatment of malignant pleural mesothelioma for nonsurgical candidates or as a single agent for locally advanced or metastatic non-small cell lung cancer	Side effects with pemetrexed plus cisplatin regimen include myelosuppression, fatigue, nausea, vomiting, chest pain, and dyspnea. Side effects were reduced with vitamin supplementation.	To reduce treatment-related hematologic and GI toxicity, administer folic acid, 350–1,000 mcg daily, starting one to three weeks prior to the first cycle and daily for three weeks after final cycle (should take at least five doses in the week prior to first treatment). In clinical trials, vitamin B_{12} injection, 1,000 mcg IM, was given one to three weeks before first cycle and repeated every nine weeks until treatment was completed. Dexamethasone 4 mg bid for three days starting the day before treatment decreases incidence of skin rash. Monitor CBC on days 8 and 15. Hold treatment if absolute neutrophil count < 1,500, platelet count < 100,000, or creatinine clearance < 45 ml/minute. Monitor renal and hepatic function. The concurrent use of ibuprofen may increase the risk of renal damage.
		Pentostatin (Nipent®)	IV	Hairy cell leukemia, CLL, lymphoma	Myelosuppression, fever, chills, nausea, vomiting, rash, renal failure, confusion, hepatic enzyme elevation, lymphocytopenia, heightened infection risk	Administer with 500–1,000 ml 5% dextrose in ½ NS solution prior to the infusion and an additional 500 ml postinfusion.
		Raltitrexed (Tomudex®)	IV (not available in the United States)	Colorectal cancer	Fatigue, diarrhea, mucositis, myelosuppression, nausea, vomiting	Ensure that the patient avoids taking multivitamins with folic acid.
		Thioguanine (6-thioguanine, 6-TG)	po, IV (investigational)	ALL, AML, CML	Myelosuppression, hyperuricemia, nausea, hepatotoxicity, diarrhea	No dose reduction is necessary when this drug is used concurrently with allopurinol. Administer on an empty stomach.

(Continued on next page)

Table 4. Characteristics of Cytotoxic Agents *(Continued)*

Classification	Mechanism of Action	Medication Name(s)	Route of Administration	Indications	Side Effects	Nursing Considerations
Antimetabolite (*cont.*)		Trimetrexate (Neutrexin®)	IV	Colorectal and head and neck cancers, non-small cell lung cancer, *Pneumocystis carinii* pneumonia, toxoplasmosis	Myelosuppression, mucositis, nausea, vomiting, alopecia, headache, rash	Use with caution in patients with abnormal renal and hepatic function.
		Uracil and tegafur (UFT®)	po	Breast, colorectal, gastric, and pancreatic cancers	Diarrhea, nausea, vomiting, fatigue, rash, neurotoxicity, myelosuppression	Make sure patient takes with a large glass of water on an empty stomach.
Antitumor antibiotic	Binds with DNA, thereby inhibiting DNA and RNA synthesis	Bleomycin (Blenoxane®)	IV, SQ, IM, intracavitary	Malignant pleural effusion; squamous cell cancer of head and neck; cervical, vulvar, penile, and testicular cancers; melanoma; Hodgkin disease; non-Hodgkin lymphoma	Hypersensitivity or anaphylactic reaction (rare), hyperpigmentation, alopecia, photosensitivity, renal toxicity, hepatotoxicity, pulmonary fibrosis, fever, chills	Patients with lymphoma have a higher incidence of anaphylaxis after receiving bleomycin than do other patients who receive the drug. Therefore, administer (per institutional protocol) a test dose of 1–2 units IV, IM, or SQ before administering the first dose of bleomycin to patients with lymphoma. Ensure that patient and family understand the lifelong necessity of disclosing previous use of bleomycin when future needs for anesthesia occur. Because of the dose-related incidence of pulmonary fibrosis, the cumulative lifetime dose should not exceed 400 units. Pulmonary function tests are recommended at initiation of bleomycin and every one to two months thereafter. Consider stopping drug if a 30%–35% decrease from pretreatment values occurs.
		Dactinomycin (Actinomycin D®, Cosmegen®)	IV	Ewing's sarcoma, Wilms' tumor, testicular cancer, gestational trophoblastic disease, rhabdomyosarcoma	Myelosuppression, nausea, vomiting, alopecia, mucositis, diarrhea, ovarian or sperm suppression, radiation recall (hyperpigmentation of previously irradiated areas)	Dactinomycin is a vesicant. This drug may be ordered in mcg, so check the dose carefully.
		Mitomycin (Mutamycin®)	IV	Pancreatic, stomach, colon, breast, lung, bladder, head and neck, and esophageal cancers	Myelosuppression, nausea, vomiting, anorexia, alopecia, mucositis, renal toxicity, pulmonary toxicity, fatigue	Mitomycin is a vesicant. Nadir occurs four to eight weeks after treatment begins. Acute shortness of breath and bronchospasm can occur very suddenly when this drug is given with a vinca alkaloid.

(Continued on next page)

Table 4. Characteristics of Cytotoxic Agents *(Continued)*

Classification	Mechanism of Action	Medication Name(s)	Route of Administration	Indications	Side Effects	Nursing Considerations
Antitumor antibiotic *(cont.)*		Mitoxantrone (Novantrone®)	IV	Breast and prostate cancers, lymphoma, acute nonlymphocytic leukemia	Myelosuppression, arrhythmia (if patient was treated with doxorubicin), nausea, vomiting, mucositis, alopecia; may turn the urine blue-green and can cause sclera to turn bluish.	Some sources classify mitoxantrone as an irritant. The cardiotoxicity of mitoxantrone is less than that of doxorubicin, but prior anthracycline use, chest irradiation, or cardiac disease can increase the patient's risk.
Antitumor antibiotic (anthracycline)	Binds with DNA, thereby inhibiting DNA and RNA synthesis	Daunorubicin (Cerubidine®, Daunomycin®)	IV	ALL in children, acute nonlymphocytic leukemia	Myelosuppression, nausea, vomiting, alopecia, cardiotoxicity, hyperuricemia, radiation recall, ovarian or sperm suppression; drug may turn the urine red.	Daunorubicin is a vesicant. Test the patient's cardiac ejection fraction via MUGA scan before starting therapy.
		Daunorubicin citrate liposomal (DaunoXome®)	IV	AIDS-related Kaposi's sarcoma	Myelosuppression, nausea, vomiting, alopecia, cardiotoxicity, hyperuricemia, radiation recall, ovarian or sperm suppression; drug may turn the urine red.	Daunorubicin citrate liposomal is not a vesicant but should be considered an irritant, and caution should be taken to avoid extravasation. Consider a dose reduction in patients with liver dysfunction. Test the patient's cardiac ejection fraction via MUGA before starting daunorubicin liposomal therapy.
		Doxorubicin (Adriamycin®)	IV	Breast, ovarian, prostate, stomach, thyroid, small-cell lung, and liver cancers; squamous cell cancer of the head and neck; multiple myeloma; Hodgkin disease; non-Hodgkin lymphoma; ALL; AML; Wilms' tumor	Myelosuppression, nausea, vomiting, alopecia, mucositis, dose-limiting cardiotoxicity, radiation recall, arrhythmia, hyperuricemia, photosensitivity; drug may turn the urine red.	Doxorubicin is a vesicant. Doxorubicin may cause a flare reaction. Test the patient's cardiac ejection fraction via MUGA scan before starting therapy. Do not exceed a lifetime cumulative dose of 550 mg/m² (450 mg/m² if the patient has had prior chest irradiation or concomitant cyclophosphamide treatment). Initiate dexrazoxane for patients who have received a cumulative dose of 300 mg/m² and are continuing doxorubicin treatment. In pediatrics, dexrazoxane may be used concurrently.
		Doxorubicin liposomal (Doxil®)	IV	AIDS-related Kaposi's sarcoma, ovarian cancer	Myelosuppression, nausea, vomiting, alopecia, mucositis, dose-limiting cardiotoxicity, arrythmia, hyperuricemia, radiation recall, hand-foot syndrome, photosensitivity; drug may turn the urine red.	Doxorubicin liposomal is not a vesicant but should be considered an irritant, and caution should be taken to avoid extravasation. The same warnings as with conventional doxorubicin apply regarding cardiovascular complications. Use only with 5% dextrose injection, USP. Do not substitute for Adriamycin. Start infusion at 1 mg/minute over at least 30 minutes.

(Continued on next page)

Table 4. Characteristics of Cytotoxic Agents *(Continued)*

Classification	Mechanism of Action	Medication Name(s)	Route of Administration	Indications	Side Effects	Nursing Considerations
Antitumor antibiotic (anthracycline) *(cont.)*		Epirubicin (Ellence®)	IV	Breast cancer	Myelosuppression, nausea, vomiting, mucositis, diarrhea, cardiotoxicity, alopecia, radiation recall; drug may turn the urine red.	Epirubicin is a vesicant. Consider a dose reduction in patients with liver dysfunction. Reduce dose by 50% in patients with SCr > 5 mg/dl. Test the patient's cardiac ejection fraction via MUGA before starting epirubicin therapy.
		Idarubicin (Idamycin®)	IV	Acute non-lymphocytic leukemia	Myelosuppression, nausea, vomiting, alopecia, vein itching, cardiomyopathy, radiation recall, rash, mucositis, diarrhea; drug may turn the urine red.	Idarubicin is a vesicant. The cardiotoxicity of idarubicin is less than that of daunorubicin. Cumulative doses > 150 mg/m² idarubicin are associated with decreased ejection fraction. Local reactions (hives at injection site) may occur.
		Valrubicin (Valstar®)	Intravesical	Intravesical therapy of BCG-refractory in situ bladder cancer	Dysuria, bladder spasm, urinary incontinence, leukopenia, neutropenia, hyperglycemia	Not used in pediatrics Valrubicin is administered as an intravesicular bladder lavage. Instruct patient that urine may be red tinged for the first 24 hours.
Hormonal therapy (antiestrogen)	Binds to estrogen receptors, forming a complex that inhibits DNA synthesis	Tamoxifen (Nolvadex®)	po	Estrogen receptor–positive breast cancer	Menstrual irregularities, vaginal bleeding or discharge, hot flashes, nausea, vomiting, edema, hypercalcemia	Not used in pediatrics Adverse reactions are relatively mild and rarely severe enough to require discontinuation of treatment. Monitor women who have an intact uterus for signs of endometrial cancer.
Hormonal therapy (estrogen)	Interferes with hormone receptors and proteins in all phases of the cell cycle	Diethylstilbestrol (DES); estramustine (Emcyt®); estrogen (Menest®); estradiol (Estrace®)	po	Prostate cancer, estrogen receptor–negative breast tumors, postmenopausal advanced breast cancer	Gynecomastia, myelosuppression, ischemic heart disease, breast tenderness, sodium and fluid retention, nausea, vomiting, hypertension, thrombophlebitis, libido change, voice changes	Not used in pediatrics Monitor women who have an intact uterus for signs of endometrial cancer. Instruct patients to avoid consuming foods containing calcium during treatment. Use with caution in patients with cerebrovascular disease, diabetes, or hypertension.
Hormonal therapy (estrogen receptor antagonist)	Selectively attaches to and blocks activity of breast cancer cell hormone receptors; causes down-regulation of estrogen receptors and inhibits tumor growth	Fulvestrant (Faslodex®)	IM	Hormone receptor–positive metastatic breast cancer in postmenopausal women with disease progression following antiestrogen therapy	Myalgia, asthenia, flu-like syndrome, hot flashes, vasodilatation, nausea, vomiting, diarrhea, constipation, anorexia, peripheral edema, bone pain, dizziness, insomnia, depression, anxiety, rash, sweating, thrombotic events, dyspnea, increased cough, headache	Store agent in refrigerator. Drug is contraindicated in patients with bleeding disorders and those on anticoagulant therapy.

(Continued on next page)

Table 4. Characteristics of Cytotoxic Agents *(Continued)*

Classification	Mechanism of Action	Medication Name(s)	Route of Administration	Indications	Side Effects	Nursing Considerations
Hormonal therapy (LHRH analog)	Inhibits pituitary gonadotropin	Goserelin (Zoladex®)	SQ	Prostate or breast cancer, endometriosis	Gynecomastia, hot flashes, impotence, nausea, vomiting, headache, bone pain	Maintaining the prescribed dose and schedule is very important. Review the side effects with patients prior to administration. Tell them that symptoms may worsen in the first few weeks of therapy.
	Suppresses secretion of FSH and LH from the pituitary gland	Leuprolide (Lupron®)	SQ, IM	Prostate or breast cancer, endometriosis	Gynecomastia, hot flashes, impotence, nausea, vomiting, headache, bone pain, sodium retention	Rotate SQ injection sites frequently. Drug may cause depression. Tell patients that symptoms may worsen in the first few weeks of therapy.
Hormonal therapy (nonsteroidal antiestrogen)	Interferes with hormone receptors and proteins in all phases of the cell cycle	Bicalutamide (Casodex®)	po	Prostate cancer	Hot flashes, diarrhea, gynecomastia	Bicalutamide interacts with warfarin. Monitor carefully if taking together.
	Binds to androgen receptors, competitively inhibiting binding of dihydrotestosterone and testosterone	Flutamide (Eulexin®)	po	Used in combination with LHRH agonists for management of locally confined stage B2, C, and D2 metastatic carcinoma of the prostate	Diarrhea, hypertension, cystitis, rectal bleeding, hot flashes, decreased libido, impotence, photosensitivity, edema, liver toxicity, gynecomastia, breast tenderness, nausea, vomiting	Flutamide increases the effects of warfarin. Contraindicated in severe hepatic impairment.
	Antiestrogenic effects compete with estrogen for binding sites in the cancer, blocking the growth-stimulating effects of estrogen in the tumor.	Toremifene (Fareston®)	po	Metastatic breast cancer in postmenopausal women with estrogen receptor–positive or hormone receptor–unknown tumors	Hot flashes, sweating, nausea, vaginal discharge, dizziness, edema, vomiting, vaginal bleeding	Patients with a history of thromboembolic diseases generally should not be treated with toremifene citrate. Patients with preexisting endometrial hyperplasia should not be given long-term treatment. Patients with bone metastases should be monitored closely for hypercalcemia during the first weeks of treatment. As with other antiestrogens, hypercalcemia and tumor flare have been reported in some patients with cancer with bone metastases during the first weeks of treatment. If hypercalcemia occurs, institute appropriate measures, and if hypercalcemia is severe, discontinue treatment. Drugs that decrease renal calcium excretion (e.g., thiazide diuretics) may increase the risk of hypercalcemia. Monitor patients on warfarin for an increased prothrombin time.

(Continued on next page)

Table 4. Characteristics of Cytotoxic Agents *(Continued)*

Classification	Mechanism of Action	Medication Name(s)	Route of Administration	Indications	Side Effects	Nursing Considerations
Hormonal therapy (nonsteroidal aromatase inhibitor)	Interferes with hormone receptors and proteins in all phases of the cell cycle	Anastrozole (Arimidex®)	po	Breast cancer	Diarrhea, asthenia, nausea, headache, hot flashes, back pain, peripheral edema	Safety and efficacy have not been established in pediatric use.
	In postmenopausal women, estrogens are mainly derived from the action of the aromatase enzyme, which converts adrenal androgens to estrone and estradiol. The suppression of estrogen biosynthesis in peripheral tissues and in cancer tissues can be achieved by inhibiting the aromatase enzyme.	Letrozole (Femara®)	po	First-line treatment of postmenopausal women with hormone receptor–positive or hormone receptor–unknown locally advanced or metastatic breast cancer; treatment of advanced cancer in postmenopausal women with disease progression following antiestrogen therapy; extended adjuvant treatment of early breast cancer in postmenopausal women who had received five years of adjuvant tamoxifen therapy	Bone pain, hot flashes, back pain, nausea, arthralgia, dyspnea, fatigue, cough, constipation, chest pain, headache	Letrozole may cause fatigue and dizziness, so patients should use caution when driving or operating machinery. Drug can be taken without regard to meals.
Hormonal therapy (steroidal aromatase inhibitor)	Acts as a false substrate for the aromatase enzyme and is processed to an intermediate that binds irreversibly to the active site of the enzyme, causing its inactivation—an effect also known as "suicide inhibition	Exemestane (Aromasin®)	po	Advanced breast cancer in postmenopausal women whose hormone-dependent cancer has progressed following tamoxifen treatment	Hot flashes, nausea, fatigue, increased sweating, increased appetite	Exemestane should not be administered to premenopausal women. Do not coadminister with estrogen-containing agents, as these could interfere with its pharmacologic action. Drug should be taken daily after a meal.
Miscellaneous	Degrades the chimeric PML/RAR alpha protein	Arsenic trioxide (Trisenox®)	IV	APL	Fatigue, prolonged QT interval, APL differentiation syndrome, leukocytosis, headache, nausea, vomiting, diarrhea, musculoskeletal pain, peripheral neuropathy	Use with caution with other agents that prolong QT interval. Use with caution in patients with renal impairment. Obtain baseline EKG prior to therapy.

(Continued on next page)

Table 4. Characteristics of Cytotoxic Agents *(Continued)*

Classification	Mechanism of Action	Medication Name(s)	Route of Administration	Indications	Side Effects	Nursing Considerations
Miscellaneous *(cont.)*	Inhibits protein synthesis	Asparaginase (Elspar®)	IV, SQ, IM	ALL	Nausea, vomiting, hepatotoxicity, fever, hyperglycemia, anaphylaxis, pancreatitis, coagulopathy, hypoalbuminemia, hypersensitivity reaction, renal toxicity	There is no reliable way to test for hypersensitivity. Treat each dose of asparaginase as one that could cause a serious reaction (Weiss, 2001). Giving the drug IM greatly reduces the incidence of anaphylaxis. In pediatrics, keep medications to treat anaphylaxis at bedside.
		Pegaspargase (Oncaspar®)	IM, IV	ALL (for those who have developed hypersensitivity to asparaginase)	Hepatotoxicity, coagulopathy, anaphylaxis	No need for test dose Presents less risk of anaphylaxis than does asparaginase
	Inhibits chymotrypsin-like activity of 26S proteasome	Bortezomib (Velcade®)	IV	Multiple myeloma	Peripheral neuropathy, hypotension, nausea, vomiting, diarrhea, blurred vision, fatigue, myelosuppression	Not used in pediatrics Use with caution in patients with severe renal or hepatic disease. Monitor hydration status and treat as necessary.
	An enzyme, derived from the yeast *Erwinia*, used to deplete the supply of asparagine for leukemic cells, particularly in acute lymphocytic leukemia, that are dependent on an exogenous source of this amino acid	*Erwinia* asparaginase	IV, IM	Indicated in patients with ALL who require L-asparaginase therapy but have developed hypersensitivity to the *E. coli* forms of L-asparaginase	Allergic reactions may include skin rashes, urticaria, respiratory distress, and acute anaphylaxis; fatal hyperthermia, pancreatitis, hyperglycemia, and coagulopathy caused by a decrease in clotting factors V, VII, VIII, and IX as well as fibrinogen, liver function enzyme abnormalities	Store agent in refrigerator but do not freeze.
	Acts in S phase as an antimetabolite	Hydroxyurea (Hydrea®, Mylocel®)	po	CML, malignant melanoma, squamous cell cancer of the head and neck, metastatic ovarian cancer, sickle cell anemia	Myelosuppression (especially severe anemia), nausea, vomiting, diarrhea, renal failure, mucositis, hyperuricemia, fever, rash	Adjust the dose according to blood counts; do not change the dose too frequently. Frequent change results in response delay. Instruct patients on strict mouth care.

(Continued on next page)

Table 4. Characteristics of Cytotoxic Agents *(Continued)*

Classification	Mechanism of Action	Medication Name(s)	Route of Administration	Indications	Side Effects	Nursing Considerations
Miscellaneous *(cont.)*	Inhibits bcr-abl tyrosine kinase, inhibiting proliferation, and induces apoptosis in bcr-abl-positive cell lines	Imatinib mesylate (Gleevec®)	po	CML in blast crisis or accelerated phase, or in chronic phase after failure of interferon alfa therapy, GI stromal tumors	Edema and fluid retention, GI irritation, nausea, vomiting, neutropenia, thrombocytopenia, hepatotoxicity	Weigh patients frequently and monitor them for signs and symptoms of fluid retention. Ensure that patients take imatinib with food and a large glass of water. Monitor CBC, differential, and LFTs. Drugs that may increase plasma concentration include ketoconazole, itraconazole, erythromycin, and clarithromycin. Drugs that may decrease plasma concentration include dexamethasone, phenytoin, carbamazepine, rifampicin, phenobarbital, and St. John's wort. Interaction is possible in patients receiving warfarin. Advise women of childbearing age not to become pregnant while taking imatinib. Researchers have not conducted studies of the drug in pregnant women.
	Inhibits adrenal steroid production	Mitotane (Lysodren®)	po	Adrenocortical cancer	Nausea, vomiting, mucositis, adrenal insufficiency	Monitor patients on warfarin therapy closely. Adrenal steroid replacement is indicated.
	May inhibit protein, RNA, and DNA synthesis	Procarbazine (Matulane®)	po	Hodgkin disease, brain tumors	Myelosuppression, nausea, vomiting	Patients should avoid foods high in tyramine, because to some degree procarbazine inhibits monoamine oxidase. Patients also should avoid alcohol for possible antabuse-like reaction.
Nitrosourea	Breaks DNA helix, interfering with DNA replication; crosses the blood-brain barrier	Carmustine (BCNU®)	IV, implantation (wafer)	Hodgkin disease, non-Hodgkin lymphoma, CNS tumors, multiple myeloma, malignant melanoma, BMT	Nausea, vomiting, myelosuppression, renal toxicity, hepatic toxicity, pulmonary fibrosis, ovarian or sperm suppression	Carmustine crosses the blood-brain barrier. Nadir occurs four to six weeks after therapy starts. Because of delayed toxicity, successive treatments usually are given no more frequently than once every six to eight weeks. Rapid infusion may cause burning along the vein and flushing of the skin. Long-term therapy can result in irreversible pulmonary fibrosis, which may present as an insidious cough and dyspnea or sudden respiratory failure.

(Continued on next page)

Table 4. Characteristics of Cytotoxic Agents *(Continued)*

Classification	Mechanism of Action	Medication Name(s)	Route of Administration	Indications	Side Effects	Nursing Considerations
Nitrosourea *(cont.)*		Lomustine (CeeNu®)	po	Pancreatic, liver, gastric, and colorectal cancers; CNS and brain tumors; multiple myeloma; Hodgkin disease; non-Hodgkin lymphoma	Myelosuppression (severe), nausea, vomiting, alopecia, renal toxicity, hepatic toxicity, mucositis, anorexia, pulmonary fibrosis	Lomustine crosses the blood-brain barrier. Because of delayed myelosuppression, do not repeat the dose more than once every six weeks. Administer on an empty stomach.
		Streptozocin (Zanosar®)	IV	Metastatic islet-cell pancreatic carcinoma, carcinoid tumor	Renal toxicity, myelosuppression, nausea, vomiting, hyperglycemia, proteinuria	Nephrotoxicity may be dose limiting. This drug may alter glucose metabolism in some patients. Rapid infusion may cause burning along the vein.
Plant alkaloid (camptothecin)	Acts in S phase; topoisomerase I inhibitors; causes double-strand DNA changes	Irinotecan (Camptosar®)	IV	Metastatic colorectal cancer	Diarrhea, myelosuppression, alopecia	Not used in pediatrics This drug can cause early and late diarrhea, which can be dose limiting. Early diarrhea can occur within 24 hours of administration and generally is cholinergic. Many institutions use atropine to treat this early diarrhea. Refer to institutional protocol regarding the dosing and administration of atropine and other antidiarrheals.
		Topotecan (Hycamtin®)	IV	Metastatic ovarian cancer, small cell lung cancer	Myelosuppression, diarrhea, alopecia, nausea, vomiting, headache	Prior to administration, dilute the appropriate volume of reconstituted solution with either 0.9% sodium chloride IV solution or 5% dextrose IV solution.
Plant alkaloid (epipodophyllotoxin)	Induces irreversible blockade of cells in premitotic phases of cell cycle (late G2 and S phases); interferes with topoisomerase II enzyme reaction	Etoposide (VP-16, Vepesid®, Etopophos®)	IV, po	ALL, breast and testicular cancers, small-cell lung cancer, Hodgkin disease, non-Hodgkin lymphoma, multiple myeloma, BMT	Myelosuppression, nausea, vomiting, alopecia, anorexia, orthostatic hypotension, hyperuricemia, hypersensitivity reaction, anaphylaxis High dose: mucositis, diarrhea	Do not administer this drug by means of rapid IV infusion; infuse it over 30–60 minutes to avoid hypotension. Monitor patient's blood pressure during infusion. Prior to use, dilute the drug to a final concentration of 0.2–0.4 mg/ml to prevent precipitation. Monitor for crystallization during infusion. Etopophos is a phosphorylated drug that can be given as a rapid IV push. Such a use is controversial if the patient is less than one year old. Etoposide is associated with the development of secondary malignancies (Pui et al., 1991). If a patient has an allergic reaction to etoposide, premedicate with diphenhydramine. Do not administer to the patient with bilirubin > 5 mg/dl.

(Continued on next page)

Table 4. Characteristics of Cytotoxic Agents *(Continued)*

Classification	Mechanism of Action	Medication Name(s)	Route of Administration	Indications	Side Effects	Nursing Considerations
Plant alkaloid (epipodophyllotoxin) *(cont.)*		Teniposide (VM-26, Vumon®)	IV	Childhood ALL	Myelosuppression, hypotension, pulmonary toxicity, anaphylaxis, nausea, vomiting	Do not administer this drug via rapid infusion. Infuse it over 30–60 minutes. To avoid hypotension, monitor the patient's blood pressure during the infusion. Drug may cause an allergic reaction. Administer through non-PVC tubing.
Plant alkaloid (taxane)	Stabilizes microtubules, inhibiting cell division; effective in G2 and M phases	Docetaxel (Taxotere®)	IV	Breast, non-small cell lung, head and neck, and metastatic ovarian cancers	Myelosuppression, hypersensitivity reaction, fluid retention, alopecia, skin and nail changes, mucositis, nausea, vomiting, paresthesia, neurotoxicity	Not used in pediatrics Premedicate as follows to reduce the severity of hypersensitivity reactions and fluid retention: dexamethasone 8 mg po bid, beginning one day prior to docetaxel treatment and continuing for the day of treatment and one day after. Refer to institutional guidelines for additional pretreatment requirements. Do not use PVC tubing or bags to administer docetaxel. Docetaxel is an irritant. Extravasation may lead to edema, erythema, and occasional pain and blister formation.
		Paclitaxel (Taxol®)	IV	Metastatic breast, ovarian, non-small cell lung, and head and neck cancers; AIDS-related Kaposi's sarcoma	Myelosuppression, alopecia, peripheral neurotoxicity, hypersensitivity reaction, facial flushing, myalgia, fatigue, cardiac arrhythmias, mucositis, diarrhea	Not used in pediatrics Pretreat as follows to help to prevent hypersensitivity reactions, including anaphylaxis, 30–60 minutes before treatment: cimetidine 300 mg IV, diphenhydramine 50 mg IV, and (unless contraindicated) dexamethasone 20 mg IV. Filter paclitaxel with a 0.2 micron in-line filter. Use glass bottles or non-PVC (polyolefin or polypropylene) bags to administer paclitaxel; do not use PVC bags or PVC tubing. Paclitaxel is an irritant and potential vesicant. Extravasation may lead to local pain, edema, and erythema at the infusion site. There are rare reports of necrosis.
		Paclitaxel protein-bound particles; albumin-bound (Abraxane™)	IV	Treatment of metastatic breast cancer after failure of combination chemotherapy or relapse within six months of adjuvant therapy	Myelosuppression, sensory neuropathy, myalgia, arthralgia, nausea, vomiting, mucositis, alopecia	Drug is free of solvents; therefore, no premedication is required to prevent hypersensitivity reactions. Consider dose reduction by about 20% for severe sensory neuropathy; resume treatment with reduced dose when neuropathy improves to grade 1 or 2. Do not use in patients with baseline neutrophil counts < 1,500.

(Continued on next page)

Table 4. Characteristics of Cytotoxic Agents *(Continued)*

Classification	Mechanism of Action	Medication Name(s)	Route of Administration	Indications	Side Effects	Nursing Considerations
Plant alkaloid (vinca alkaloid)	Acts in late G2 phase, blocking DNA production, and in M phase, preventing cell division	Vinblastine (Velban®)	IV	Testicular cancer, squamous-cell cancer of the head and neck, Hodgkin disease, Kaposi's sarcoma, histiocytosis	Myelosuppression, alopecia, anorexia, jaw pain, peripheral neuropathy, constipation, paralytic ileus	Vinblastine is a vesicant. Generally, neurotoxicity occurs less frequently with vinblastine than with vincristine; however, it can occur with high doses. Drug is fatal if given intrathecally.
		Vincristine (Oncovin®)	IV	ALL, Hodgkin disease, non-Hodgkin lymphoma, CML, sarcoma, breast cancer, small-cell lung cancer, neuroblastoma, Wilms' tumor	Peripheral neuropathy, alopecia, constipation, paralytic ileus, jaw pain, foot drop	Vincristine is a vesicant. Neurotoxicity is cumulative but often reversible; conduct a neurologic evaluation before each dose. Withhold dose if severe paresthesia, motor weakness, or other abnormality develops. Reduce dose in the presence of significant liver disease. Stool softeners and/or a stimulant laxative may help to prevent severe constipation. In pediatrics, acetaminophen or an opioid is used for jaw pain. Drug is fatal if given intrathecally.
		Vinorelbine (Navelbine®)	IV	Non-small cell lung cancer, breast and ovarian cancers, Hodgkin disease	Myelosuppression, nausea, vomiting, neurotoxicity, peripheral neuropathy, alopecia	Not used in pediatrics Vinorelbine is a vesicant. Administer via IV push over 6–10 minutes through the side port of a free-flowing IV, then flush with 75–125 ml solution. Drug is fatal if given intrathecally.

ALL—acute lymphocytic leukemia; AML—acute myelogenous leukemia; APL—acute promyelocytic leukemia; BCG—Bacillus Calmette-Guérin; bid—twice daily; BMT—bone marrow transplant; CBC—complete blood count; CLL—chronic lymphocytic leukemia; CML—chronic myelogenous leukemia; CNS—central nervous system; DNA—deoxyribonucleic acid; EGFR—epidermal growth factor receptor; EKG—electrocardiogram; FSH—follicle-stimulating hormone; GI—gastrointestinal; IM—intramuscular; IT—intrathecal; IV—intravenous; LFT—liver function test; LH—luteinizing hormone; LHRH—luteinizing hormone releasing hormone; MUGA—multiple gated acquisition scan; NS—normal saline; po—oral; RNA—ribonucleic acid; SCr—serum creatinine; SQ—subcutaneous; VEGF—vascular endothelial growth factor

Note. Based on information from Ascherman et al., 2000; Camp et al., 2001; Chu, 2003; Cleri, 2002; Solimando, 2003; and manufacturers' prescribing information.

IV. Principles of Biotherapy

Biotherapy: The use of agents derived from biologic sources or agents that affect biologic responses (Rieger, 2001)

A. Theory of immune surveillance: The transformation of a cell from normal to malignant involves a number of genetic mutations over a span of years. As cells differentiate, they produce proteins (antigens) on their surface that the immune system recognizes as nonself; an immune response can be mounted in defense (Rieger, 2001).

B. Methods of biotherapeutic action: Experts propose that biotherapeutic agents work by doing one or more of the following (Rieger, 2001).
   1. Enhancing the patient's own immune response
   2. Altering the milieu in which cancer cells grow by modifying the actions of the normal cells in the area of the tumor
   3. Increasing the vulnerability of cancer cells to the body's own immune system
   4. Altering the pathway by which normal cells transform into malignant cells, which may be more preventive than therapeutic
   5. Preventing the metastasis of cancer cells
   6. Enhancing the repair of normal cells damaged by treatment
   7. Changing cancer cells so they behave like healthy cells

C. Categories of biotherapy (Rieger, 2001; Rosenberg, 2000)
   1. Cytokines
      a) Interferons
      b) Interleukins
      c) Hematopoietic growth factors
   2. Monoclonal antibodies (for nomenclature, see Figure 3)
      a) Unconjugated
         (1) Murine (derived from mouse antibody)
         (2) Chimeric (combination of mouse and human antibodies)
         (3) Humanized (small part mouse fused with human)
         (4) Human (only human antibodies)
      b) Armed or conjugated antibodies
         (1) Immune toxin conjugates (antibodies fused with a toxin)
            (a) Gemtuzumab ozogamicin
            (b) Denileukin diftitox
         (2) Radioisotope conjugates (antibodies labeled with a radioisotope) (Groch, 2002)
            (a) Ibritumomab tiuxetan
            (b) I-131 tositumomab
      c) Cellular therapies
         (1) Dendritic cells
         (2) Tumor-infiltrating lymphocytes
         (3) Antibody-activated T cells
      d) Vaccines
      e) Gene therapy

D. Therapeutic uses for biotherapeutic agents (see Table 5). Biotherapeutic agents have been shown to
   1. Cure, when used as a primary or adjuvant therapy.
   2. Improve overall response or increase disease-free survival when used in conjunction with conventional therapies (Rieger, 2001; Rosenberg, 2000).
   3. Control or stabilize disease.
   4. Maintain or enhance quality of life.

E. Supportive uses for biotherapeutic agents: Biotherapeutic agents can decrease the severity of toxicities associated with other therapeutic modalities (e.g., hematopoietic growth factors can lessen the side effects of chemotherapy).

F. Uses for biotherapeutic agents in research: Numerous biotherapy agents are in clinical trials, including

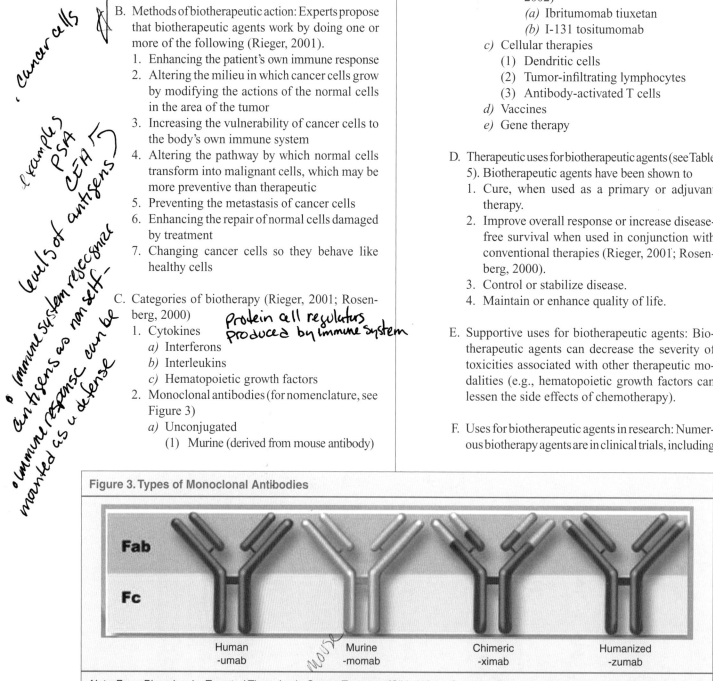

Figure 3. Types of Monoclonal Antibodies

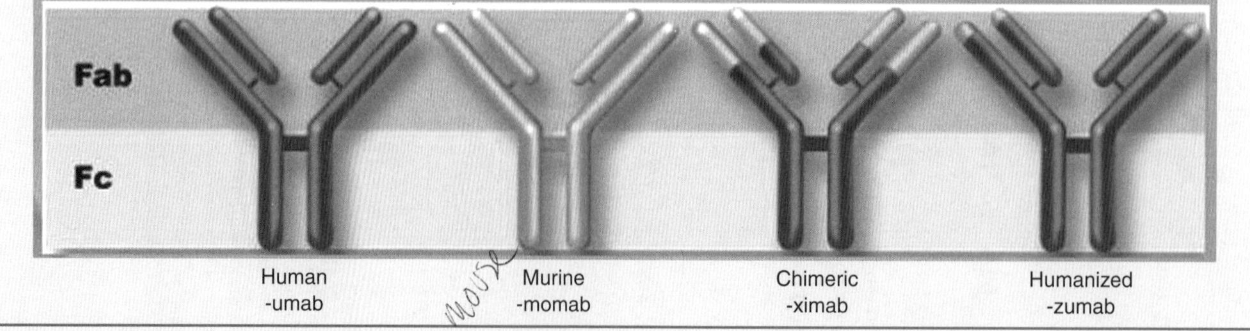

Note. From *Biomolecular Targeted Therapies in Cancer Treatment* [Slide kit], by Oncology Education Services, Inc., 2003, Pittsburgh, PA: Author. Copyright 2003 by Oncology Education Services, Inc. Reprinted with permission.

Table 5. Characteristics of Biologic Agents

Classification	Mechanism of Action	Medication Name(s)	Route of Administration	Indications	Side Effects	Nursing Considerations
Anticoagulant	A recombinant hirudin that is a direct inhibitor of thrombin	Lepirudin (Refludan®)	IV	Anticoagulation for prevention and treatment of thromboembolic disease and complications in patients with heparin-induced thrombocytopenia	Bleeding, fever, bronchospasm, dyspnea, hypersensitivity	Monitor via PTT. Adjust dose in renal insufficiency. Carefully assess patients with an increased risk of bleeding.
Enzyme	Recombinant urate-oxidase enzyme produced by the yeast *Saccharomyces cerevisiae* that converts uric acid into allantoin, a soluble metabolite	Rasburicase (Elitek®)	IV	Used to manage elevations in plasma uric acid that may be associated with tumor lysis syndrome, in pediatric patients treated with chemotherapy for leukemia, lymphoma, and solid tumor malignancies	Anaphylaxis, hemolysis in G6PD deficient patients, methemoglobinemia, fever, respiratory distress, vomiting, headache, nausea	Agent is contraindicated in patients with G6PD deficiency. Patient should receive standard therapy for tumor lysis syndrome in addition to rasburicase. Monitoring of uric acid during rasburicase therapy must be in samples of plasma. Blood is recommended to be collected into pre-chilled tubes, and samples must be immediately immersed in an ice water bath because active rasburicase in the samples can result in incorrect assay readings. Plasma samples also must be prepared in a pre-cooled centrifuge at 4°C. Store agent in refrigerator but do not freeze. Protect from light. Do not shake reconstituted product. Reconstituted solution can be stored under refrigeration and must be administered within 24 hours.
Granulocyte–colony-stimulating factor	Promotes proliferation and differentiation of neutrophils and enhances functional properties of mature neutrophils	Filgrastim (Neupogen®); pegfilgrastim (Neulasta®)	SQ, IV	Facilitate neutrophilic recovery or maintain neutrophil levels in patients with cancer, including AML and those receiving chemotherapy; following BMT; idiopathic, cyclic or congenital neutropenia; for peripheral blood progenitor cell mobilization; decrease the incidence of infection/febrile neutropenia in patients with nonmyeloid malignancies receiving myelosuppressive anticancer drugs associated with a clinically significant incidence of febrile neutropenia	Bone pain, flu-like symptoms	Filgrastim is dosed daily. The drug may be diluted in 5% dextrose in water for IV administration. Store both agents in refrigerator but do not freeze. Pegfilgrastim is dosed as a single 6 mg dose given once per chemotherapy cycle.

(Continued on next page)

Table 5. Characteristics of Biologic Agents *(Continued)*

Classification	Mechanism of Action	Medication Name(s)	Route of Administration	Indications	Side Effects	Nursing Considerations
Granulocyte macrophage–colony-stimulating factor	Stimulates granulocyte and macrophage proliferation; enhances functional properties of mature granulocytes and macrophages	Sargramostim (Leukine®)	SQ, IV	Facilitate granulocyte and macrophage recovery following induction chemotherapy in AML, myeloid reconstitution after allogeneic/autologous BMT, enhance peripheral stem cell mobilization, use in BMT failure or engraftment delay	Fever, bone pain, flushing	Store agent in refrigerator but do not freeze. Dilute with NS for IV use.
Hematopoietic growth factor	Stimulates growth and differentiation of stem cells in bone marrow to increase red blood cell production	Darbepoetin (Aranesp®)	SQ, IV	Anemia caused by cancer chemotherapy or chronic renal failure (on dialysis) or chronic renal insufficiency (not on dialysis)	Pain at injection site, hypertension, myalgia	Darbepoetin is an analog of epoetin alfa with a longer half-life that allows for less frequent dosing.
		Erythropoietin (epoetin alfa, Procrit®, Epogen)	SQ, IV	Anemia caused by cancer, chemotherapy, chronic renal failure, or zidovudine treatment; to reduce need for transfusion during elective, noncardiac, nonvascular surgery	Pain at injection site, hypertension, myalgia	Do not shake product. Store agent in refrigerator but do not freeze. Expect Hgb/HCT response in 2–4 weeks. Check Hgb and/or HCT regularly.
	Stimulates growth and development of megakaryocytes and platelets	Oprelvekin (IL-11, Neumega®)	SQ	Prevent severe chemotherapy-induced thrombocytopenia and reduce need for platelet transfusions	Reduced HCT, edema, fluid retention, dyspnea, exacerbation of CHF, arrhythmias, dizziness, fever, headache, insomnia, rash, anorexia, vomiting	Store agent in refrigerator but do not freeze. Do not shake. Use within three hours of reconstitution. Anemia, possibly caused by a dilutional effect, appears within three days of starting therapy and resolves about two weeks after discontinuation.
	Binds to the keratinocyte growth factor receptor, resulting in proliferation, differentiation, and migration of epithelial cells	Palifermin (Kepivance™)	IV	To decrease the incidence and duration of severe oral mucositis in patients with hematologic malignancies receiving myelotoxic therapy requiring hematopoietic stem cell support	Skin rash (erythema, edema, pruritus), oral toxicities, pain, arthralgias, dysesthesia, hypertension, proteinuria, reversible elevation in serum lipase and amylase	Flush IV line with normal saline before and after palifermin administration. Do not administer palifermin within 24 hours before, during infusion of, or within 24 hours after administration of myelotoxic chemotherapy.

(Continued on next page)

Table 5. Characteristics of Biologic Agents *(Continued)*

Classification	Mechanism of Action	Medication Name(s)	Route of Administration	Indications	Side Effects	Nursing Considerations
HER1/EGFR tyrosine kinase inhibitor	Inhibits the intracellular phosphorylation of tyrosine kinase associated with EGFR	Erlotinib (Tarceva™)	po	Locally advanced or metastatic non-small cell lung cancer after failure of at least one prior chemotherapy regimen	Rash and diarrhea (may be severe [grade 3–4]), abnormal liver function tests (may be transient or associated with liver metastases), GI bleeding, conjunctivitis, keratitis, rare reports of serious interstitial lung disease	Educate patients to report severe or persistent diarrhea, nausea, anorexia or vomiting, worsening of unexplained shortness of breath or cough, and eye irritation. Cotreatment with ketoconazole or other potent CYP3A4 inhibitors may increase erlotinib levels, requiring a lower dose. Pretreatment with rifampin and other CYP3A4 inducers (includes phenytoin, phenobarbital, and St. John's wort) may decrease erlotinib activity, requiring an increased dose. Monitor patient for signs of GI bleeding and elevated INR. Patients on anticoagulants should be monitored for changes in PT and INR. Diarrhea usually can be managed with loperamide. Both diarrhea and severe skin reactions may require dose reduction or temporary interruption of therapy. In patients who develop an acute onset of new or progressive pulmonary symptoms (e.g., dyspnea, cough, fever), therapy should be interrupted pending diagnostic evaluation. If interstitial lung disease is diagnosed, discontinue therapy and treat as needed.
Interferon	Mechanisms of activity are not clearly understood but include inhibition of viral replication, direct antiproliferation of tumor cells, and modulation of host immune response.	Interferon alfa-2a (Roferon-A®)	SQ, IM	Hairy cell leukemia, chronic hepatitis C, AIDS-related Kaposi's sarcoma, chronic-phase Philadelphia chromosome–positive CML	Fever, chills, malaise, headache, anorexia, fatigue, depression, nausea, vomiting, diarrhea, dizziness, impaired memory, agitation, leucopenia, injection site reactions	Store agent in refrigerator but do not freeze. Do not shake product. Product is stable for 30 days after reconstitution when stored in refrigerator. Advise patients to report feelings of depression or suicidal thoughts to a physician.

(Continued on next page)

Table 5. Characteristics of Biologic Agents *(Continued)*

Classification	Mechanism of Action	Medication Name(s)	Route of Administration	Indications	Side Effects	Nursing Considerations
Interferon *(cont.)*		Interferon alfa-2B (Intron A®)	SQ, IM, IV	Hairy cell leukemia, malignant melanoma, follicular lymphoma, condylomata acuminata, AIDS-related Kaposi's sarcoma, chronic hepatitis B and C	Fever, chills, malaise, myalgia, headache, anorexia, fatigue, depression, nausea, vomiting, diarrhea, nephrotic syndrome, pancreatitis, psychosis, hallucinations, renal failure, renal insufficiency	Store agent in refrigerator but do not freeze. Do not shake product. Product is stable for 30 days after reconstitution when stored in refrigerator.
	Mechanisms of activity are not clearly understood but include inhibition of viral replication, direct antiproliferation of tumor cells, and modulation of host immune response; also exhibits a potent phagocyte-activating effect that mediates killing of select microorganisms	Interferon gamma (IFN-γ, Actimmune®)	SQ	Chronic granulomatous disease	Fever, rash, chills, malaise, headache, anorexia, fatigue, depression, nausea, vomiting, diarrhea, injection site erythema	Store agent in refrigerator but do not freeze. Do not shake product.
Interleukin	Promotes proliferation, differentiation, and recruitment of T and B cells, NK cells, LAK cells, and tumor-infiltrating lymphocytes that enhance tumor fighting capabilities	Aldesleukin (IL-2, Proleukin®)	SQ, IV	Renal cell carcinoma, metastatic melanoma	Fever, rigors, malaise, headache, myalgia, arthralgia, tachycardia, hypotension, cardiomyopathy, arrhythmias, capillary leak syndrome, dyspnea, nausea, vomiting, diarrhea, dizziness, anemia, thrombocytopenia, leukopenia, elevated transaminases	Do not use with an in-line filter. Do not mix with NS or bacteriostatic water. Do not mix with other medications. Hypotension is dose limiting and mimics septic shock, and treatment may require vasopressor support.

(Continued on next page)

Table 5. Characteristics of Biologic Agents *(Continued)*

Classification	Mechanism of Action	Medication Name(s)	Route of Administration	Indications	Side Effects	Nursing Considerations
Monoclonal antibody	Binds to CD52 present on the surface of B and T cells, monocytes, macrophages, NK cells, and some granulocytes resulting in antibody-dependent lysis	Alemtuzumab (anti-CD52, Campath®)	IV, SQ	B-cell CLL in patients who have been treated with alkylating agents and who have failed fludarabine therapy	Thrombocytopenia, anemia, neutropenia, hypotension, fever, fatigue, rash, urticaria, nausea, vomiting, diarrhea, rigors, dyspnea	Investigational use is being studied to treat rheumatoid arthritis, graft-versus-host disease, and multiple myeloma. Premedicate with diphenhydramine and acetaminophen. Anti-infective prophylaxis should be considered.
	Monoclonal antibody fragment labeled with Technetium-Tc 99m that binds to the CEA surface antigen found on colorectal carcinomas	Arcitumomab (CEA-Scan®)	IV	Nuclear imaging agent used in conjunction with other diagnostic tools to detect the presence, location, and extent of recurrent or metastatic colorectal cancer	Nausea, urticaria, pruritus, fever	Agent is not used in colorectal cancer screening. It must be used as part of a complete diagnostic evaluation. Contents of vial are not radioactive prior to preparation. Take appropriate measures to minimize radioactive exposure once product is made radioactive. Store agent in refrigerator but do not freeze. Agent can be stored at room temperature and used within four hours of reconstitution.
	Binds to and inhibits the activity of human vascular endothelial growth factor blocking proliferation and formation of new blood vessels	Bevacizumab (anti-VEGF, Avastin®)	IV	Used in combination with fluorouracil-containing regimens as first-line treatment for patients with metastatic carcinoma of the colon or rectum	Hemorrhage, hypertension, proteinuria, CHF, asthenia, diarrhea, leucopenia, thromboembolism, hyponatremia	Avoid use for at least 28 days after major surgery, and surgical incision should be fully healed. Suspend treatment with bevacizumab several weeks before surgery. Store agent in refrigerator but do not freeze. Do not shake. Protect vials from light. Diluted solution may be stored for up to eight hours under refrigeration. Do not mix or administer with dextrose-containing solutions. Blood pressure should be monitored during treatment. Permanently discontinue medication if patient develops GI perforation, wound dehiscence requiring medical intervention, serious bleeding, nephrotic syndrome, or hypertensive crisis. Temporarily suspend if evidence of moderate to severe proteinuria and severe hypertension until evaluation and treatment are provided. See Table 8 for additional product-specific information.

(Continued on next page)

Table 5. Characteristics of Biologic Agents *(Continued)*

Classification	Mechanism of Action	Medication Name(s)	Route of Administration	Indications	Side Effects	Nursing Considerations
Monoclonal antibody *(cont.)*	Binds to extracellular domain of the EGFR, resulting in inhibition of cell growth and induction of apoptosis and decreasing matrix metalloproteinase and vascular endothelial growth factor production	Cetuximab (Erbitux®)	IV	Used with irinotecan or in patients with metastatic colorectal cancer who are refractory to or intolerant of irinotecan	Infusion-related reactions may include bronchospasm, urticaria, hypotension, stridor, and hoarseness; pulmonary toxicity, rash, dry skin and fissuring, diarrhea, malaise, asthenia, fever, diarrhea, nausea, vomiting, anorexia, leucopenia, acneform rash	Instruct patients to wear sunscreen and hats and limit sun exposure. Premedicate with H_1 antagonist. Administer through 0.22-micron in-line filter. Flush line with NS after infusion. Store agent in refrigerator but do not freeze. Do not shake. Do not dilute. Unused portion should be discarded after 8 hours at room temperature or 12 hours under refrigeration.
	Directs cytotoxic action of diphtheria toxin to cells that express the IL-2 receptor, resulting in inhibition of intracellular protein synthesis leading to cell death	Denileukin diftitox (Ontak®)	IV	Treatment of patients with persistent or recurrent cutaneous T-cell lymphoma whose malignant cells express the CD25 component of the IL-2 receptor	Hypersensitivity, vascular leak syndrome, hypotension, edema, hypoalbuminemia, fever, chills, headache, rash, anorexia, reduced lymphocytes, increased transaminases, asthenia	The incidence of adverse effects diminishes after the first two treatment courses. Store at or below −10°C. Agent cannot be refrozen after thawing and must be brought to room temperature before preparing dose. Vials should not be heated. Avoid vigorous agitation. Prepared solution should be used within six hours. Do not infuse through a filter.
	Binds to CD33 on leukemic cells resulting in internalization of antibody-antigen complex and subsequent release of calicheamicin toxin that binds to DNA resulting in double strand breaks and cell death.	Gemtuzumab ozogamicin (anti-CD33, Mylotarg®)	IV	CD33-positive AML in patients age 60 years or older in first relapse who are not considered candidates for standard chemotherapy	Severe neutropenia, anemia, thrombocytopenia, chills, fever, hypotension, peripheral edema, headache, rash, nausea, vomiting, diarrhea, anorexia, hyperbilirubinemia, weakness	Administer only by IV infusion. Store agent in refrigerator but do not freeze. Protect from light during reconstitution until completion of infusion. Premedicate with diphenhydramine and acetaminophen. Neutropenia and thrombocytopenia are severe and prolonged.

(Continued on next page)

Table 5. Characteristics of Biologic Agents *(Continued)*

Classification	Mechanism of Action	Medication Name(s)	Route of Administration	Indications	Side Effects	Nursing Considerations
Monoclonal antibody *(cont.)*	Binds to CD20 on B cells resulting in direct delivery of the radioactive isotope indium-111 or yttrium-90 that induces cell damage through the formation of free radicals	Ibritumomab tiuxetan (Zevalin®)	IV	Relapsed or refractory low-grade, follicular, or transformed B-cell non-Hodgkin lymphoma	Severe and potentially life-threatening allergic reactions during infusion; fever, chills, rigors, headache, bronchospasm, dyspnea, myalgia, arthralgia, prolonged B-cell lymphocytopenia, leucopenia, thrombocytopenia, neutropenia	Drug is combined with rituximab. Administered dose cannot exceed 32 mCi regardless of patient's weight. Drug is not transported with radioisotope; radiolabeling must be done by appropriate personnel in a specialized facility.
	Binds to CD20 on B cells resulting in activation of complement-dependent cytotoxicity as well as antibody-dependent cellular toxicity	Rituximab (anti-CD20, Rituxan®)	IV	Relapsed or refractory CD20-positive non-Hodgkin lymphoma	Fever, chills, rigors, headache, bronchospasm, dyspnea, myalgia, arthralgia, prolonged B-cell lymphopenia, leucopenia, infection, asthenia, nausea, rash	Administer only by IV infusion. Store agent in refrigerator but do not freeze. Do not shake product. Stable for 24 hours under refrigeration or 12 hours at room temperature. Consider premedication with acetaminophen and diphenhydramine. Infusion-related side effects may resolve with slowing or suspending infusion. The incidence of infusion-related side effects is reduced with subsequent infusions.
	Binds to CD20 on pre-B and mature lymphocytes resulting in apoptosis, and antibody-dependent cellular cytotoxicity; ionizing radiation caused by I-131 results in additional cell death	Tositumomab I-131 (Bexxar®)	IV	Patients with CD20-positive follicular non-Hodgkin lymphoma whose cancer is refractory to rituximab and has relapsed following chemotherapy	Anaphylaxis, hypothyroidism, cytopenias, allergic reactions, asthenia, fever, infection, chills, nausea, rash, secondary leukemia/myelodysplastic syndrome	Not indicated for initial treatment of CD20 positive non-Hodgkin lymphoma. Thyroid-blocking agents should be given 24 hours prior to tositumomab I-131 therapy and continued for 14 days after. Instruct patients how to minimize exposure of other people to radioactivity that will remain in their system for several days. Only personnel trained in handling of radioactive agents should prepare and administer this agent.

(Continued on next page)

Table 5. Characteristics of Biologic Agents *(Continued)*

Classification	Mechanism of Action	Medication Name(s)	Route of Administration	Indications	Side Effects	Nursing Considerations
Monoclonal antibody *(cont.)*	Binds to the extra-cellular domain of HER2, resulting in mediation of anti-body-dependent cellular toxicity against cells that overproduce HER2	Trastuzumab (anti-HER2/neu, Herceptin®)	IV	Metastatic breast cancer tumors that overexpress the HER2/neu protein	Chills, fever, cardiomyopathy, hypersensitivity reactions, diarrhea, chills, headache, rash, leucopenia, anemia	Administer only by IV infusion. Store agent in refrigerator but do not freeze. Solution reconstituted with bacteriostatic water is stable for 28 days under refrigeration. Solution reconstituted with sterile water must be used immediately and not saved. Do not shake product. Agent usually is combined with chemotherapy. HER2 protein overexpression is seen in 25%–30% of primary breast cancers.

ALL—acute lymphocytic leukemia; AML—acute myelogenous leukemia; BMT—bone marrow transplant; CEA—carcinoembryonic antigen; CHF—congestive heart failure; CLL—chronic lymphocytic leukemia; CML—chronic myelogenous leukemia; EGFR—human epidermal growth factor receptor; G6PD—glucose-6-phosphate dehydrogenase; HCT—hematocrit; HER2—human epidermal growth factor receptor 2 protein; Hgb—hemoglobin; IM—intramuscular; IV—intravenous; LAK—lymphokine-activated killer; NK—natural killer; NS—normal saline; PEG—polyethylene glycol; PTT—partial thromboplastin time; SQ—subcutaneous

Note. Based on information from Amgen Inc., 2002, 2003, 2004; Berlex Laboratories, 2002a, 2002b, 2002c; Biogen Idec, 2003; Chiron Corp., 2000; Corixa Corp. & GlaxoSmithKline, 2003; Enzon, 1998; Genentech, Inc., 2004a, 2004b, 2004c; ImClone Systems & Bristol-Myers Squibb, 2004; Immunomedics, Inc., 1999; InterMune, Inc., 2004; Ligand Pharmaceuticals, 2002; Merck & Co., 2002; Ortho Biotech, 2004; Roche Laboratories, Inc., 2004; Sanofi Synthelabo, 2002; Schering Corp., 2004; Sweetman, 2004; Wyeth Pharmaceuticals, Inc., 2004a, 2004b.

cancer vaccines, dendritic cells, tumor- infiltrating lymphocytes, other interleukins, and antiangiogenic agents (Rosenberg, 2000) (see Table 6).

G. Biotherapeutic strategies: The majority of biotherapeutic agents are approved for single-agent therapy for therapeutic or supportive purposes. The strategy of combining monoclonal antibodies with chemotherapy is well recognized as an effective therapeutic approach to malignancy. Significantly improved survival and response in patients with breast cancer (trastuzumab and paclitaxel) and lymphoma (CHOP/rituximab) has been reported. More recently, the FDA has approved bevacizumab in combination with IV 5-FU–based chemotherapies as first-line treatment for metastatic colorectal cancer (Genentech, Inc., 2004a).

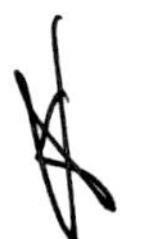

H. Actions of the immune system: The immune system (see Figure 4) is a highly specialized and adaptive system that protects an individual by providing
   1. Defense against foreign organisms.
   2. Homeostasis: Destruction of worn or damaged cells.
   3. Surveillance: Identification of foreign, or nonself, substances (Hyde, 2000).

I. Types of immune response: An immune response is the reaction of the immune system against a foreign substance. Any substance capable of producing such a response is called an antigen. There are two types of immune response (see Table 7).
   1. Innate, or nonspecific, immunity (see Figure 5) involves the following.
      a) Physical barriers (skin and mucous membranes)
      b) Mechanical barriers (coughing, sneezing, and blinking)
      c) Chemical barriers (tears and sweat)
      d) Inflammatory responses (production of monocytes, macrophages, and polymorphonuclear cells)
      e) Complement activation
      f) Acute-phase protein production (e.g., IL-2)
      g) Production of large granular lymphocytes (natural killer [NK] or NK and NKT cells)
   2. Adaptive, or specific, immunity involves the following (Hyde, 2000).
      a) Immunologic memory and specificity
      b) Collaboration of B cells and T cells
      c) Three types of adaptive immunity are the following.

Table 6. Investigational Biologic Agents

Agent	Manufacturer	Phase of Investigation	Mechanism of Action	Potential Indications
Advexin (INGN 201, Ad-SCMVp53)	Introgen Therapeutics	Phase II/III	p53 gene on an adenoviral vector	Head and neck, breast, lung, and pancreatic cancers; transitional cell carcinoma
AG-858 (HSPPC-70)	Antigenics, Inc.	Phase II	Autologous derived heat-shock proteins complexed with malignant antigens designed to stimulate an anticancer immune response	CML
Ampligen® (AMP 719)	Hemispherx Biopharma, Inc.	Phase II/III	Interferon	Renal cell cancer, malignant melanoma
Epratuzumab (Lymphocide®, AMG-412)	Amgen Inc.	Phase III	Humanized anti-CD22 monoclonal antibody	Non-Hodgkin lymphoma
Genasense® (Oblimersen sodium, G-3139)	Genta, Inc.	Phase II/III	Anti-sense oligonucleotide that prevents synthesis of Bcl-2 protein to facilitate apoptosis	CLL, AML, melanoma, multiple myeloma, prostate cancer
GVAX	Cell Genesys, Inc.	Phase II/III	Vaccine of irradiated tumor cells modified to secrete GM-CSF and induce a systemic immune response against the tumor	Prostate, lung, and pancreatic cancers; multiple myeloma, AML
Multikine® (leukocyte interleukin injection)	CEL-SCI Corp.	Phase II	Mixture of interferons, interleukins, and colony-stimulating factors	Prostate and head and neck cancers
Oncophage (HSPPC-96)	Antigenics, Inc.	Phase III	Autologous tumor-derived heat shock protein-peptide complex designed to stimulate an anticancer immune response	Lung and stomach cancers, renal cell carcinoma, lymphoma
OncoVAX®	Intracel, LLC	Phase II	Autologous cells attached to BCG vaccine	Colon cancer, renal cell carcinoma
Onyx-015 (CI-1042)	Onyx Pharmaceuticals, Inc.	Phase III	Genetically modified adenovirus that destroys cancer cells containing abnormal p53 tumor-suppressing proteins	Head and neck, pancreatic, colorectal, and lung cancers
Palifermin	Amgen Inc.	Phase III	Recombinant human keratinocyte growth factor	Reduce duration and incidence of severe oral mucositis in bone marrow transplantation
Panitumumab (formerly ABX-EGF)	Amgen Inc. and Abegenix, Inc.	Phase II/III	Humanized monoclonal antibody against the epidermal growth factor receptor	Renal cell cancer
		Phase III	Recombinant antibody that targets the epidermal growth factor receptor, required for normal and tumor cell growth	Solid tumors
Provenge® (APC-8015)	Dendreon Corp.	Phase III	Vaccine to sensitize dendritic cells to attack tumor cells expressing prostate acid phosphatase protein	Prostate cancer
Ranpirnase (Onconase®)	Alfacell	Phase III	Degrades tRNA, leading to direct cell death or signaling of a cell to stop replicating	Malignant mesothelioma

AML—acute myelogenous leukemia; BCG—Bacillus Calmette-Guérin; CML—chronic myelogenous leukemia; GM-CSF—granulocyte macrophage–colony-stimulating factor; tRNA—transfer ribonucleic acid

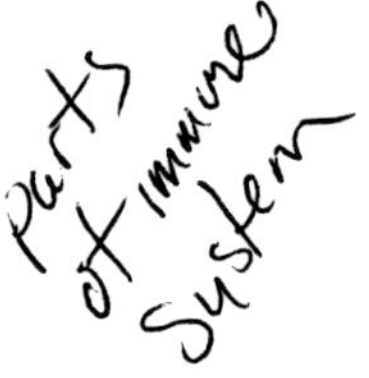

Figure 4. Primary and Secondary Lymphoid Organs

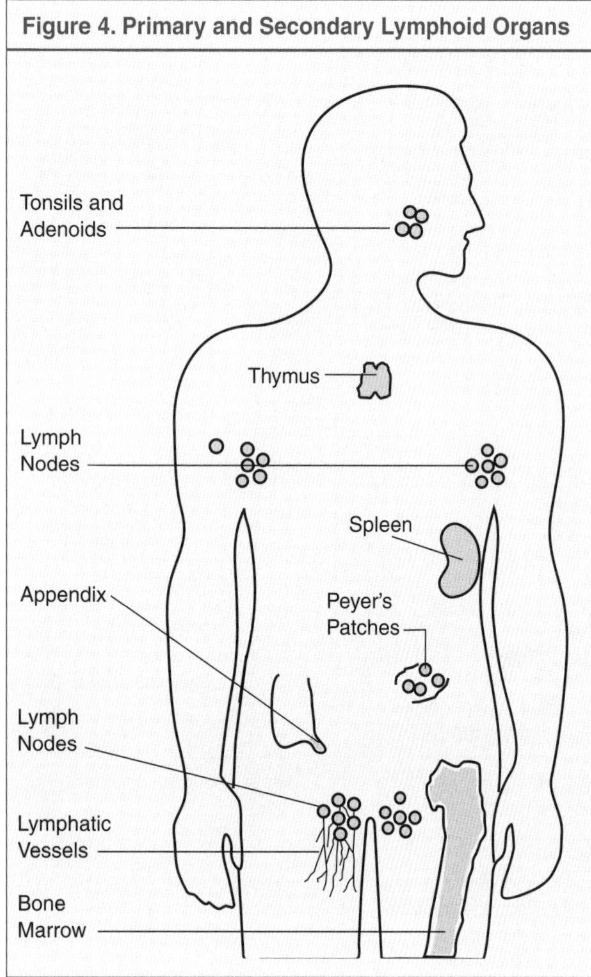

(1) Humoral immunity (see Figure 6): B lymphocytes, memory B cells, and plasma cells mediate humoral immunity. The result is the production of immunoglobulins.

(2) Cell-mediated immunity (see Figure 7): Cell-mediated immunity is mediated by T cells and their cytokine products. This type of immunity does not involve an antibody; it does involve the following.
   (a) Cytotoxic T cells (T_C)
   (b) Helper T cells (T_H)
   (c) Suppressor T cells (T_S)

(3) Antibody-dependent cellular cytotoxicity (ADCC): This type of response is believed to involve a three-step process.
   (a) The antibody binds to the antigen of the tumor cell.
   (b) NK cells recognize the antibody-covered tumor cells.
   (c) Cytotoxic proteins are released to destroy tumor cells.

... system (see Figure 8): The ... volves the intricate interaction ... and proteins (Hyde, 2000).

... ng cells (APCs): Cells (e.g., macrophages, B cells, dendritic cells) that efficiently present antigen to T cells; only dendritic cells are capable of initiating a primary immune response.

2. T cells (Hyde, 2000)
   a) Helper (T_H cells): Cells that coordinate the immune response and cell-mediated immunity. They are required to maintain cytotoxic T cell responses.
   b) Cytotoxic (T_C cells): Cells that kill foreign cells, virally infected cells, or cells with new surface antigens
   c) Suppressor (T_S cells): Cells that interfere with development of immune reaction when recognizing antigen; their primary role is to modulate the severity of inflammation produced by infection but also play an important role to prevent autoimmunity and may be involved in malignancy.
   d) Memory T cells (T_M cells): Cells that recognize specific antigens and induce recall responses
3. NK cells: Cells that are cytotoxic to tumor cells and virally infected autologous cells by producing substances that can bind to and destroy foreign invaders, without having to identify a specific antigen
4. NKT cells: Cells that have markers both of NK cells and T cells
5. B lymphocytes: Plasma cells that manufacture immunoglobulin or an antibody specific to an initiating antigen
6. Antibodies: Protein products of plasma cells; known as immunoglobulins, they enhance effector-cell functions. One type of antibody is immunoglobulin G (IgG). Other types include IgM, IgA, IgD, and IgE.

Table 7. Innate and Acquired Immune Responses

Immune Response	Mechanism of Action	Cells Primarily Involved
Innate	Primary line of defense Nonspecific No memory	Neutrophils Monocytes, macrophages Large granular lymphocytes (natural killer cells)
Adaptive	Secondary line of defense Specific memory	Lymphocytes T cells (in cell-mediated immunity) B cells (in humoral immunity)

Figure 5. Innate (Nonspecific) Immune Response

Natural killer cells
Lyse
Tumor cells
Engulf
Phagocytes
Polymorphonuclear leukocytes
Monocytes
Macrophages
Engulf

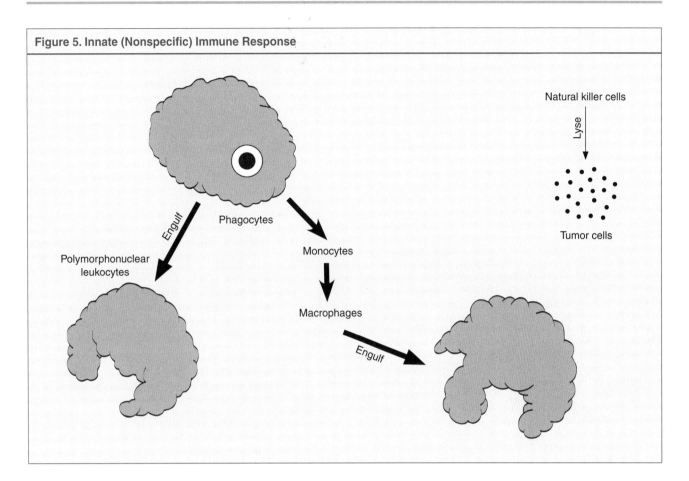

Figure 6. Adaptive (Specific) Immune Response: B Cells and Humoral Immunity

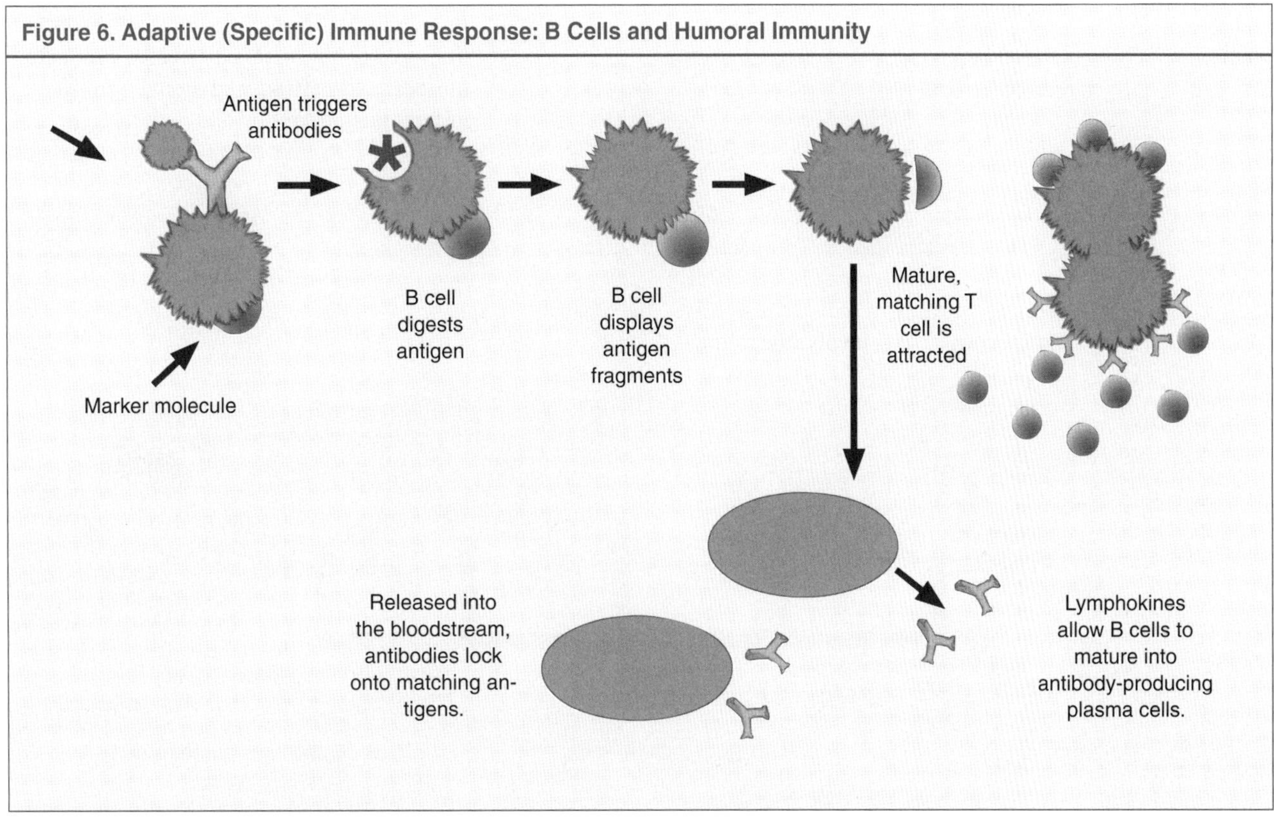

7. Cytokines: Glycoprotein products of immune cells such as lymphocytes and macrophages. Cytokines mediate effector defense functions. Cytokines themselves usually are not cytotoxic.

K. Tumor escape mechanisms: When immune surveillance fails, tumor formation occurs. The theories set forth to explain this process include the following (Muehlbauer & Schwartzentruber, 2003).

1. Altered immunogenicity: Tumors can be targeted by the immune system either through cell surface molecules that function as targets for antibody responses or intracellular molecules that are presented within the context of the major histocompatibility complex (MHC) molecules. Antigen expression on the tumor-cell surface is altered, allowing the antigen to go unrecognized by the humoral immune system. Alternatively, cell-mediated immune response can be blunted through loss or alteration of the MHC molecules or loss or mutation of the peptide epitope that binds to the MHC molecule and is recognized by the T cells.
2. Antigen modulation: Antibodies produced as part of the immune response cause antigens to enter the tumor cell or leave it completely. This further limits the ability of the immune cells to recognize the tumor cell as nonself.
3. Immune suppression: The tumor itself produces substances that alter or inhibit the body's immune response.
4. Acquired deficiencies to immune sensitivity: This includes age- and disease-associated alterations such as decreased or increased apoptosis and signaling defects of T cells.
5. Immunologic aging: Alterations in T-cell functions cause declines in T-cell proliferation, generation of T killer cells, production of interleukin (IL)-2 and signal transduction of lymphocytes.

Figure 7. Adaptive (Specific) Immune Response: Cell-Mediated Immunity

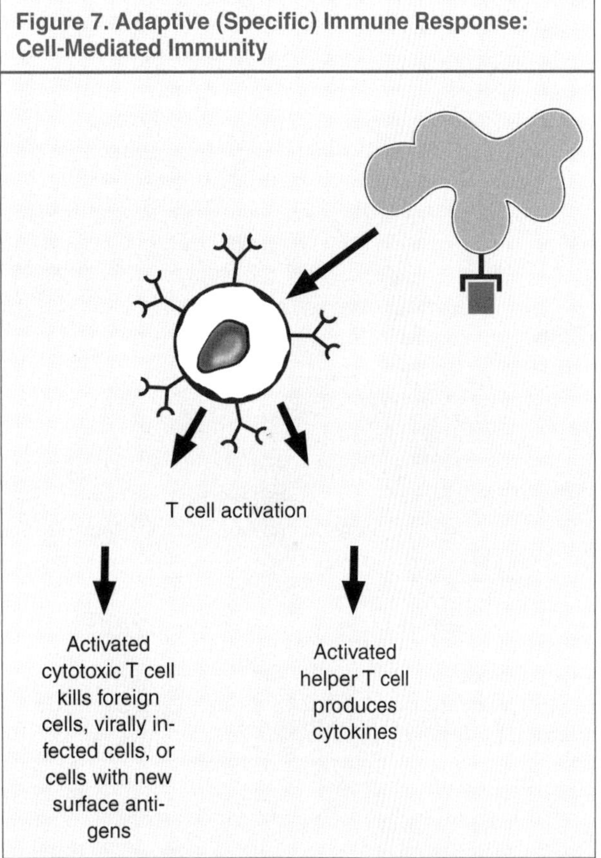

Figure 8. Cells of the Immune System

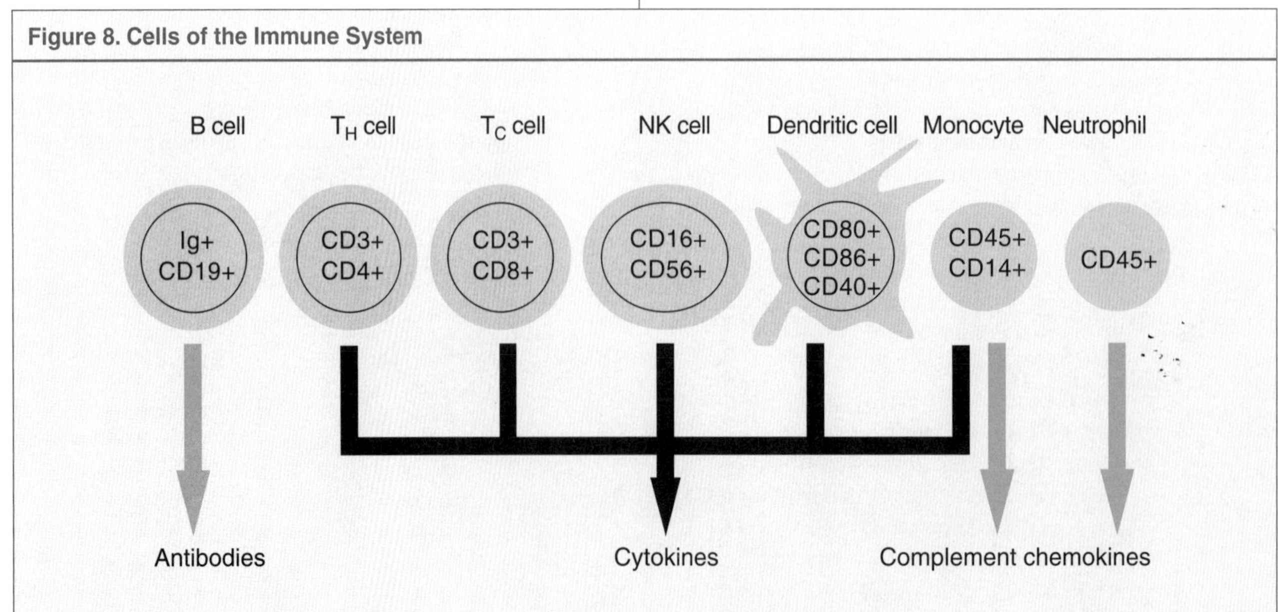

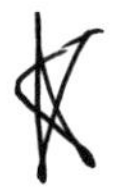

flammatory warning mune response.

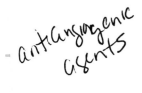

L. Angiogenesis and antiangiogenic agents (Carmeliet & Jain, 2000; Gasparini, 1999; Libutti & Pluda, 2000; Muehlbauer, 2003; Papetti & Herman, 2002; Risau, 1995; Yancopoulos et al., 2000)

1. Angiogenesis is the development of new blood vessels. It is a complex, multistep process that is required for a host of normal functions, including wound healing, tissue repair, reproduction, growth, and development.
2. Under normal circumstances, angiogenesis is tightly controlled by a balance of stimulators and inhibitors.
3. In malignant angiogenesis, that balance is upset, leading to a cascade of irregular molecular and cellular events that contribute to tumor neovascularization.
4. In the context of tumor growth, angiogenesis refers to the growth of new vessels within a tumor. The new vessels develop from the existing vascular network and provide a blood supply for the tumor.
    - *a)* Vascular endothelial growth factor (VEGF) and basic fibroblast growth factor (bFGF) are circulating growth factors known to induce angiogenesis. Their presence has been reported to correlate with extent of disease, clinical status, and survival.
    - *b)* Endothelial cells line the vasculature of normal tissues. In a resting state, they provide a homeostatic barrier that prevents the uncontrolled extravasation of intravascular components and inhibits coagulation.
    - *c)* When a tumor begins to grow in normal tissue, tumor cells release factors that elicit responses from the surrounding endothelium. The result is vascular growth from normal tissue into the tumor.
    - *d)* Neovascularization contributes to tumor invasion and metastasis.
5. Antiangiogenic agents
    - *a)* Mechanism of action: Antiangiogenic agents target the neovasculature of tumors to halt their growth, prevent tumor invasion, and preclude metastatic diffusion. Potentially, antiangiogenic agents are ideal for use with other cancer therapy modalities because antiangiogenic agents maximize the efficacy of the other therapies.
    - *b)* Side effects: Table 8 presents a list of some of the side effects of antiangiogenic agents.
6. Administration: Always review the clinical research protocol before administering an antiangiogenic agent. Know the side effects, interventions, and diagnostic studies that apply to the agent that will be used.

M. Principles of radioimmunotherapy (RIT): See Bruner, Gosselin-Acomb, and Haas (2005) for an in-depth discussion. RIT is a radiopharmaceutical cancer treatment that employs unsealed radionuclide-labeled, or radiolabeled, monoclonal antibodies. These antibodies, which are administered systemically by injection, recognize tumor-associated antigens to deliver radioactivity to tumor cells selectively (Kaminski et al., 1996). Radiolabeled monoclonal antibodies have an important and growing role in cancer therapy (Groch, 2002; Hainsworth, 2003; Larson, Divgi, Sgouros, Cheung, & Scheinberg, 2000; Wahl et al., 1998).

1. The goal of RIT is to destroy or inactivate cancer cells while preserving the integrity of normal tissues (Dunne-Daly, 1999).
2. Radioactive isotopes may emit one or more type of radiation.
    - *a)* Alpha particles
    - *b)* Beta particles
    - *c)* Gamma rays
3. Each radionuclide emits radiation particles and/or rays with energies that are characteristic of that specific radionuclide (Bruner et al., 2005).
4. Immunoconjugated radioactive biologicals should be handled according to guidelines for the specific isotope used.
5. Radioactive isotopes must be administered by professionals licensed to do so.

N. Toxin-conjugated molecules: Toxins such as diphtheria or pseudomonas exotoxin are potent inhibitors of cell viability. One molecule of diphtheria toxin delivered intracellularly is capable of inhibiting protein synthesis that results in the death of the cells. Antibodies and cytokines can be used to target these toxic molecules to cancer cells and depend upon the uptake of these toxins by the cells to cause their death. The strategy of delivering toxins intracellularly has resulted in the

Table 8. Antiangiogenic and Immunomodulating Agents

Medication Name(s)	Mechanism of Action	Route of Administration	Indication	Side Effects	Product-Specific Information
Bevacizumab (anti-VEGF, Avastin®)	Binds to and inhibits the activity of human vascular endothelial growth factor, blocking proliferation and formation of new blood vessels	IV	Used in combination with IV fluorouracil-containing regimens as first-line treatment for patients with metastatic carcinoma of the colon or rectum	Hemorrhage, hypertension, proteinuria, congestive heart failure, asthenia, diarrhea, leucopenia, thromboembolism, hyponatremia	Avoid use for at least 28 days after major surgery, and surgical incision should be fully healed. Suspend treatment with bevacizumab several weeks before surgery. Store agent in refrigerator but do not freeze. Do not shake. Protect vials from light. Diluted solution may be stored for up to eight hours under refrigeration. Patients should notify their physician if headache persists or worsens despite treatment. Patients should notify their physician if hemoptysis, shortness of breath, or signs of bleeding occur. Patients should notify their physician if fever persists for more than three days following dose. Patients should be aware of signs of disease progression (e.g., new or worsening bone pain, a change in the level of consciousness). Patients should be informed that the benefits of therapy may not immediately become apparent. Use antipyretics as needed for constitutional symptoms. If hemolysis or epistaxis develops, hold therapy pending evaluation. If infusion-related symptoms appear, premedicate subsequent doses. Before each dose, assess • Monthly complete blood count with differential and electrolytes, liver function, and urinalysis • Presence of epistaxis, hemolysis, or bleeding • Nutritional status • Presence of constipation or diarrhea • Pain that may include muscle or joint aches • Skin for rash • Level of consciousness • Disease status.
Levamisole (Ergamisol®)	Restores depressed immune function; stimulates antibodies to various antigens; stimulates T cell activation and proliferation; potentiates monocyte and macrophage functions; and increases neutrophil mobility, adherence, and chemotaxis	po	In combination with fluorouracil in the treatment of colon cancer	Nausea, diarrhea, vomiting, dermatitis, fatigue, taste perversion, arthralgia, agranulocytosis	Because of risk of agranulocytosis, routine hematologic monitoring should be performed. Flu-like syndrome often accompanies agranulocytosis; instruct patients to report any symptoms. An Antabuse-like effect may occur when taken concomitantly with alcohol. Monitor INR in patients taking warfarin and adjust accordingly when taking concomitantly with levamisole.

(Continued on next page)

Table 8. Antiangiogenic and Immunomodulating Agents *(Continued)*

Medication Name(s)	Mechanism of Action	Route of Administration	Indication	Side Effects	Product-Specific Information
Thalidomide (Thalomid®)	Poorly understood immunomodulation	po	Multiple myeloma (non–FDA-approved indication)	Birth defects, drowsiness or somnolence, peripheral neuropathy, dizziness, rash, anorexia, increase in appetite and/or weight gain, constipation, neutropenia, headache	Administer weekly pregnancy test during first four weeks of therapy, then monthly if menses are regular or every two weeks if irregular. Patients may develop numbness, tingling, or pain in hands or feet. Evaluate monthly during first three months then every three months thereafter. Obtain monthly CBC with differential. Perform monthly body weight check. Evaluate for presence of constipation and level of fatigue. Evaluate for episodes of dizziness or orthostatic hypotension and notify physician if symptoms develop. Both male and female patients must be appropriately educated on birth control necessity during therapy. Per FDA requirement, patients must view manufacturer's gender-specific video regarding thalidomide-associated birth defects. Patients must be provided with S.T.E.P.S.™ (System for Thalidomide Education and Prescribing Safety) literature and sign an informed consent form regarding proper birth control from Celgene, the manufacturer of thalidomide. Immediately stop thalidomide therapy and notify physician if patient becomes pregnant. Discontinue therapy and notify physician if patient develops peripheral neuropathy, and consider restarting therapy at a reduced dose when symptoms resolve. If ANC < 750/mm^3, hold therapy. If allergic reaction occurs, hold therapy. Provide nutritional counseling. Provide information about signs and symptoms of disease progression. Contact physician if suspicious symptoms appear during therapy.

ANC—absolute neutrophil count; CBC—complete blood count; FDA—U.S. Food and Drug Administration; INR—international normalized ratio approval of two agents by the FDA for the treatment of malignancy: gemtuzumab ozogamicin for the treatment of leukemia and denileukin diftitox for the treatment of mycosis fungoides.

References

Amgen Inc. (2002). Neupogen [Package insert]. Thousand Oaks, CA: Author.

Amgen Inc. (2003). Aranesp [Package insert]. Amgen, Inc., Thousand Oaks, CA: Author.

Amgen Inc. (2004). Neulasta [Package insert]. Thousand Oaks, CA: Author.

Berlex Laboratories. (2002a). Campath [Package insert]. Richmond, CA: Author.

Berlex Laboratories. (2002b). Leukine [Package insert]. Richmond, CA: Author.

Berlex Laboratories. (2002c). Refludan [Package insert]. Richmond, CA: Author.

Biogen Idec. (2003). Zevalin [Package insert]. Cambridge, MA: Author.

Bruner, D.W., Gosselin-Acomb, T., & Haas, M. (Eds.). (2005). *Manual for radiation oncology nursing practice and education* (3rd ed.). Pittsburgh, PA: Oncology Nursing Society.

Carmeliet, P., & Jain, R.K. (2000). Angiogenesis in cancer and other diseases. *Nature, 407,* 249–257.

Chiron Corp. (2000). Proleukin [Package insert]. Emeryville, CA: Author.

Corixa Corp. & GlaxoSmithKline. (2003). Bexxar [Package insert]. Seattle, WA, & Philadelphia: Author.

Dunne-Daly, C.F. (1999). Principles of radiotherapy and radiobiology. *Seminars in Oncology Nursing, 15,* 250–259.

Enzon. (1998). Oncaspar [Package insert]. Piscataway, NJ: Author.

Gasparini, G. (1999). The rationale and future potential of angiogenesis inhibitors in neoplasia. *Drugs, 58,* 17–38.

Genentech, Inc. (2004a). Avastin [Package insert]. South San Francisco, CA: Author.

Genentech, Inc. (2004b). Herceptin [Package insert]. South San Francisco, CA: Author

Genentech, Inc. (2004c). Rituxan [Package insert]. South San Francisco, CA: Author.

Groch, M.W. (2002, February 9–10). *New perspectives on PET.* Paper presented at the Mid-Winter Educational Symposium, Society of Nuclear Medicine, Scottsdale, AZ. Retrieved December 7, 2004, from http://www.medscape.com/viewarticle/440520

Hainsworth, J.D. (2003, May 31–June 3). *Non-Hodgkin's lymphoma: Where do we stand today?* Paper presented at the 39th Annual Meeting of the American Society of Clinical Oncology, Chicago, IL. Retrieved December 7, 2004, from http://www.medscape.com/viewarticle/457534

Hyde, R.M. (Ed.). (2000). *Immunology* (4th ed.). Philadelphia: Lippincott Williams & Wilkins.

ImClone Systems & Bristol-Myers Squibb. (2004). Erbitux [Package insert]. Branchburg, NJ, & Princeton, NJ: Author.

Immunomedics, Inc. (1999). CEA-Scan [Package insert]. Morris Plains, NJ: Author.

InterMune, Inc. (2004). Actimmune [Package insert]. Brisbane, CA: Author.

Kaminski, M.S., Zasakny, K.R., Francis, I.R., Fenner, M.C., Ross, C.W., Milik, A.W., et al. (1996). Iodine-131-anti-B1 radioimmunotherapy for B-cell lymphoma. *Journal of Clinical Oncology, 4,* 1974–1981.

Larson, S.M., Divgi, C., Sgouros, G., Cheung, N-K.V., & Scheinberg, D.A. (2000). Monoclonal antibodies: Basic principles: Radioisotope conjugates. In S.A. Rosenberg (Ed.), *Principles and practice of the biologic therapy of cancer* (2nd ed., pp. 396–412). Philadelphia: Lippincott Williams & Wilkins.

Libutti, S.K., & Pluda, J.M. (2000). Antiangiogenesis: Clinical applications. In S.A. Rosenberg (Ed.), *Principles and practice of the biologic therapy of cancer* (2nd ed., pp. 844–861). Philadelphia: Lippincott Williams & Wilkins.

Ligand Pharmaceuticals. (2002). Ontak [Package insert]. San Diego, CA: Author.

Merck & Co. (2002). Elspar [Package insert]. West Point, PA: Author.

Muehlbauer, P.M. (2003). Anti-angiogenesis in cancer therapy. *Seminars in Oncology Nursing, 19,* 180–192.

Muehlbauer, P.M., & Schwartzentruber, D.J. (2003). Cancer vaccines. *Seminars in Oncology Nursing, 19,* 206–216.

Ortho Biotech. (2004). Procrit [Package insert]. Raritan, NJ: Author.

Papetti, M., & Herman, I.M. (2002). Mechanisms of normal and tumor derived angiogenesis. *American Journal of Cell Physiology, 282,* C947–C970.

Rieger, P.T. (2001). Biotherapy. In P.T. Rieger (Ed.), *Biotherapy: A comprehensive overview* (pp. 3–37). Sudbury, MA: Jones and Bartlett.

Risau, W. (1995). Differentiation of endothelium. *Federation of American Societies for Experimental Biology Journal, 9,* 926–933.

Roche Laboratories, Inc. (2004). Roferon- A [Package insert]. Nutley, NJ: Author.

Rosenberg, S.A. (Ed.). (2000). *Principles and practice of the biologic therapy of cancer.* Philadelphia: Lippincott Williams & Wilkins.

Sanofi Synthelabo. (2002). Elitek [Package insert]. New York: Author.

Schering Corp. (2004). Intron-A [Package insert]. Kenilworth, NJ: Author.

Sweetman, S. (Ed.). (2004). *Martindale: The complete drug reference* [Electronic version]. Green Village, CO: Thompson MICROMEDEX.

Wahl, R.L., Zasadny, K.R., MacFarlane, D., Francis, I.R., Ross, C.W., Estes, J., et al. (1998). Iodine-131 anti-B1 antibody for B-cell lymphoma: An update on the Michigan phase I experience. *Journal of Nuclear Medicine, 39*(Suppl. 8), 21S–27S.

Wyeth Pharmaceuticals, Inc. (2004a). Mylotarg [Package insert]. Philadelphia: Author.

Wyeth Pharmaceuticals, Inc. (2004b). Neumega [Package insert]. Philadelphia: Author.

Yancopoulos, G.D., Davis, S., Gale, N.W., Rudge, J.S., Wiegand, S.J., & Holash, J. (2000). Vascular-specific growth factors and blood vessel formation. *Nature, 407,* 242–248.

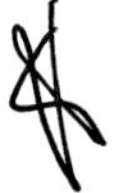

V. Fundamentals of Administration

A. Safe handling: Many drugs used in the treatment of cancer are considered to be hazardous to healthcare workers. The term *hazardous* refers to drugs that require special handling because of potential health risks. These risks are a result of the inherent toxicities of the drugs (American Society of Hospital Pharmacists, 1990; National Institute for Occupational Safety and Health [NIOSH], 2004). According to the Occupational Safety and Health Administration (OSHA, 1995), safe levels of occupational exposure to hazardous agents cannot be determined, and no reliable method of monitoring exposure exists. Therefore, it is imperative that those who work with hazardous drugs adhere to practices designed to minimize occupational exposure.

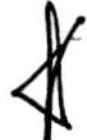

1. Definition of hazardous drugs: The American Society of Hospital Pharmacists (1990) provided the first definition of hazardous drugs; NIOSH (2004) refined the definition. Drugs are considered hazardous if they meet one or more of the following criteria.
   - *a)* Carcinogenicity
   - *b)* Teratogenicity or developmental toxicity
   - *c)* Reproductive toxicity
   - *d)* Organ toxicity at low doses
   - *e)* Genotoxicity
   - *f)* Drugs similar in structure or toxicity to drugs classified as hazardous using these criteria

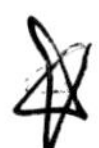

2. Potential occupational health risks of hazardous drugs
   - *a)* The International Agency for Research on Cancer (IARC) publishes independent assessments of the carcinogenic risks of chemicals. The IARC lists nine drugs used in the treatment of cancer as known human carcinogens, whereas other antineoplastic agents are classified as probable or possible carcinogens (see Table 9) (IARC, 2004).
   - *b)* Exposure during pregnancy may cause structural defects in fetuses (Hemminki, Kyyrönen, & Lindbohm, 1985; Peelen, Roeleveld, Heederik, Kromhout, & de Kort, 1999).
   - *c)* Adverse reproductive outcomes, such as spontaneous abortions (Stucker et al., 1990; Valanis, Vollmer, & Steele, 1999) and infertility (Valanis, Vollmer, Labuhn, & Glass, 1997), have been reported in healthcare workers exposed to cytotoxic agents.
   - *d)* Many cytotoxic drugs are known to be toxic to the skin, mucous membranes, and corneas. Some drugs are known to cause organ damage.
   - *e)* Chromosomal damage has been documented in healthcare workers following exposure to cytotoxic agents (Fuchs et al., 1995; Harrison, 2001; Sessink et al., 1994).
   - *f)* Acute symptoms have occurred from accidental exposure. Symptoms depend on the drug involved and may include headache, nausea, dizziness, or skin, eye, or throat irritation (Harrison, 2001; Valanis et al., 1997).

3. Potential occupational health risks associated with biotherapy agents
   - *a)* Limited data are available regarding the effects of handling biologic agents.
   - *b)* Most biologic agents do not affect DNA and do not cause genetic changes.
   - *c)* Interferon is considered a hazardous drug because of its reproductive toxicity (OSHA, 1995).
4. Potential routes of exposure to hazardous drugs

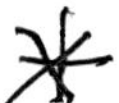

   - *a)* Absorption through skin or mucous membranes after direct contact with drug or from surfaces or objects that are contaminated with hazardous drugs: Several studies have documented cytotoxic contamination of workers (Labuhn, Valanis, Schoeny,

Table 9. Carcinogens

Exposure Risk	Antineoplastic Drugs
Group 1: Carcinogenic to humans	• Azathioprine • Busulfan • Chlorambucil • Cyclophosphamide • Melphalan • MOPP • Semustine • Tamoxifen • Thiotepa
Group 2A: Probably carcinogenic to humans	• Carmustine • Cisplatin • Doxorubicin • Etoposide • Lomustine • Nitrogen mustard • Procarbazine • Teniposide
Group 2B: Possibly carcinogenic to humans	• Amsacrine • Bleomycin • Dacarbazine • Daunorubicin • Mitomycin • Mitoxantrone • Streptozocin

Note. Based on information from International Agency for Research on Cancer, 2004.

Loveday, & Vollmer, 1998; Pethran et al., 2003). Multiple studies have demonstrated contamination of the environment in drug preparation and administration areas (Connor, Anderson, Sessink, Broadfield, & Power, 1999; NIOSH, 2004; Polovich, 2003).

b) Injection by inadvertent injury from a needle stick or contaminated sharps (Dorr & Alberts, 1992; Harrison & Schultz, 2000)

c) Inhalation of drug aerosols, dust, or droplets (Dorr & Alberts, 1992; Harrison & Schultz, 2000)

d) Ingestion through contaminated food, beverage, tobacco products, or other hand-to-mouth behavior (NIOSH, 2004)

5. Guidelines regarding personal protective equipment (PPE)

a) Types of apparel

(1) Gloves: Wear disposable gloves that are powder-free and have been tested for use with hazardous drugs. Inspect gloves for physical defects before use. Latex gloves provide protection but should be used with caution because of the risk of latex sensitivity. Gloves made of other materials, such as nitrile (Singleton & Connor, 1999), polyurethane, or neoprene, provide protection (Connor, 1999). Double gloves are recommended for all handling activities (NIOSH, 2004). Change gloves immediately after each use; if a tear, puncture, or drug spill occurs; or after 30 minutes of wear (American Society of Hospital Pharmacists, 1990; NIOSH, 2004).

(2) Gowns: Wear a disposable, lint-free gown made of a low-permeability fabric, such as polyethylene-coated materials (Connor, 1993; Harrison & Kloos, 1999). The gown should have a solid front, long sleeves, tight cuffs, and a back closure. Inner glove cuffs should be worn under the gown cuffs; outer glove cuffs should extend over the gown cuffs. Discard the gown if it is visibly contaminated, before leaving drug preparation areas, and after handling hazardous drugs. Gowns should not be re-used (NIOSH, 2004).

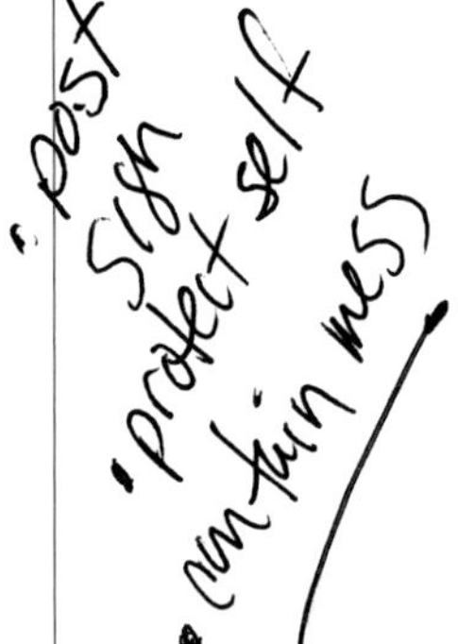

(3) Respirators: Wear a NIOSH-approved respirator mask (such as a nonpowered, air-purifying, particulate-filter respirator) when cleaning hazardous drug spills. Consult the material safety data sheet (MSDS) for the respirator appropriate to the situation (NIOSH, 1996). Surgical masks do not provide respiratory protection.

(4) Eye and face protection: Wear a face shield whenever there is a possibility of splashing.

b) Situations requiring PPE: Wear PPE whenever there is a risk of hazardous drugs being released into the environment, such as in the following situations (NIOSH, 2004).

(1) Introducing or withdrawing needles from vials
(2) Transferring drugs using needles or syringes
(3) Opening ampules
(4) Expelling air from a drug-filled syringe
(5) Administering hazardous drugs by any route
(6) Spiking IV bags and changing IV tubing
(7) Priming IV tubing
(8) Handling leakage from tubing, syringe, and connection sites
(9) Disposing of hazardous drugs and items contaminated by hazardous drugs
(10) Handling the body fluids of a patient who received hazardous agents in the past 48 hours
(11) Cleaning hazardous drug spills

6. Storage and labeling of chemotherapeutic agents

a) On the clinical unit

(1) Store chemotherapy drug containers in a location that permits appropriate temperature and safety regulation.
(2) Label all drug containers to indicate the hazardous nature of their contents (OSHA, 1995).
(3) Have access to instructions (e.g., MSDS) regarding what to do in the event of accidental exposure.

(4) Check hazardous drug containers before taking them from the storage area to ensure that the packaging is intact and to detect any breakage.

b) In the home (Polovich, 2003) (see Appendix 3)

(1) Keep all hazardous drugs out of the reach of children and pets.

(2) Store drugs in containers that provide adequate protection from puncture or breakage.

(3) Label containers to indicate the hazardous nature of their contents.

(4) Provide instructions listing proper procedure for handling a damaged container.

(5) Store hazardous drugs in an area free of moisture and temperature extremes.

(6) Provide spill kits and instructions for their use.

(7) Give verbal and written instructions about handling and storing hazardous drugs and hazardous drug waste.

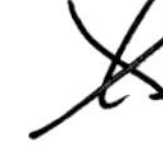

7. Safe handling while mixing hazardous drugs: Maintain sterile technique during the preparation of parenteral drugs.

a) Chemotherapeutic drugs

(1) Prepare cytotoxic drugs, including oral drugs that must be compounded or crushed, in a biological safety cabinet (BSC) (American Society of Hospital Pharmacists, 1990; NIOSH, 2004). The BSC should

(a) Provide vertical laminar airflow. Vertical airflow carries contaminated air away from the BSC operator and out of the environment.

(b) Eliminate exhaust through a high-efficiency particulate air (HEPA) filter. Ideally, a BSC should be vented to the outside (NIOSH, 2004).

(c) Have a blower that operates continuously (American Society of Hospital Pharmacists, 1990).

(d) Be located in a low-traffic area to reduce interference with airflow.

(e) Be used by individuals trained to employ techniques that reduce interference with airflow.

(f) Be serviced according to the manufacturer's recommendations.

(g) Be recertified every six months (American Society of Hospital Pharmacists, 1990).

(2) Wash hands before donning PPE.

(3) Wear appropriate PPE.

(4) If desired, place a sterile, plastic-backed absorbent pad on the work surface. Such pads may interfere with airflow in the BSC (Minoia et al., 1998).

(5) Use safe technique when opening ampules (American Society of Hospital Pharmacists, 1990).

(a) Clear fluid from the ampule neck.

(b) Tilt the ampule away from yourself.

(c) Wrap gauze or an alcohol pad around the neck of the ampule.

(d) Break the ampule in the direction away from yourself.

(e) Use a filtered needle to withdraw fluid.

(6) When reconstituting drugs packaged in vials, avoid pressure buildup, which can result in the release of drug aerosols. Use a closed-system device (e.g., PhaSeal® [Baxa Corp., Englewood, CO]) if available (NIOSH, 2004).

(7) Use tubing and syringes with Luer lock fittings.

(8) Avoid overfilling syringes. A syringe that is too full may separate from the plunger end (OSHA, 1995).

(9) Prime all tubing with fluid that does not contain the drug before adding cytotoxic drugs, preferably in a BSC (American Society of Hospital Pharmacists 1990; OSHA, 1995) or use a closed-system device to minimize the risk of exposure (Connor, Anderson, Sessink, & Spivey, 2002; Wick, Slawson, Jorgenson, & Tyler, 2003).

(10) Place a label on each container that says "Cytotoxic Drug" or a similar warning.

(11) Wipe the outside of the container with moist gauze before placing it in a sealable bag for transport.

(12) Dispose of all material that has come into contact with a cytotoxic drug by placing the material into a waste container designated for cytotoxic waste.

(13) Remove and discard outer gloves and gown. Then remove inner gloves.

(14) Wash hands before leaving the work area.

b) Safe handling while mixing biotherapy drugs

(1) Use safe handling precautions for biotherapy agents that are considered hazardous (e.g., interferon) (NIOSH, 2004).

(2) Wear gloves when mixing biotherapy agents that are irritating to skin (e.g., rituximab [Genentech, Inc., 2000]).

(3) A nuclear pharmacist prepares radiolabeled monoclonal antibodies for infusion. Note: Federal and state laws require that radiation-safety warning signs designate the areas in which radioisotopes are stored or used (Bruner, Haas, & Gosselin-Acomb, 2005).

8. Transporting chemotherapeutic drugs (OSHA, 1995)

a) Transport syringes containing hazardous drugs in a sealed container, with the Luer lock end of the syringe capped. Do not transport syringes with needles in place.

b) Select a transport receptacle that can contain spillage if dropped (e.g., a leakproof, sealable bag) and additional impervious packing material as necessary to avoid damage during transport.

c) Label the outermost receptacle to indicate that its contents are hazardous.

d) Ensure that whoever will be transporting the drugs has a spill kit and knows how to use it.

9. Safe handling considerations during administration of hazardous drugs (American Society of Hospital Pharmacists, 1990; OSHA, 1995)

a) Always wear PPE.

b) Work below eye level.

c) Ensure that a spill kit and hazardous waste container are available.

d) Use a closed-system device (NIOSH, 2004), or place a disposable, absorbent, plastic-backed pad underneath the work area to absorb droplets of the drug that may spill.

e) Use a closed-system device, or place a gauze pad under the syringe at injection ports to catch droplets during administration.

f) Use needles, syringes, and tubing with Luer lock connectors.

g) If priming occurs at the administration site, prime IV tubing with a fluid that does not contain the drug or by using the backflow method.

h) After drug administration, remove the IV bag or bottle with the tubing attached (NIOSH, 2004; Polovich, 2003). Do not remove the spike from IV containers or reuse tubing.

i) Use detergent and water to wash surfaces that come into contact with hazardous drugs (Polovich, 2003).

j) Discard all contaminated material and PPE in a hazardous waste container.

10. Safety precautions are necessary to protect healthcare workers from exposures while caring for patients receiving some types of radiation therapy. Radiation protection standards and regulations are determined by the U.S. Nuclear Regulatory Commission (NRC), the FDA (radiopharmaceuticals), and state radiation regulatory agencies. The next section provides information about radiation precautions. Principles of radiation precautions:

a) Occupational radiation exposure should be kept as low as reasonably achievable (ALARA). This requires close collaboration between the healthcare team and the radiation safety officer (RSO). Three factors help to provide protection (Dunne-Daly, 1999).

(1) Time: The amount of time spent near the radioactive source. The amount of exposure received is directly proportional to the amount of time spent near the source. (After a patient receives RIT, the patient is the radioactive source.)

(2) Distance: The amount of space between a point and the radioactive

source. As the distance from the radioactive source increases, its radiation exposure decreases.

(3) Shielding: A protective shield placed between the radioactive source (usually the patient) and what is to be protected (known as the point). The type of shielding used depends on the type of radiation.

b) Radiation monitoring devices are used to monitor occupational exposure.

(1) Monitoring of personnel: Personnel monitoring is required by law regardless of whether the patient is treated as an inpatient or outpatient. The film badge is the most widely used monitoring device. Each person caring for a patient receiving radiation should be assigned a film badge that is only worn within the work environment, is changed according to institutional guidelines, and is not shared with anyone else (Bruner et al., 2005). A dosimeter is another monitoring device. It can be a personal device or one that is shared after being reset.

(2) Monitoring of the environment: Environmental monitoring is done with a Geiger-Müller counter, which reacts to the presence of ionizing particles. After a course of inpatient RIT is completed and before the room is cleaned, the RSO surveys the room, linens, and garbage with the Geiger-Müller counter.

c) Type of radiation emission: A radionuclide, depending on its type, can emit one, two, or three types of emissions (Bruner et al., 2005).

(1) Alpha particles: These particles travel at great speed but have poor penetrating ability. Alpha particles cannot penetrate the outermost layers of skin, and they travel a maximum distance of 5 cm. A sheet of paper between the radiation source and the point or a distance of 5 cm between the radiation source and the point will shield the radiation. The skin of an alpha-irradiated patient is adequate to protect others from radiation exposure; in other words, alpha particles are not external hazards. However, contact with an irradiated patient's excreted body fluids may be hazardous.

(2) Beta particles: Beta particles have greater penetration abilities than do alpha particles. Like alpha particles, beta particles are not external hazards. The patient's skin or thick plastic shielding is usually adequate protection from beta particles. Yttrium-90 (such as Zevalin®) emits beta particles. After RIT, the following apply.

(a) The patient's body fluids are temporarily radioactive.

(b) The patient should receive specific discharge instructions to limit family exposure.

(3) Gamma rays

(a) High-energy gamma-emitting radionuclides: Protection from these rays is achieved by maintaining a specific distance from the radioactive source and the point (the distance is specific to the radioisotope used) and using appropriate shielding. Patients receiving this type of radionuclide may have to be in radiation isolation and behind lead shields (Bruner et al., 2005).

i) Iodine-131 emits high-energy beta particles and gamma rays.

ii) Care should include the following (Bruner et al., 2005).

- Restrict people entering the room during infusion
- Observe time and distance limitations based on recommendations of the RSO or nuclear pharmacist.
- Release patient after administration based on specific guidelines that vary by state.
- Pregnant women and children should avoid contact with the patient.
- Body fluids are radioactive for a period of time depend-

ing on the half-life and elimination of the isotope.
- Provide patient-specific discharge instructions to limit family exposure.

(b) Low-energy, or weak, gamma-emitting radionuclides: Special precautions usually are not necessary (Bruner et al., 2005).

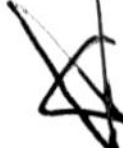

11. Handling a patient's body fluids
   a) After chemotherapy
      (1) Institute universal (standard) precautions (double gloves and disposable gown) when handling the blood, emesis, or excreta of a patient who has received chemotherapy within the previous 48 hours. Wear a face shield if splashing is possible (NIOSH, 2004).
      (2) For an incontinent child or adult: Clean the patient's skin well with each diaper change. Apply a protective barrier ointment to the skin of the patient's diaper area to decrease the chance of skin irritation from contact with urinary metabolites (Polovich, 2003).
      (3) Flush the toilet with the lid down after disposing of excreta from a patient who has received cytotoxic agents within the past 48 hours. There is no research to support the effectiveness of double flushing. Double flushing has been suggested in the literature (Brown et al., 2001; Welch & Silveira, 1997) and may be helpful with low volume per flush toilets (Polovich, 2003).
   b) After RIT (Bruner et al., 2005)
      (1) Institute universal (standard) precautions as above when handling the patient's body fluids (e.g., sweat, saliva, urine, feces, blood, semen, vaginal fluid). The duration of precautions varies depending on the radionuclide's half-life.
      (2) Consult the RSO or nuclear pharmacist.
12. Handling a patient's linens
   a) After chemotherapy (Polovich, 2003)
      (1) To the extent possible, preclude the need for laundering linens and clothing by using disposable linens or leakproof pads to contain body fluids.
      (2) If body fluids are present, use universal (standard) precautions when handling the linens of a patient who has received chemotherapy within 48 hours.
      (3) Handle bed linens and clothing according to the setting.
         (a) In the hospital setting
            i) Place linens into a plastic bag.
            ii) Prewash linens before they are added to other hospital laundry for a second washing (OSHA, 1995).
         (b) In the home setting (Polovich, 2003) (see Appendix 3)
            i) Wearing gloves, place contaminated linens into a washable pillowcase, separate from other items.
            ii) Machine wash linens and cloth diapers twice in hot water, with regular detergent, separately from other household items (Gullo, 1995).
            iii) Discard disposable diapers with other hazardous wastes by placing them in appropriately labeled plastic bags intended for hazardous waste disposal.
            iv) Discard used gloves and gowns in an appropriately labeled hazardous waste container.
   b) After RIT (Bruner et al., 2005)
      (1) If body fluids are present, use universal (standard) precautions when handling the linens of a patient who has received RIT.
      (2) Keep linens in the hospital room until scanned and cleared by the RSO or nuclear pharmacist.
13. Disposal of hazardous drugs and materials contaminated with hazardous drugs
   a) In a hospital setting (NIOSH, 2004)

(1) Place soft contaminated materials into a sealable, leakproof plastic bag or a rigid cytotoxic waste container marked with a brightly colored label that cites the hazardous nature of the contents.

(2) Use puncture-proof containers for sharp or breakable items. Dispose of needles and syringes intact; do not break or recap needles or crush syringes.

(3) Seal containers when full.

(4) Do not dispose of drug-contaminated items in infectious waste (red) containers. Some facilities autoclave or microwave these materials (NIOSH, 2004).

(5) Only housekeeping personnel who have received instruction in safe-handling procedures should handle waste containers. These personnel should wear gowns with cuffs and a back closure and two pairs of disposable latex or nitrile gloves.

b) In a home setting (Polovich, 2003) (see Appendix 3)

(1) Follow all the instructions applicable to a hospital setting excep[illegible] to handling the filled v[illegible]

(2) Designate an area awa[illegible] and pets where filled [illegible] await pickup.

(3) Follow county and st[illegible] regarding the disposa[illegible] wastes.

(4) Many agencies that [illegible] drug(s) will arrange f[illegible] disposal of contaminated equipment.

14. Procedures following acute accidental cytotoxic exposure: Improper technique, faulty equipment, or negligence in BSC operation can lead to exposure (OSHA, 1995).

a) Cleansing

(1) In the event of skin exposure: Remove any contaminated garments and immediately wash contaminated skin with soap and water. Refer to the MSDS for agent-specific interventions.

(2) In case of eye exposure: Immediately flush the eye with saline solution or water for at least 15 minutes (OSHA, 1995). Then seek emergency treatment. Ideally, each area designated for the handling of cytotoxic agents should contain an eyewash station. An acceptable alternative is sterile saline connected to IV tubing.

b) Reporting (Polovich, 2003)

(1) In case of employee exposure: Report the exposure to the employee health department or as institutional policy requires.

(2) In case of patient exposure: Report the exposure as institutional policy requires. In addition, inform the patient's healthcare providers.

15. Spill management

a) Radioactive spills: In case of a spill of radiolabeled antibody or contamination with the radioactive body fluid of a patient recently treated with RIT (Bruner et al., 2005)

(1) Restrict access to the area, and contact the RSO immediately. Never try to clean the area or touch the radioactive source. Adhere to the principles of time, distance, and shielding (see section V.A.10, Principles of Radiation Precautions).

(2) Follow other applicable NRC guidelines.

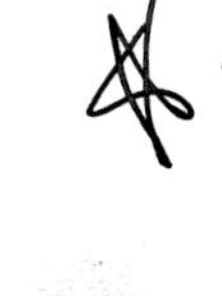

b) Cytotoxic spills: Spill kits should be available wherever hazardous drugs are stored, transported, prepared, or administered (see Figure 9). Everyone who works with hazardous drugs should be trained in spill cleanup. Individuals trained in handling hazardous materials (such as a Hazardous Materials Response Team) should clean up large spills whenever possible (OSHA, 2004b). In case of a spill involving a cytotoxic agent, follow these procedures.

(1) Immediately post a sign or signs that warn others of the presence of a hazardous spill. This will prevent others from being exposed.

(2) Don two pairs of gloves, a disposable gown, and a face shield.

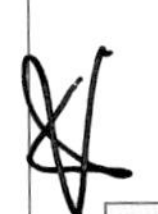

Figure 9. Contents of an Antineoplastic Spill Kit

- Two pairs of disposable gloves (one outer pair of utility gloves and one inner latex pair)
- Low permeability, disposable protective garments (coveralls or gown and shoe covers)
- Safety glasses or splash goggles
- Respirator
- Absorbent, plastic-backed sheets or spill pads
- Disposable toweling
- At least two sealable thick plastic hazardous waste disposal bags (prelabeled with an appropriate warning label)
- A disposable scoop for collecting glass fragments
- A puncture-resistant container for glass fragments

Note. Based on information from American Society of Hospital Pharmacists, 1990.

(3) Wear a NIOSH-approved respirator (OSHA, 2004c).

(4) Use appropriate items in the spill-control kit to contain the spill.

(5) Clean up the spill according to its location and type. Do not use chemical inactivators, with the exception of sodium thiosulfate. (Sodium thiosulfate is used to inactivate mechlorethamine, also known as nitrogen mustard.) Inactivators other than sodium thiosulfate may react with the spilled material to form potentially dangerous by-products (Harrison, 2001).

(a) To clean up a spill on a hard surface (American Society of Hospital Pharmacists, 1990)

i) Wipe up liquids by using absorbent gauze pads or spill-control pillows. Wipe up solids by using wet absorbent gauze pads.

ii) Pick up glass fragments by using a small scoop or utility gloves worn over chemotherapy gloves. Place the glass in a puncture-proof container.

iii) Place puncture-proof container and contaminated materials into a leakproof waste bag. Seal the bag. Place the sealed bag inside another bag, appropriately labeled as hazardous waste. For the moment, leave the outer bag open.

iv) Clean the spill area thoroughly, from least contaminated to most contaminated areas, using a detergent solution followed by clean water.

v) Use fresh detergent solution to wash any reusable items used to clean up the spill and items located in the spill area (e.g., a volumetric pump). Use water to rinse the washed items. Repeat the washing and rinsing.

vi) Remove PPE and place disposable items in the unsealed cytotoxic waste disposal bag.

vii) Seal the outer cytotoxic waste disposal bag and place it in a puncture-proof container.

viii) Follow institutional guidelines regarding cleaning or maintenance of equipment.

ix) Dispose of all material used in the cleanup process according to institutional policy and federal, state, and local laws (OSHA, 1995).

(b) To clean up a spill on a carpeted surface (note that carpet is not recommended in drug administration areas), OSHA (1995) and American Society of Hospital Pharmacists (1990) recommend the following.

i) Don PPE, including a NIOSH-approved respirator.

ii) Use absorbent powder, not absorbent towels, to absorb the spill.

iii) Use a small vacuum cleaner, reserved for hazardous-drug cleanup only, to remove the powder.

iv) Clean the carpet as usual.

v) Follow guidelines for a spill on a hard surface to clean and dispose of other contaminated items.

(c) To clean up a spill in a BSC (American Society of Hospital Pharmacists, 1990; OSHA, 1995)

i) If the volume of the spill is < 150 ml: Clean up the spill according to the guidelines for a spill on a hard surface.

ii) If the volume of the spill is > 150 ml: Clean up the spill as if it were a spill on a hard surface. Include the drain spillage trough in washing efforts. Then complete the following additional steps.

- If the spill was not contained in a small area or the drain spillage trough: Wash the affected areas with a

cleaning agent designed to remove chemicals from stainless steel.
- If the spill contaminated the HEPA filter: Seal the BSC in plastic and label it as contaminated equipment. Schedule a BSC service technician to change the HEPA filter. Ensure that the BSC is not used before the filter is changed.
- Clean and/or dispose of contaminated items as described in the guidelines for spills on a hard surface.

(d) To clean up a spill in the home setting: See Figure 10.

(6) Report and document the spill according to institutional policy: Each time a spill of more than 5 ml occurs, complete a report about the spill and forward it to those specified by institutional policy (Harrison, 2001). Document the following.

(a) The name of the drug and the approximate volume spilled
(b) How the spill occurred
(c) Spill management procedures followed
(d) The names of personnel, patients, and others exposed to the spill
(e) A list of personnel notified of the spill

16. Requirements for policies regarding the handling of hazardous drugs: OSHA (2004a) requires that employers provide a safe or healthful workplace. Employers must implement policies and procedures related to the safe handling of hazardous drugs. Policies should address all aspects of handling these hazardous materials to protect employees, patients, customers, and the environment from exposure. Such policies must (NIOSH, 2004)

a) Outline procedures to ensure the safe storage, transport, administration, and disposal of hazardous agents.
b) Describe the procedure for identifying and updating the list of the hazardous drugs used in the facility (NIOSH, 2004).
c) Require that all employees who handle hazardous drugs wear PPE.
d) Mandate that hazardous drugs be prepared in a BSC.
e) Prohibit staff from eating, drinking, smoking, chewing gum, using tobacco, storing food, and applying cosmetics in areas where hazardous drugs are prepared or used.
f) Mandate training for all employees who prepare, transport, or administer hazardous

Figure 10. Spill Kit Procedure for Home Use

(Please review this procedure with your nurse.)

1. Do not touch the spill with unprotected hands.
2. Open the spill kit and put on both pairs of gloves. If the bag or syringe with chemotherapy drugs has been broken or is leaking and you have a catheter or implantable access system (e.g., Port-a-Cath device) in place, before cleaning the spill disconnect the catheter from the tubing and rinse and cap it according to normal procedure.
3. Put on the gown (closes in back), splash goggles, and respirator.
4. Use spill pillows to contain spill—put around puddle to form a V.
5. Use the absorbent sheets to blot up as much of the drug as possible.
6. Put contaminated clean-up materials directly into the plastic bag contained in the kit. Do not lay them on unprotected surfaces.
7. Use the scoop and brush to collect any broken glass, sweeping toward the V'd spill pillows, and dispose of the glass in the box of the kit.
8. While still wearing the protective gear, wash the area with dishwashing or laundry detergent and warm water, using disposable rags or paper towels, and put them in the plastic bag with other waste. Rinse the area with clean water and dispose of the towels in the same plastic bag.
9. Remove gloves, goggles, respirator, and gown and place them in plastic bag. Put all contaminated materials, including the spill kit box, into the second large plastic bag, and label the bag with the hazardous waste label in the kit.
10. Wash your hands with soap and water.
11. Call the home health nurse, clinic, or doctor's office promptly to report the spill. Plans need to be made to replace the spilled chemotherapy so the treatment can be completed. Arrangements will be made to have the waste material picked up or have you bring it to the hospital for proper disposal.
12. If the spill occurs on sheets or clothing, wash the items in hot water, separate from other wash. Wash clothing or bed linen contaminated with body wastes in the same manner.
13. Patients on 24-hour infusions should use a plastic-backed mattress pad to protect the mattress from contamination.

Following these procedures prevents undue exposure and ensures your safety. Call your nurse if you have any questions. Thank you.

Note. From "Home Chemotherapy Safety Procedures," by C. Blecke, 1989, *Oncology Nursing Forum, 16*, p. 721. Copyright 1989 by the Oncology Nursing Society. Adapted with permission.

drugs or care for patients receiving these drugs. Document the training program.

g) Make documents such as MSDS available to healthcare workers who handle hazardous drugs.

h) State that spills should be managed according to the institution's hazardous drug spill policy and procedure.

i) Set forth a plan for medical surveillance of personnel handling hazardous drugs.

j) Allow employees who are pregnant, actively trying to conceive, or breast-feeding or who have other medical reasons for not being exposed to hazardous drugs to refrain from preparing or administering those agents or caring for patients during their treatment with them upon request. (No information is available regarding the reproductive risks of workers who use currently recommended precautions [OSHA, 1995; Polovich, 2003; Welch & Silveira, 1997].) Alternate duty that does not include hazardous drug preparation or administration must be made available to both men and women involved in planning a pregnancy when requested.

k) Define quality improvement programs that monitor compliance with safe-handling policies and procedures (Maxson & Wolk, 1998).

References

American Society of Hospital Pharmacists. (1990). ASHP technical assistance bulletin on handling cytotoxic and hazardous drugs. *American Journal of Hospital Pharmacists, 47,* 1033–1049.

Brown, K.A., Esper, P., Kelleher, L.O., O'Neill, J.E.B., Polovich, M., & White, J.M. (Eds.). (2001). *Chemotherapy and biotherapy guidelines and recommendations for practice.* Pittsburgh, PA: Oncology Nursing Society.

Bruner, D.W., Haas, M., & Gosselin-Acomb, T.K. (Eds.). (2005). *Manual for radiation oncology nursing practice and education* (3rd ed.). Pittsburgh, PA: Oncology Nursing Society.

Connor, T.H. (1993). An evaluation of the permeability of disposable polypropylene-based protective gowns to a battery of cancer chemotherapy drugs. *Applied Occupational and Environmental Hygiene, 8,* 785–789.

Connor, T.H. (1999). Permeability of nitrile rubber, latex, polyurethane, and neoprene gloves to 18 antineoplastic drugs. *American Journal of Health-System Pharmacists, 56,* 2450–2453.

Connor, T.H., Anderson, R.W., Sessink, P.J., Broadfield, L., & Power, L.A. (1999). Surface contamination with antineoplastic agents in six cancer treatment centers in Canada and the United States. *American Journal of Health-System Pharmacists, 56,* 1427–1432.

Connor, T.H., Anderson, R.W., Sessink, P.J., & Spivey, S.M. (2002). Effectiveness of a closed-system device in containing surface contamination with cyclophosphamide and ifosfamide in an IV admixture area. *American Journal of Health-System Pharmacists, 59,* 68–72.

Dorr, R.T., & Alberts, D.S. (1992). Topical absorption and inactivation of cytotoxic anticancer drugs in vitro. *Cancer, 70*(Suppl. 4), 983–987.

Dunne-Daly, C.F. (1999). Principles of radiotherapy and radiobiology. *Seminars in Oncology Nursing, 15,* 250–259.

Fuchs, J., Hengstler, J.G., Jung, D., Hiltl, G., Konietzko, J., & Oesch, F. (1995). DNA damage in nurses handling antineoplastic agents. *Mutation Research, 342,* 17–23.

Genentech, Inc. (2000). Rituxan [Material safety data sheet]. South San Francisco, CA: Author.

Gullo, S.M. (1995). Safe handling of antineoplastic agents: Translating the recommendations into practice. *Oncology Nursing Forum, 22,* 19–24.

Harrison, B. (2001). Risks of handling cytotoxic drugs: A review. In M.C. Perry (Ed.), *The chemotherapy source book* (3rd ed., pp. 566–582). Philadelphia: Lippincott Williams & Wilkins.

Harrison, B.R., & Kloos, M.D. (1999). Penetration and splash protection of six disposable gown materials against fifteen antineoplastic drugs. *Journal of Oncology Pharmacy Practice, 5*(2), 61–66.

Harrison, B.R., & Schultz, C.D. (2000). Determination of tablet trituration dust in work zone air. *Journal of Oncology Pharmacy Practice, 6,* 23.

Hemminki, K., Kyyrönen, P., & Lindbohm, M.L. (1985). Spontaneous abortions and malformations in the offspring of nurses exposed to anesthetic gases, cytostatic drugs, and other potential hazards in hospitals, based on registered information of outcome. *Journal of Epidemiology and Community Health, 39,* 141–147.

International Agency for Research on Cancer. (2004). *Overall evaluations of carcinogenicity to humans.* Retrieved December 27, 2004, from http://www-cie.iarc.fr/monoeval/crthall.html

Labuhn, K., Valanis, B., Schoeny, R., Loveday, K., & Vollmer, W.M. (1998). Nurses and pharmacists exposure to antineoplastic drugs: Findings from industrial hygiene scans and urine mutagenicity tests. *Cancer Nursing, 21,* 79–89.

Maxson, J.H., & Wolk, J.E. (1998). Principles of preparation, administration, and disposal of antineoplastic agents. In J.K. Itano & K.N. Taoka (Eds.), *Core curriculum for oncology nursing* (3rd ed., pp. 657–661). Philadelphia: Saunders.

Minoia, C., Turci, R., Sottaui, C., Schiavi, A., Perbellini, L., Angeleri, S., et al. (1998). Application of high performance liquid chromatography/tandem mass spectrometry in the environmental and biological monitoring of health care personnel occupationally exposed to cyclophosphamide and ifosfamide. *Rapid Communications in Mass Spectrometry, 12,* 1485–1493.

National Institute for Occupational Safety and Health. (1996). *Summary for respirator users.* Retrieved March 28, 2004, from http://www.cdc.gov/niosh/respsumm.html

National Institute for Occupational Safety and Health. (2004). *Preventing occupational exposure to antineoplastic and other hazardous drugs in health care settings.* Retrieved December 14, 2004, from http://www.cdc.gov/niosh/docs/2004-165/

Occupational Safety and Health Administration. (1995). *Controlling occupational exposure to hazardous drugs* (OSHA Instruction CPL 2-2.20B). Washington, DC: Author.

Occupational Safety and Health Administration. (2004a). *Code of federal regulations. Title 29, Labor: Subpart: General: Definitions* (Title 29, Part (29CFR 1910.2). Washington, DC: U.S. Government Printing Office. Retrieved April 18, 2004, from http://www.access.gpo.gov/nara/cfr/waisidx_04/29cfr1910_04.html

Occupational Safety and Health Administration. (2004b). *Code of federal regulations. Title 29, Labor: Subpart: Hazardous waste operations and emergency response: Hazardous materials* (29CFR1910.120). Washington, DC: U.S. Government Printing

Office. Retrieved April 18, 2004, from http://www.access.gpo.gov/nara/cfr/waisidx_04/29cfr1910_04.html

Occupational Safety and Health Administration. (2004c). *Code of federal regulations. Title 29, Labor: Subpart: Personal protection equipment: Respiratory protection* (29 CFR1910.134). Washington, DC: U.S. Government Printing Office. Retrieved April 18, 2004, from http://www.access.gpo.gov/nara/cfr/waisidx_04/29cfr1910_04.html

Peelen, S., Roeleveld, N., Heederik, D., Kromhout, H., & de Kort, W. (1999). Toxic effects on reproduction in hospital personnel. *Reproductie-toxische effecten bij ziekenhuispersonel*. Amsterdam: Elsivier.

Pethran, A., Schierl, R., Hauff, K., Grimm, C.H., Boos, K.S., & Nowak, D. (2003). Uptake of antineoplastic agents in pharmacy and hospital personnel. Part I: monitoring of urinary concentrations. *International Archives of Occupational and Environmental Health, 76,* 5–10.

Polovich, M. (Ed). (2003). *Safe handling of hazardous drugs*. Pittsburgh, PA: Oncology Nursing Society.

Sessink, P.J.M., Cerna, M., Rossner, P., Pastorkova, A., Bavarova, H., Frankova, K., et al. (1994). Urinary cyclophosphamide excretion and chromosomal aberrations in peripheral blood lymphocytes after occupational exposure to antineoplastic agents. *Mutation Research, 309,* 193–199.

Singleton, L.C., & Connor, T.H. (1999). An evaluation of the permeability of chemotherapy gloves to three cancer chemotherapy drugs. *Oncology Nursing Forum, 26,* 1491–1496.

Stucker, I., Caillard, J.F., Collin, R., Gout, M., Poyen, D., & Hemon, D. (1990). Risk of spontaneous abortion among nurses handling antineoplastic drugs. *Scandinavian Journal of Work and Environmental Health, 16*(2), 102–107.

Valanis, B., Vollmer, W., Labuhn, K., & Glass, A. (1997). Occupational exposure to antineoplastic agents and self-reported infertility among nurses and pharmacists. *Journal of Occupational and Environmental Medicine, 39,* 574–580.

Valanis, B., Vollmer, W.M., & Steele, P. (1999). Occupational exposure to antineoplastic agents: Self-reported miscarriages and stillbirths among nurses and pharmacists. *Journal of Occupational and Environmental Medicine, 41,* 632–638.

Welch, J., & Silveira, J.M. (Eds.). (1997). *Safe handling of cytotoxic drugs: An independent study module* (2nd ed.). Pittsburgh, PA: Oncology Nursing Society.

Wick, C., Slawson, M.H., Jorgenson, J.A., & Tyler, L.S. (2003). Using a closed-system protective device to reduce personnel to antineoplastic agents. *American Journal of Health-System Pharmacists, 60,* 2314–2320.

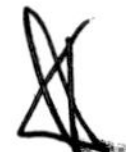

B. Treatment schedule

1. Dosing category

a) Standard-dose therapy

(1) Standard is the most frequent type of treatment schedule used.

(2) A patient may receive lower than standard dose because of

(a) Dose delays: Chemotherapy may be delayed for an additional week because of inadequate neutrophil counts or oral mucositis toxicities.

(b) Reduced dosing: Doses may be reduced by 25%–75% according to platelet levels. A 20% dose reduction can result in about 50% less cure rate (Chu & DeVita, 2001).

(c) Inadvertent miscalculation of dose (Biganzoli & Piccart, 1997).

(3) Decreased cytotoxic effect occurs in more than 30% of people receiving standard regimens (Gurney, 2002).

(4) Inadequate dosing may be a problem in

(a) The elderly (Hood & Mucenski, 2003; Piccart, Biganzoli, & Di Leo, 2000; Repetto, 2003). Doses in the elderly often are not evidence based (Gillespie, 2001).

(b) People who have curable disease (Felici, Verweij, & Sparreboom, 2002).

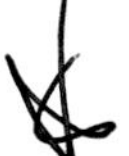

b) High-dose therapy

(1) High-dose involves administration of a dose that is potentially sufficient to eradicate the tumor and may cause severe, even lethal, side effects that warrant supportive therapy (e.g., stem cell transplant).

(2) It usually includes an alkylating agent–based regimen such as cyclophosphamide (Vose, 1996).

(3) High-dose therapy usually is used in patients with acute leukemias or aggressive lymphomas (Gurney, 2002).

(4) It includes use of colony-stimulating factors.

(5) One of the most important variables influencing successful stem cell transplant is a patient's enduring response to standard-dose chemotherapy before the high-dose therapy (Philip et al., 1987; Pico, Fadel, Ibrahim, Bourhis, & Droz, 1995; Wahlin, Eriksson, & Huttden, 2004).

(6) Some cancers, and certain chemotherapy regimens, have not involved high enough doses to obtain the best survival response. Standard, but sub-

optimal, doses may achieve a clinical complete remission, but because the tumor is still present, relapse is almost certain. Dose intensity is beneficial in these situations where standard doses have not been optimal (Biganzoli & Piccart, 1997). However, there seems to be a critical level below which the lack of optimal dosing compromises survival outcome and above which there is little therapeutic benefit and only increased toxicity (Gurney, 2002).

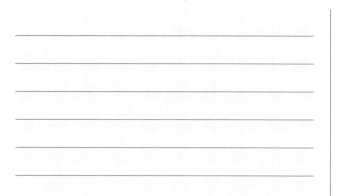

(7) It may require supportive therapy (e.g., colony-stimulating factors, transfusions, antiemetics, analgesia).

(8) Hryniuk (1987) criticized the technique of dose intensity, administering smaller doses more frequently, for delivering suboptimal doses and, thus, never exposing the cancer to therapeutic and lethal levels that will eradicate the cancer.

2. Dosing modifications

a) Dose intensity

(1) Dose intensity provides unit-based measurement to compare efficacies of different chemotherapies with different dosing approaches.

(2) It is measured as milligrams per meter squared per week.

(3) With multiple drug regimens, each drug is compared to standard or relative drug intensity (Chu & DeVita, 2004; Foote, 1998; Gianni & Piccart, 2000; Gradishar, Tallman, & Abrams, 1996; Hryniuk, 1987; Piccart et al., 2000).

b) Dose density: This is based on dose per source, interval between doses, and/or the total amount of dose given (Biganzoli & Di Leo, 2000; Piccart et al., 2000).

c) Combined modality therapy

(1) Combined modality is chemotherapy (including biotherapy) administered before (neoadjuvant), after (adjuvant), or concurrently with surgery or radiation therapy (Works, 2000).

(2) An example of chemotherapy and biotherapy, or targeted therapy, is gefitinib and gemcitabine for non-small cell lung cancer, which is in phase III clinical trial.

(3) Chemotherapy may be used as a radiosensitizer that enhances the lethal effects of radiation therapy.

(a) The primary goal is to prevent radiation resistance and enhance local and regional control of disease by eliminating radiation-resistant cancer cells and increasing the oxygen supply to the tumor as it shrinks in response to the chemotherapy (Tortorice, 2000).

(b) An example is carboplatin and radiation for non-small cell lung cancer.

(c) Cisplatin, methotrexate, doxorubicin, vinblastine, etoposide, fluorouracil, actinomycin, and bleomycin are other examples of chemotherapy that have been used in combined modality regimens.

(d) The most frequent toxicities occur in the gastrointestinal (GI) tract, skin and mucosa, and bone marrow.

3. Dose determination

a) Each method contains variance. To reduce iatrogenic variance and increase accuracy, use a systematic approach that includes the following.

(1) Current and accurate (not stated) weights, heights, age, and lab values (e.g., creatinine, aspartate aminotransferase [AST], platelets, absolute neutrophil count [ANC])

(2) Multiple checks and balances that include dose verification by at least two healthcare professionals prepared in cancer chemotherapy administration

(3) Some organizations have determined that a 5%–10% variance in BSA, area under the plasma concentration versus time curve (AUC), and mg per kg dose calculations is acceptable, but no evidence has been found in the literature to support this. Establish institutional policies and procedures for resolving issues related to dose variance.

(4) Standardized and systematic dose calculations and tools to determine these calculations

b) Dosing procedure (Chen et al., 1997; Cotton et al., 2003)

(1) Determine accurate method and tools to arrive at BSA (m^2), AUC (using estimated creatinine clearance), mg/kg (weight in kilograms), or other measure.

(2) Multiply the value obtained in (1) by the prescribed unit dose according to the reference (e.g., clinical trials protocol information, drug product insert, current drug books and software, evidence-based articles in reputable medical journals) that describes the chemotherapy regimen. This determines patient-specific dose (see Table 10 for examples of how to determine the final dose).

(3) Verify safe dose based on a reliable source that lists dose ranges approved for each chemotherapy drug. If the patient is on a research study, clinical trial protocol recommendations supersede all other referenced information. "Safe" doses still can be inaccurate. It is important to verify accurate dosing by examining the source that contains the chemotherapy protocol.

c) Methods

(1) Milligrams per kilogram

(a) This method is more commonly used in children younger than one year or weighing less than 10 kg.

(b) BSA estimation based only on weight is being studied in children, especially for infants weighing less than 10 kg (Sharkey et al., 2001).

(c) Many biologic agents use mg/kg dosing, including bevacizumab, epoetin alfa, trastuzumab, and darbepoetin alfa.

(2) BSA or m^2

(a) Many methods exist for determining BSA. Mosteller's (1987) formula requires only a pocket calculator with square root function (see Figure 11). Many BSA calculators now are available on the Internet.

(b) Use of a nomogram is not recommended because of inaccuracy that can result from copy machine distortion of the chart and inability to accurately read the BSA value on the chart. Briars and Bailey (1994) suggested an 8% error rate when using nomograms.

(c) Accuracy of BSA has been questioned, citing 5% underestimation (Wang, Moss, & Thisted, 1992) to 40% inaccuracy (Gurney, 2002). Other than AUC or kg/mg for selected drugs, no other standardized and practical approach has been determined.

(d) Modifications to final administered dose are based on the variables in Table 11. Consider establishing an institutional policy on approach to modifications made to chemotherapy doses.

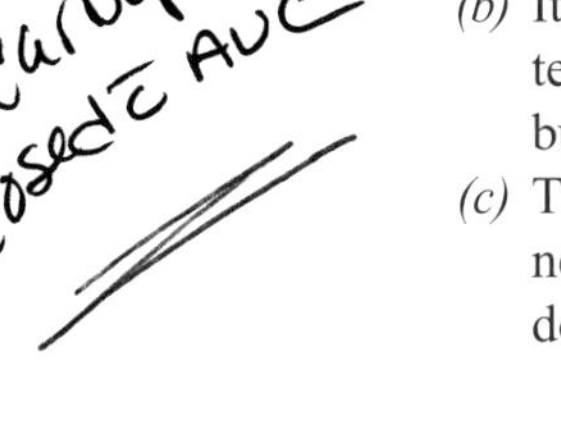

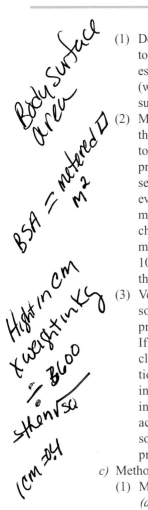

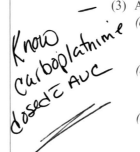

(3) AUC

(a) The Calvert formula is used most frequently for AUC dosing (Calvert et al., 1989).

(b) It is the standard of practice for determining carboplatin dosing only but still contains error variance.

(c) The following information is needed to determine carboplatin dose based on AUC.

Figure 11. Formula for Calculating Body Surface Area

$$\sqrt{\frac{\text{height in cm x weight in kg}}{3,600}}$$

Note. Based on information from Mosteller, 1987.

Table 10. Verification of Chemotherapy Dosing

Factor	BSA (m^2)	AUC (Cockcroft-Gault method for estimated creatinine clearance)	mg/kg (current actual weight in kg)
Example of value obtained	1.86 m^2	159 ml/minute using Cockcroft-Gault formula	57 kg
Prescribed unit dose per protocol	125 mg/m^2	Target AUC of 6	35 mg/kg
Dose to be given according to formula and protocol source	1.86 x 125 = 232.5 mg	Calvert formula: mg dose = target AUC x (est. creatinine clearance + 25) or 6 x (159 + 25) = 1,104 mg	57 x 35 = 1,995 mg

Table 11. Variables That Contribute to Alteration of Chemotherapy Dosing

Variable	Comments	Alteration Suggested	Evidence
Obesity	Some cap body surface area (BSA) at 2.0 m².	If BSA is more than 2.0 m², use average of ideal and actual weight in BSA formula.	Livingston & Lee, 2001; Madarnas et al., 2001
Children	If less than 10 kg or BSA is less than 1.3 m², dose may be underestimated.	Use mg/kg dosing.	Sawyer & Ratain, 2001; Sharkey et al., 2001
Cachexia	Overdosing may occur when using BSA if patient has recently lost a significant amount of weight.	Determine BSA of individual and then use proportional dose reduction to the person's weight loss. Example: 165.1 cm tall individual whose weight has been 85 kg has a BSA of 1.97. Dosing recommended is 125 mg/m² or 247 mg. Now weight is 56.8 kg, so BSA is 1.61. Normally you would give 201 mg, but because this person had a 33% weight loss, you would reduce the dose by 33% to 166 mg.	O'Marcaigh & Gilchrist, 1997
Altered liver function	BSA dosing does not account for altered liver function, so reductions should be made based on liver function abnormalities if the drug is metabolized by the liver.	Follow recommendations of clinical research protocol or drug package insert.	Canal, Chatelut, & Guichard, 1998; Felici, Verweij, & Sparreboom, 2002; Gurney, 1996; Masson & Zamboni, 1997
Altered renal function	BSA dosing does not account for altered renal function, so reductions should be made based on renal function abnormalities if the drug is metabolized by the kidneys.	Follow recommendations of clinical research protocol or drug package insert.	Canal et al., 1998; Felici et al., 2002; Gurney, 1996; Masson & Zamboni, 1997
Drug–drug interaction	Many people, especially the elderly, are on other medications that can affect the effectiveness of chemotherapy. Many chemotherapy sources can help to identify which drugs cause interactions and how to adjust dosing.	The dose of the chemotherapy agent may need to be reduced or increased, or the dose of the patient's other drug(s) may need to be altered or discontinued.	Gurney, 1996
Elderly	Factors that make the elderly vulnerable to altered chemotherapy effectiveness include comorbidities, polypharmacy, and altered physiologic functioning.	Consider less-toxic chemotherapy drugs, such as vinorelbine or gemcitabine, weekly docetaxel, carboplatin instead of cisplatin (less hydration required), idarubicin or epirubicin instead of doxorubicin, and the use of chemoprotectants.	Hood & Mucenski, 2003; Repetto, 2003

i) Formula used to determine estimated creatinine clearance

ii) Formula used to determine AUC dose

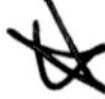

iii) Target AUC. This is ordered by the physician and found in the chemotherapy protocol resource. It most often falls between 5 and 7 mg/ml/minute in pretreated patients and is based on research recommendations (Alberts & Dorr, 1998).

iv) Rationale for changes in recommended dose. Examples of variables that could contribute to alterations in computed dose include platelet level, using combination chemotherapy, abnormally high or low creatinine, obesity, and previous treatment with renal toxic drugs. A pediatric patient would require a modified formula (Marina et al., 1993; Thomas et al., 2000).

(d) Why use AUC for carboplatin dosing? (De Jonge, Mathot, Van Dam, Beijnen, & Rodenhuis, 2002; Donahue al., 2001; van den Bongard, Mathot, Beijnen, & Schellens, 2000)
   i) 70%–90% of carboplatin is excreted in urine chemically unchanged.
   ii) Renal function, especially glomerular filtration rate (GFR), plays a major role in determining efficacy and toxicities of carboplatin and is a major variable in determining the dose of carboplatin to administer.

(e) Begin by estimating creatinine clearance based on a serum creatinine, unless you have an actual nuclear GFR value. The most commonly used formula is the Cockcroft-Gault (see Figure 12). Other formulas also are available, such as the Jelliffe formula (see Figure 13).

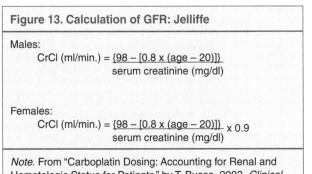

Figure 12. Calculation of GFR: Cockcroft-Gault

Males:

$$\text{CrCl (ml/min.)} = \frac{(140\text{–age}) \times (\text{weight in kg})}{72 \times \text{serum creatinine (mg/dl)}}$$

Females:

$$\text{CrCl (ml/min.)} = \frac{(140\text{–age}) \times (\text{weight in kg})}{72 \times \text{serum creatinine (mg/dl)}} \times (0.85)$$

Note. From "Carboplatin Dosing: Accounting for Renal and Hematologic Status for Patients," by T. Busse, 2003, *Clinical Journal of Oncology Nursing, 7,* p. 105. Copyright 2003 by the Oncology Nursing Society. Reprinted with permission.

Figure 13. Calculation of GFR: Jelliffe

Males:

$$\text{CrCl (ml/min.)} = \frac{\{98 - [0.8 \times (\text{age} - 20)]\}}{\text{serum creatinine (mg/dl)}}$$

Females:

$$\text{CrCl (ml/min.)} = \frac{\{98 - [0.8 \times (\text{age} - 20)]\}}{\text{serum creatinine (mg/dl)}} \times 0.9$$

Note. From "Carboplatin Dosing: Accounting for Renal and Hematologic Status for Patients," by T. Busse, 2003, *Clinical Journal of Oncology Nursing, 7,* p. 105. Copyright 2003 by the Oncology Nursing Society. Reprinted with permission.

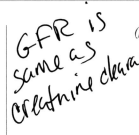

(f) Use the estimated creatinine clearance value obtained from the Cockcroft-Gault formula to complete the Calvert formula. This will determine the final recommended dose of carboplatin to administer to the patient (see Figure 14). The 25 is a formula constant that denotes unexcreted drug bound to protein and drug that is secreted by the renal tubules (van Warmerdam, 1997).

Figure 14. Calvert Formula

Dose of carboplatin (mg) = (Target AUC) x (GFR + 25)

Note. Total dose calculated is in mg, not mg/m².

References

Alberts, D.S., & Dorr, R.T. (1998). New perspectives on an old friend: Optimizing carboplatin for the treatment of solid tumors. *Oncologist, 3,* 15–34.

Biganzoli, L., & Di Leo, A. (2000). The impact of chemotherapy dose density and dose intensity on breast cancer outcome: What have we learned? *European Journal of Cancer, 36*(Suppl. 1), S4–S10.

Biganzoli, L., & Piccart, M.J. (1997). The bigger the better? . . . Or what we know and what we still need to learn about anthracycline dose per course, dose density and cumulative dose in the treatment of breast cancer. *Annals of Oncology, 8,* 1177–1182.

Briars, G.L., & Bailey, B.J. (1994). Surface area estimation: Pocket calculator v nomogram. *Archives of Disease in Childhood, 70,* 246–247.

Calvert, A.H., Newell, D.R., Gumbrell, L.A., O'Reilly, S., Burnell, M., Boxall, F.E., et al. (1989). Carboplatin dosage: Prospective evaluation of a simple formula based on renal function. *Journal of Clinical Oncology, 7,* 1748–1756.

Canal, P., Chatelut, E., & Guichard, S. (1998). Practical treatment guide for dose individualisation in cancer chemotherapy. *Drugs, 56,* 1019–1038.

Chen, C.S., Seidel, K., Armitage, J.O., Fay, J.W., Appelbaum, F.R., Horowitz, M., et al. (1997). Safeguarding the administration of high-dose chemotherapy: A national practice survey by the American Society for Blood and Marrow Transplantation. *Biology of Blood and Marrow Transplantation, 3,* 331–340.

Chu, E., & DeVita, V.T. (2001). Principles of cancer management: Chemotherapy. In V.T. DeVita, S. Hellman, & S.A. Rosenberg (Eds.), *Cancer: Principles and practice of oncology* (6th ed., pp. 289–306). Philadelphia: Lippincott-Raven.

Chu, E., & DeVita, V.T. (2004). *Physician's cancer chemotherapy manual.* Sudbury, MA: Jones and Bartlett.

Cotton, L., Johnson, K., Keith, B., Malloy, P.S., Moore-Higgs, G.J., Nesbitt, M., et al. (2003). *ONS cancer chemotherapy and biotherapy course renewal: An independent study module.* Pittsburgh, PA: Oncology Nursing Society.

De Jonge, M., Mathot, R., Van Dam, S., Beijnen, J., & Rodenhuis, S. (2002). Extremely high exposure in an obese patient receiving high-dose cyclophosphamide, thiotepa and carboplatin. *Cancer Chemotherapy and Pharmacology, 507,* 251–255.

Donahue, A., McCune, J.S., Faucette, S., Gillenwater, H.H., Kowalski, E., Socinski, M.A., et al., (2001). Measured versus estimated glomerular filtration rate in the Calvert equation: Influence on carboplatin dosing. *Cancer Chemotherapy and Pharmacology, 47,* 373–379.

Felici, A., Verweij, J., & Sparreboom, A. (2002). Dosing strategies for anticancer drugs: The good, the bad and the body-surface area. *European Journal of Cancer, 38,* 1677–1684.

Foote, M. (1998). The importance of planned dose of chemotherapy on time: Do we need to change our clinical practice? *Oncologist, 3,* 365–368.

Gianni, A.M., & Piccart, M.J. (2000). Optimizing chemotherapy dose density and dose intensity: New strategies to improve outcomes in adjuvant therapy for breast cancer. *European Journal of Cancer, 36,* S1–S3.

Gillespie, R.W. (2001). Chemotherapy dose and dose intensity: Analyzing data to guide therapeutic decisions. *Oncology Nursing Forum, 28*(Suppl. 2), 5–10.

Gradishar, W.J., Tallman, M.S., & Abrams, J.S. (1996). High-dose chemotherapy for breast cancer. *Annals of Internal Medicine, 125,* 599–604.

Gurney, H. (1996). Dose calculation of anticancer drugs: A review of the current practice and introduction of an alternative. *Journal of Clinical Oncology, 14,* 2590–2611.

Gurney, H. (2002). How to calculate the dose of chemotherapy. *British Journal of Cancer, 86,* 1297–1302.

Hood, L.E., & Mucenski, J. (2003). *Management of elderly patients with cancer: Treatment of chemotherapy-induced neutropenia and anemia. An independent study program accredited for nurses and pharmacists.* Chicago: Discovery International.

Hryniuk, W.M. (1987). Average relative dose intensity and the impact on design of clinical trials. *Seminars in Oncology, 14,* 65–74.

Livingston, E.H., & Lee, S. (2001). Body surface area prediction in normal-weight and obese patients. *American Journal of Physiology, Endocrinology and Metabolism, 281,* E586–E591.

Madarnas, Y., Sawka, C.A., Franssen, E., & Bjarnason, G.A. (2001). Are medical oncologists biased in their treatment of the large woman with breast cancer? *Breast Cancer Research and Treatment, 66,* 123–133.

Marina, N.M., Rodman, J., Shema, S.J., Bowman, L.C., Douglass, E., Furman, W., et al. (1993). Phase I study of escalating targeted doses of carboplatin combined ifosfamide and etoposide in children with solid tumors. *Journal of Clinical Oncology, 11,* 554–560.

Masson, E., & Zamboni, W.C. (1997). Pharmacokinetic optimization of cancer chemotherapy: Effect on outcomes. *Clinical Pharmacokinetics, 32,* 324–343.

Mosteller, R.D. (1987). Simplified calculation of body surface area. *New England Journal of Medicine, 317,* 1098.

O'Marcaigh, A.S., & Gilchrist, G.S. (1997). Dose reduction of chemotherapeutic agents after weight loss. *American Journal of Clinical Oncology, 20,* 193–195.

Philip, T., Armitage, J.O., Spitzer, G., Chauvin, F., Jagannath, S., Cahn, J., et al. (1987). High-dose therapy and autologous bone marrow transplantation after failure of conventional chemotherapy in adults and intermediate-grade or high-grade non-Hodgkin's lymphoma. *New England Journal of Medicine, 316,* 1493–1498.

Piccart, M.J., Biganzoli, L., & Di Leo, A. (2000). The impact of chemotherapy dose density and dose intensity on breast cancer outcome: What have we learned? *European Journal of Cancer, 36,* S4–S10.

Pico, J.L., Fadel, E., Ibrahim, A., Bourhis, H.H., & Droz, J.D. (1995). High-dose chemotherapy followed by hematological support: Experience in the treatment of germ cell tumors. *Bulletin du Cancer, 82*(Suppl. 1), 56S–60S.

Repetto, L. (2003). Greater risks of chemotherapy toxicity in elderly patients with cancer. *Journal of Supportive Oncology, 1*(4 Suppl. 2), 18–24.

Sawyer, M., & Ratain, M.J. (2001). Body surface area as a determinant of pharmacokinetics and drug dosing. *Investigational New Drugs, 19,* 171–177.

Sharkey, I., Boddy, A.V., Wallace, H., Mycroft, J., Hollis, R., & Picton, S. (2001). Body surface area estimation in children using weight alone: Application in pædiatric oncology. *British Journal of Cancer, 85,* 23–28.

Thomas, H., Boddy, A., English, M., Hobson, R., Imeson, J., Lewis, I., et al. (2000). Prospective validation of renal function-based carboplatin dosing in children with cancer: A United Kingdom Children's Cancer Study Group trial. *Journal of Clinical Oncology, 18,* 3614–3621.

Tortorice, P.V. (2000). Chemotherapy: Principles of therapy. In C.H. Yarbro, M.H. Frogge, M. Goodman, & S.L. Groenwald (Eds.), *Cancer nursing: Principles and practice* (5th ed., pp. 352–382). Sudbury, MA: Jones and Bartlett.

van den Bongard, H.J., Mathot, R.A., Beijnen, J.H., & Schellens, H.H. (2000). Pharmacokinetically guided administration of chemotherapeutic agents. *Clinical Pharmacokinetics, 39,* 345–367.

van Warmerdam, L.J. (1997). Tailor-made chemotherapy for cancer patients. *The Netherlands Journal of Medicine, 51,* 30–35.

Vose, J.M. (1996). Dose-intensive ifosfamide for the treatment of non-Hodgkin's lymphoma. *Seminars in Oncology, 23*(Suppl. 6), 33–37.

Wahlin, A., Eriksson, M., & Hultden, M. (2004). Relation between harvest success and outcome after autologous peripheral blood cell transplantation in multiple myeloma. *European Journal of Haematology, 73,* 263–268.

Wang, Y., Moss, J., & Thisted, R. (1992). Predictors of body surface area. *Journal of Clinical Anesthesia, 4,* 4–10.

Works, C.R. (2000). Principles of treatment planning and research. In C.H. Yarbro, M.H. Frogge, M. Goodman, & S.L. Groenwald (Eds.), *Cancer nursing: Principles and practice* (5th ed., pp. 259–271). Sudbury, MA: Jones and Bartlett.

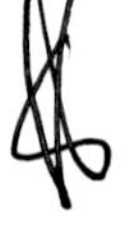

C. Pretreatment

Follow institutional guidelines regarding documentation of assessment and provision of care. Appendices 1 and 2 provide sample flow sheets.

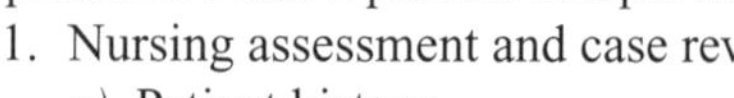

1. Nursing assessment and case review
   - *a)* Patient history
     - (1) Review recent treatment(s), including surgery, radiation therapy, prior cytotoxic therapy, hormonal therapy, and complementary therapies (e.g., acupuncture, chiropractic, nutritional).
     - (2) Review and document medical, psychiatric, and nononcologic surgical history.
     - (3) Document drug, food, and environmental allergies.
     - (4) Obtain an accurate list of all medications that the patient uses, including

prescription, over-the-counter, herbs, and vitamins. More than 40% of the American public use complementary and alternative medicine. Patients may disclose use of these products only when directly questioned in a non-judgmental fashion (Oliveira, 2001; Reuters Health, 2000).

(5) *Age-specific concerns:* The elderly often have multiple comorbidities for which they take multiple medications. Be aware of the potential for drug interactions with chemotherapy agents (Hood, 2003).

b) Signs and symptoms of underlying disease process and any previous treatments

(1) Symptom screening during the pretreatment phase is crucial to successful symptom management.

(2) Poorly controlled symptoms impact the quality of life for the patient and can interfere with delivery of chemotherapy and other treatment modalities (Dodd, Miaskowski, & Paul, 2001; Houldin, 2000).

2. Screening tools

a) Assess performance status by using scales such as the Karnofsky, Zubrod, or ECOG (see Table 3).

b) Assess pain using an age-appropriate scale (e.g., numeric 0–10 scale, facial expressions, visual analog).

c) Assess for fatigue using an appropriate scale, such as the Brief Fatigue Inventory (Mendoza et al., 1999), the Piper Fatigue Scale (Piper et al.,1998), or the Schwartz Cancer Fatigue Scale (Schwartz, 1998).

3. Patient data

a) Obtain and document the patient's actual height and weight; compare with previous visits.

b) Compare current and previous lab values. *Age-specific concern:* Assess for age-related changes in pulmonary, renal, and cardiac function in the elderly.

c) Review diagnoses, tumor type, grade, and staging.

d) Obtain treatment records from past encounters to determine symptom management strategies that were employed.

e) Assess cultural and spiritual issues that may affect the treatment plan.

f) Assess how the patient and family are coping with the cancer experience.

g) Determine the need for referral to a social worker, spiritual care provider, dietitian, physical therapist, and other member of the multidisciplinary team as needed. *Age-specific concerns*: When caring for pediatric patients, consult play therapists and child-life specialists. If a school-age youth is going to be out of school for a prolonged time, explore options for continued study available through the appropriate school district (e.g., home study, online programs).

4. Information and learning needs of patient and family (Houldin, 2000, p. 51)

a) Determine the preferred language.

b) Assess speaking fluency and reading literacy.

c) Assess level of understanding of the disease and treatment.

d) Identify the patient's preferred learning style.

e) Provide information regarding

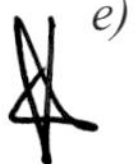

(1) Drugs, side effects, and symptom management

(2) When and how to call the nurse and/or doctor

(3) Follow-up care and labs

(4) How to access support services.

5. Treatment plan (Santell, Protzel, & Cousins, 2004)

a) Read the written orders in their entirety, then scrutinize each line for

(1) Name of drug ordered

(2) Drug dose

(3) Method of determining dose

(4) Route of administration

(5) Rate of administration

(6) Frequency and/or date(s) of administration

(7) Premedications

(8) Hydration, if applicable

(9) Protocol or reference.

b) Assess orders for completeness (e.g., hydration, premedications).

c) Review the patient's actual height and weight; double-check the patient's BSA.

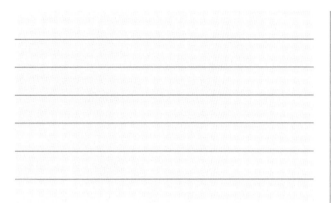

d) Have two individuals independently recalculate the drug dose and compare to the ordered dose (ASHP, 2002). Follow institutional policy for who can double-check doses (e.g., two RNs, RN and pharmacist).

e) Verify that the dose is appropriate for the patient, diagnosis, and treatment plan. If in doubt, clarify. Consult a pharmacist and/or physician.

f) Determine the vesicant and irritant potential of the drug(s).

g) Follow institutional policy regarding obtaining consent.

h) Assess the patient's prior experience with cytotoxic therapy (e.g., adequacy of symptom management, delayed side effects, willingness to proceed).

i) Immediately before administration, verify the order, the drug names, calculations, expiration dates and times, appearance of the drugs, and accuracy of two different patient identifiers (Joint Commission on Accreditation of Healthcare Organizations [JCAHO], 2004).

References

American Society of Health-System Pharmacists. (2002). ASHP guidelines on preventing medication errors with antineoplastic agents. *American Journal of Health-System Pharmacists, 59,* 1648–1668.

Dodd, M.J., Miaskowski, C., & Paul, S.M. (2001). Symptom clusters and their effect on the functional status of patients with cancer. *Oncology Nursing Forum, 28,* 465–470.

Hood, L.E. (2003). Chemotherapy in the elderly: Supportive measures for chemotherapy-induced myelotoxicity. *Clinical Journal of Oncology Nursing, 7,* 185–190.

Houldin, A.D. (2000). *Patients with cancer: Understanding the psychological pain.* Philadelphia: Lippincott Williams and Wilkins.

Joint Commission on Accreditation of Healthcare Organizations. (2004). *Comprehensive accreditation manual for hospitals: The official handbook.* Oakbrook Terrace, IL: Author.

Mendoza, T.R., Wang, X.S., Cleeland, C.S., Morrissey, M., Johnson, B.A., Wendt, J.K., et al. (1999). The rapid assessment of fatigue severity in cancer patients: Use of the Brief Fatigue Inventory. *Cancer, 85,* 1186–1196.

National Association of Children's Hospitals and Related Institutions. (1999). *Enhancing the chemotherapy process in oncology services.* Alexandria, VA: Author.

Oliveira, N. (2001). *Herbal and non-herbal supplement use in the cancer patient.* Retrieved March 26, 2004, from http://www.cancersourcern.com/search/getcontent.cfm?DiseaseID=1&Contentid=25904

Piper, B.F., Dibble, S.L., Dodd, M.J., Weiss, M.C., Slaughter, R.E., & Paul, S.M. (1998). The revised Piper Fatigue Scale: Psychometric evaluation in women with breast cancer. *Oncology Nursing Forum, 25,* 677–684.

Reuters Health. (2000). *Cancer patients only reveal alternative therapies when pressed.* Retrieved March 26, 2004, from http://www.cancersourcern.com/news/detail.cfm?DiseaseID=1&Contentid=19447

Santell, J.P., Protzel, M.M., & Cousins, D. (2004). Medication errors in oncology practice. *U.S. Pharmacist, 29:04.* Retrieved January 14, 2005, from http://www.uspharmacist.com/index.asp?show=article&page=8_1259.htm

Schwartz, A.L. (1998). The Schwartz Cancer Fatigue Scale: Testing reliability and validity. *Oncology Nursing Forum, 25,* 711–717.

D. Treatment

1. Patient preparation

a) Explain to the patient and family/caregivers who will administer the chemotherapy, the route, and the planned sequence of events.

b) Describe the plan for symptom management. Provide information regarding (Vandegrift, 2001)

(1) Premedications

(2) Hydration

(3) Intake and output assessment

(4) Laboratory monitoring

(5) Diet during chemotherapy

(6) Potential side effects of chemotherapeutic and adjunct medications

(7) Baseline vital signs as indicated.

2. Staff preparation

a) Review all physician orders.

b) Have a spill kit, extravasation equipment, and emergency drugs/equipment available as needed (Otto, 2004). *Age-specific concerns:* If administering chemotherapy to a child, patient-specific dosing information and emergency equipment must be available. Calculate emergency drug doses before they are needed.

c) Obtain monitoring equipment as indicated.

d) Obtain infusion pumps and other devices as needed. *Age-specific concerns:* Use a volumetric pump to administer chemotherapy to pediatric patients (Frey, 2001; Infusion Nurses Society [INS], 2000).

3. Routes of administration
   a) Oral: The role of oral chemotherapy agents is expanding, with many new drugs in development, reflecting a new paradigm in which cancer is treated as a chronic disease with long-term management (Bedell, 2003).
      (1) Advantages
         (a) Ease and portability of administration
         (b) Increased sense of patient independence
      (2) Disadvantages
         (a) Inconsistency of absorption
         (b) Potential loss of drug in the event of emesis
         (c) Potential for drug/herb/diet interactions
         (d) Issue of medication adherence
         (e) Cost/reimbursement concerns (Birner, 2003)
      (3) Potential complications
         (a) Drug-specific
         (b) Related to drug–drug interactions
         (c) Related to swallowing difficulties
      (4) Nursing implications
         (a) *Age-specific concerns:* Young children may require liquid preparations. For elderly patients, evaluate ability to swallow pills intact, plus ability to self-manage medication regimen (Hartigan, 2000).
         (b) Patient education is key to promoting medication regimen adherence. Provide verbal and written instructions, including name of the medication, dose/schedule, how taken, and safety (storage and handling).
   b) SQ or IM injection (see Table 12 for maximum volumes for IM injections for children) (Camp-Sorrell, 2004; Goodman, 2000)
      (1) Advantages
         (a) Ease of administration
         (b) Decreased side effects
      (2) Disadvantages
         (a) Inconsistency of absorption
         (b) Requires adequate muscle mass and tissue for absorption
      (3) Potential complications
         (a) Pain/discomfort
         (b) Infection
         (c) Bleeding
      (4) Nursing implications
         (a) Monitor platelet count and ANC.
         (b) Use smallest needle possible; some solutions may come with pre-prepared syringes (follow manufacturer's instructions).
         (c) Follow institutional policy for site antisepsis and documentation.
         (d) Assess previous injection sites for signs and symptoms of infection or bleeding.
   c) Intra-arterial: Delivers medication directly into an organ (e.g., brain, liver, head and neck, pelvis) or tumor by means of three types of access devices. Refer to the ONS *Access Device Guidelines and Recommendations for Practice* (Camp-Sorrell, 2004) for more detailed information.
      (1) Types of devices

Table 12. Guidelines for Maximum Safe Volumes for Intramuscular Injections

Age	Site			
	Deltoid	Ventro-Gluteal	Dorso-Gluteal	Vastus Lateralis
Premature	–	–	–	0.5 ml
Neonate	–	–	–	0.5 ml
Infant	–	–	–	1 ml
Young child (3–6 years)	–	1.5 ml	1 ml	1.5 ml
Older child (6–14 years)	0.5 ml	1.5–2 ml	1.5–2 ml	1.5 ml
Adolescent (15 years to adult)	1 ml	1–2.5 ml	2–2.5 ml	1.5–2 ml

Note. From "Medicating Infants and Children" (p. 403) in J.W. Ashwill and S.C. Droske (Eds.), *Nursing Care of Children: Principles and Practice,* 2002, Philadelphia: W.B. Saunders. Copyright 2002 by W.B. Saunders. Reprinted with permission.

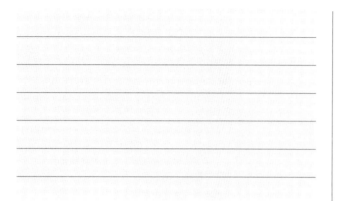

(a) Short-term percutaneous catheters inserted via femoral or brachial artery (frequently placed by interventional radiologists)
(b) Long-term catheters placed during surgery and used as an external catheter or attached to an implanted pump
(c) Implanted ports for long-term therapy

(2) Advantages
(a) Increased exposure of tumor to drug results in greater tumor response with less systemic side effects.
(b) This therapy is considered a local treatment, as the drug's first major site of action is the target lesion, thereby avoiding the first pass effect.

(3) Disadvantages
(a) Less systemic circulation of the chemotherapy increases the risk for distant metastasis.
(b) Requires surgical procedure or special radiography equipment for catheter or port placement.
(c) Requires specialized nursing education for arterial pumps.
(d) When treatment is given by percutaneous catheter, the patient may have sharply limited mobility for three to seven days.

(4) Potential complications
(a) Bleeding
(b) Embolism
(c) Pain
(d) Pump occlusion or malfunction
(e) Hepatic artery injury
(f) Arterial catheter leak or break
(g) Skin reaction to tape or dressing
(h) Catheter migration/dislodgment

(5) Nursing implications
(a) Monitor for signs/symptoms of bleeding, including monitoring prothrombin time (PT)/partial thromboplastin time (PTT).
(b) Monitor catheter site for infection, bleeding, signs of catheter migration/dislodgment, including epigastric pain, nausea/vomiting/diarrhea, edema, diminished peripheral pulse, and inability to infuse.
(c) Monitor for signs of occlusion, including inability to flush or withdraw fluid, abdominal pain, or change in color/pulse/temperature of involved extremity. If patient is going home with infusion, provide patient education regarding pump and catheter care. Follow pump manufacturer's recommendations for implanted pumps (Barber & Fabugais-Nazario, 2003; Hagle, 2003).

d) Intrathecal/intraventricular (Camp-Sorrell, 2000; Gullatte, 2001)

(1) Advantages
(a) Affords more consistent drug levels in cerebrospinal fluid
(b) Bypasses the blood-brain barrier
(c) Also can be used to sample cerebrospinal fluid and to administer opiates and antibiotics

(2) Disadvantages
(a) Requires lumbar puncture or surgical placement of implanted intraventricular device (e.g., Ommaya reservoir)
(b) Generally requires a physician or specially trained RN to access and administer chemotherapy via this route

(3) Potential complications: Increased intracranial pressure, headaches, confusion, lethargy, nausea and vomiting, seizures, and infection

(4) Nursing implications
(a) Observe site for signs of infection.
(b) Assess patient for headache or other signs of increased intracranial pressure (Kosier & Minkler, 1999).
(c) Accessing the Ommaya reservoir is a sterile procedure. Medication to be instilled must be preservative free.

(d) Do not use a Vacutainer® (Beckton Dickinson & Co., Franklin Lakes, NJ) to withdraw CSF: Rapid withdrawal of fluid could damage the choroids plexus of the ventricle. Avoid air embolism.

e) Intraperitoneal (Camp-Sorrell, 2004; Goodman, 2000).
(1) Advantages
(a) Provides direct exposure of intra-abdominal metastases to the drug(s)
(b) Also may instill radioactive or colloid materials intraperitoneally
(2) Disadvantages: Requires placement of a peritoneal catheter or intraperitoneal port
(3) Potential complications
(a) Abdominal pain
(b) Distention
(c) Bleeding
(d) Ileus
(e) Intestinal perforation
(f) Infection
(4) Nursing implications
(a) Warm chemotherapy to body temperature (Otto, 2004).
(b) Check patency of catheter or port according to institutional policy.
(c) Instill solution according to protocol: Infuse drug, reposition patient for maximum surface exposure to drug, and drain if ordered.

f) Intrapleural: Instills sclerosing agents such as nitrogen mustard, bleomycin, or 5-FU, or sterile talc into the pleural space (Goodman, 2000); also may instill radioactive colloidal materials
(1) Advantage: Scleroses the pleural lining to prevent recurrence of effusions
(2) Disadvantages
(a) Requires insertion of a thoracotomy tube
(b) Physicians must administer the intrapleural agents.
(3) Potential complications
(a) Pain
(b) Infection
(4) Nursing implications
(a) The effusion must be completely drained from the pleural cavity before instillation of the drug (thoracentesis).
(b) Following instillation, clamp the tubing and reposition the patient every 10–15 minutes for two hours, or as ordered (Otto, 2004).
(c) Assess for and treat pain and anxiety.

g) Intravesicular (Goodman, 2000)
(1) Advantage: Provides direct exposure of superficial, localized cancers of the bladder surfaces to drugs, such as thiotepa, mitomycin, epirubicin, doxorubicin, and mitoxantrone
(2) Disadvantages: Requires placement of a Foley catheter
(3) Potential complications
(a) Urinary tract infection
(b) Cystitis
(c) Bladder contracture
(d) Urinary urgency
(4) Nursing implications
(a) Maintain sterile technique during Foley insertion.
(b) Follow physician orders or protocol for schedule of repositioning the patient and clamping and unclamping the catheter after instilling the chemotherapy.

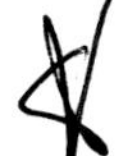

h) IV (Camp-Sorrell, 2004; Goodman, 2000)
(1) Advantages
(a) Consistent absorption
(b) Required for vesicant and many other agents
(2) Disadvantages
(a) Requires considerable nursing and patient time in a healthcare facility
(b) Interferes with patient's activities; sclerosing of veins over time
(c) May require surgical procedure for central line placement
(3) Potential complications
(a) Infection
(b) Phlebitis
(c) Infiltration
(d) Extravasation (INS, 2000)
(e) Local discomfort

(f) Drug-specific concerns

(4) Nursing implications will be discussed in the following section.

4. IV cytotoxic administration: Most cytotoxic agents are given intravenously. Refer to *Access Device Guidelines: Recommendations for Nursing Practice and Education* (Camp-Sorrell, 2004) for a complete discussion of obtaining IV access.

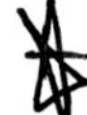

a) Peripheral IV access

(1) Existing IV site

(a) Avoid using a site that is more than 24 hours old.

(b) Assess the insertion site for signs of inflammation and infiltration, and consider the patient's statements about comfort. Use another access site if there is any doubt about the integrity of the IV site.

(c) Assess blood return and patency.

(2) New IV site: Avoid use of steel needles for vesicant administration (Centers for Disease Control and Prevention [CDC], 2002). Select the smallest gauge and shortest length catheter to accommodate the prescribed therapy (INS, 2000). Consider use of dermal anesthesia to minimize pain during IV insertion.

(a) In adults (Camp-Sorrell, 2004; Goodman, 2000)

i) Identify an appropriate IV site by assessing the patient's arms carefully. Veins of choice are smooth and pliable; the large veins of the forearm are preferred.

ii) Avoid establishing an IV site in the following.

- Injured or sclerosed veins
- Areas of flexion
- Small, fragile, tortuous veins
- An extremity with altered venous return or lymphedema
- An extremity with decreased sensation or paresthesia
- The lower extremities

iii) Perform venipuncture per institutional policy and procedure.

iv) Establish blood return and patency.

v) Secure the IV device appropriately, in a manner that allows a clear view of the site.

vi) If venipuncture is unsuccessful, utilize the opposite arm for the next attempt. If it is not possible to use the opposite arm, select a site proximal to the first venipuncture.

(b) In children, select an appropriate site, following institutional policies and the guidelines that follow (Hankins, Lonsway, Hedrick, & Perdue, 2001).

i) If possible, do not use the feet or dominant hand of an infant or toddler as an IV site.

ii) The veins of the scalp of a child younger than 12 months old can be used as an IV site; however, do not use a scalp vein to administer a vesicant.

iii) Stabilize the extremity, if necessary, while inserting and securing the IV.

b) Central venous catheters (CVCs): CVCs include percutaneous subclavian catheters, tunneled subclavian catheters, and peripherally inserted central catheters (PICCs). (A midline catheter is considered a peripheral line because it ends in the middle of the upper arm.) An implanted port, although technically a CVC, is unique and will be addressed later. Note: Most CVCs require the use of syringes larger than 10 cc to minimize pressure (pounds per square inch [psi]) on delicate catheter walls (Camp-Sorrell, 2004). Follow manufacturer's and institutional guidelines carefully to avoid catheter rupture. After CVC insertion and before administering the agent, perform the following.

(1) Verify that the catheter's placement is correct prior to initial use per institutional guidelines.

(2) Inspect exit site for evidence of erythema, swelling, drainage, and leakage.

(3) Inspect ipsilateral chest for signs of venous thrombosis (Mayo & Pearson, 1995).

(4) Aspirate the line to verify blood return. If blood return is not evident,

(a) Flush the catheter with saline, gently using the push-pull method.

(b) Reposition the patient as appropriate.

(c) Ask the patient to cough.

(d) Explain to the patient why delaying therapy is necessary. Although patients may report that lack of blood return from their catheter is common, do not administer cytotoxic therapy.

(e) Obtain a physician's order for a declotting procedure; follow institutional protocol.

(f) Use x-rays or dye studies to confirm proper CVC placement and rule out catheter malfunction or migration in the absence of a blood return.

c) Implanted ports: Implanted ports are available that allow venous, peritoneal, arterial, and epidural access. Ascertain which type is being used. Some patients have more than one type.

(1) Assess initial line placement by using the results of x-ray or fluoroscopic dye studies.

(2) Choose a noncoring needle (Goodman, 2000) with a length that is appropriate to the

(a) Depth of the port

(b) Size of the patient (i.e., the amount of SQ tissue or fat located above the port).

(3) Prepare the patient's skin according to institutional policy.

(4) Access the port, ensuring proper placement of the needle in the reservoir.

(5) Establish blood return and patency. If blood return is not evident, repeat steps listed for CVCs. (Blood return is not expected with epidural or peritoneal access devices.)

(6) Inspect the needle insertion site for needle dislodgment, leakage of IV fluid, drainage, or edema.

(7) Examine the ipsilateral chest for venous thrombosis.

(8) Apply an occlusive dressing to stabilize the needle. The dressing should be transparent, to allow a clear view of the insertion site. Experts disagree about other dressing characteristics that are desirable (Camp-Sorrell, 2004). When working with children, padding the undersides of the butterfly wings of the access needle may be necessary if the needle does not lie securely on the skin.

d) Piggy-back or short-term infusion

(1) Verify blood return and IV patency prior to hanging the infusion. Do not pinch the IV catheter to determine blood return because of the resulting dramatic change in pressure within the vein. Preferred methods of verifying patency are the following.

(a) Use a syringe inserted at the injection port closest to the patient to gently aspirate the line, while pinching off fluid from the bag.

(b) Use a gravity check by removing the bag from the pump, lowering it below the patient's IV site, and watch for blood return.

(2) Attach the secondary tubing to the appropriate injection port, using a needleless, Luer lock connector (INS, 2000).

(3) Initiate flow rate according to the physician's orders and observe the patient closely for any reactions.

(4) When administering a vesicant drug by short infusion using a peripheral vein,

(a) Avoid using an IV pump in order to decrease pressure on the veins.

(b) Remain with the patient during the infusion. Visually monitor the site for signs of extravasation while

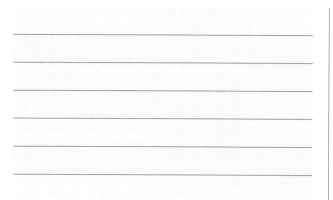

verifying blood return every 5–10 minutes.

(c) Avoid infusing vesicant agents peripherally for more than 30–60 minutes.

(5) Once the short infusion is complete, check vein patency and flush the line with a compatible IV solution.

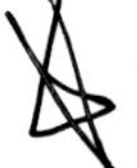

e) Continuous infusion

(1) Follow guidelines for checking blood return and IV patency.

(2) The cytotoxic agent may be connected directly to the IV catheter, or into a compatible line of maintenance solution, according to institutional policy.

(3) Secure all connections with locking devices.

(4) Monitor the IV site throughout the infusion according to institutional policy and procedure. Monitor the patient closely for any reactions, such as signs or symptoms of hypersensitivity (Otto, 2004). *Age-specific concerns:* For pediatric patients with continuous infusions, monitor the IV site hourly or according to institutional policy (Shutak, 2000).

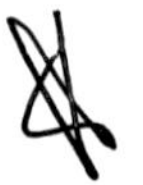

(5) When administering a vesicant, (Chu & DeVita, 2005; Vandergrift, 2001)

(a) DO NOT use a peripheral IV site for continuous vesicant administration.

(b) Use a central venous access catheter or implanted access device to administer any vesicant infusing for longer than 30–60 minutes.

(c) Check for blood return and patency periodically, according to institutional policy.

(6) Once the infusion is complete, check vein patency and flush the line with a compatible IV solution (Otto, 2004).

f) IV push: Refer to physician orders and/or pharmacy guidelines for suggested IV push rates, diluents, and other drug-specific details (Goodman, 2000; Vandergrift, 2001).

(1) Free-flow method (side-arm technique)

(a) Attach the syringe with the drug at the injection port closest to the patient.

(b) Aspirate the line in order to verify IV patency.

(c) Allow IV solution to flow freely.

(d) Slowly administer the chemotherapy agent as an IV push, allowing the flush solution to dilute the drug. Unless otherwise indicated, administer the agent at a rate of 1–2 ml/minute.

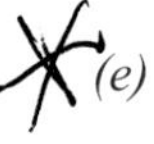

(e) When administering a vesicant, verify blood return every 2–5 ml.

(f) Once the IV push is completed, check vein patency and flush the line with a compatible IV solution.

(2) Direct push method: Some institutions may require that certain cytotoxic agents be administered as an IV push directly into the IV device (Goodman, 2000; Temple & Poniatowski, 2005; Vandergrift, 2001).

(a) Select an appropriate vein and prep the skin according to policy.

(b) Establish a patent IV, flushing the new line with sterile IV solution (typically normal saline [NS] or 5% dextrose in water [D5W])

(c) Verify blood return by aspirating the line gently.

(d) Detach the flush syringe, and attach the syringe containing the cytotoxic agent. Maintain sterile technique and minimize blood loss.

(e) Slowly administer the agent, aspirating for blood return every 2–5 ml.

(f) Upon completion of the IV push, disconnect the cytotoxic syringe. Avoid blood loss; the blood will contain the cytotoxic agent.

(g) Connect a syringe containing sterile flush solution; gently flush the catheter.

(h) Cap or discontinue the IV access device, as indicated.

References

Barber, F.D., & Fabugais-Nazario, L.E. (2003). What's old is new again: Patients receiving hepatic arterial infusion chemotherapy. *Clinical Journal of Oncology Nursing, 7,* 647–652.

Bedell, C.H. (2003). A changing paradigm for cancer treatment: The advent of new oral chemotherapy agents. *Clinical Journal of Oncology Nursing, 7*(Suppl. 6), 5–9.

Birner, A. (2003). Safe administration of oral chemotherapy. *Clinical Journal of Oncology Nursing, 7,* 158–162.

Camp-Sorrell, D. (Ed.). (2004). *Access device guidelines: Recommendations for nursing practice and education.* Pittsburgh, PA: Oncology Nursing Society.

Centers for Disease Control and Prevention. (2002). Guidelines for prevention of intravascular catheter-related infections. *Morbidity and Mortality Weekly Report, 51*(32), 1–29.

Chu, E., & DeVita, V.T. (2005). *Physicians' cancer chemotherapy drug manual.* Sudbury, MA: Jones and Bartlett.

Frey, A.M. (2001). Intravenous therapy in children. In J. Hankins, R.A.W. Lonsway, C. Hedrick, & M. Perdue (Eds.), *Infusion therapy in clinical practice* (2nd ed., pp. 561–591). St. Louis, MO: Saunders.

Goodman, M. (2000). Chemotherapy: Principles of administration. In C.H. Yarbro, M.H. Frogge, M. Goodman, & S.L. Groenwald (Eds.), *Cancer nursing: Principles and practice* (5th ed., pp. 385–443). Sudbury, MA: Jones and Bartlett.

Gullatte, M.M. (2001). Principles and standards of chemotherapy administration. In M.M. Gullatte (Ed.), *Clinical guide to antineoplastic therapy: A chemotherapy handbook* (pp. 31–46). Pittsburgh, PA: Oncology Nursing Society.

Hagle, M.E. (2003). Arterial access devices. *Clinical Journal of Oncology Nursing, 7,* 669–674.

Hankins, J., Lonsway, R.A., Hedrick, C., & Perdue, M. (Eds.). (2001). *Infusion therapy in clinical practice* (2nd ed.). Philadelphia: Saunders.

Hartigan, K. (2000). Patient education: The cornerstone of successful oral chemotherapy treatment. *Clinical Journal of Oncology Nursing, 7*(Suppl. 6), 21–24.

Infusion Nurses Society. (2000). Infusion nursing standards of practice. *Journal of Intravenous Nursing, 23*(Suppl. 6), S1–S88.

Kosier, M.B., & Minkler, P. (1999). Nursing management of patients with an implanted Ommaya reservoir. *Clinical Journal of Oncology Nursing, 3,* 63–67.

Mayo, D.J., & Pearson, D.C. (1995). Chemotherapy extravasation: A consequence of fibrin sheath formation around venous access devices. *Oncology Nursing Forum, 22,* 675–680.

Otto, S. (2004). *Oncology nursing clinical reference.* St. Louis, MO: Mosby.

Shutak, V.P. (2000). Pediatrics. In A.M. Corrigan, G. Pelletier, & M. Alexander (Eds.), *Core curriculum for intravenous nursing* (2nd ed., pp. 231–275). Philadelphia: Lippincott Williams & Wilkins.

Temple, S.V., & Poniatowski, B.D. (2005). Nursing implications of antineoplastic therapy. In J.K. Itano & K.N. Taoka (Eds.), *Core curriculum for oncology nursing* (4th ed., pp. 785–802). St. Louis, MO: Elsevier.

Vandergrift, K.V. (2001). Oncologic therapy. In J. Hankins, R.A.W. Lonsway, C. Hedrick, & M.B. Perdue (Eds.), *Infusion therapy in clinical practice* (2nd ed., pp. 248–275). St. Louis, MO: Saunders.

VI. Immediate Complications of Cytotoxic Therapy

- The oncology nurse must be alert for immediate complications of cytotoxic therapy. The information in this section covers those complications most frequently experienced by patients during the chemotherapy infusion or shortly thereafter. Terms used in this section include

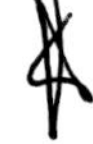

- *Extravasation:* "Passage or escape into tissue of antineoplastic drugs. Tissue slough and necrosis may occur if the condition is severe" (*Mosby's*, 2002, p. 648).

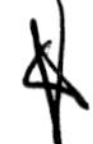

- *Vesicant:* Any agent that has the potential to cause blistering, severe tissue injury or tissue necrosis when extravasated (Langhorne & Barton-Burke, 2001; *Mosby's* 2002)

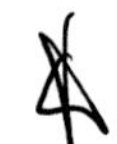

- *Irritant:* Any agent that causes aching, tightness, and phlebitis along the vein or at the injection site, with or without a local inflammatory reaction but does not cause tissue necrosis (Langhorne & Barton-Burke, 2001; Otto, 2001)

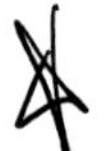

- *Flare reaction:* A local allergic reaction to an agent, manifested by streaking or red blotches along the vein, but without pain (Clamon, 2001; Langhorne & Barton-Burke, 2001; Steele, 2001)

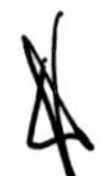

- *Anaphylaxis:* Dramatic, acute systemic reaction that may be marked by the sudden onset of rapidly progressing hives, itching, or respiratory distress. May precipitate vascular collapse, leading to shock and death (Labovich, 1999; Mone & Summers, 1998).

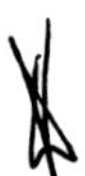

- *Hypersensitivity:* Exaggerated or inappropriate immune response that may be localized or systemic, occurring during or within hours of drug administration (Shepherd, 2003; Weiss, 2001).

A. Extravasation: Table 13 lists the vesicants, irritants, and nursing measures.

1. Pathophysiology: Tissue damage secondary to drug infiltration occurs as a result of one of two major mechanisms (Clamon, 2001).
   a) The drug is absorbed by local cells in the tissue and binds to critical structures (e.g., DNA, microtubules), causing cell death. It then is released into the surrounding tissue. Healing is inhibited because the process is repeated as the drug is taken up by other cells (Albanell & Baselga, 2000; Dorr, 1994).
   b) The drug does not bind to cellular DNA. Local tissue damage is caused by the solvents used in the drug formulations and is more readily neutralized (Albanell & Baselga, 2000; Dorr, 1994).
2. Extent of tissue damage: Factors that affect the amount of tissue damage include the site of infiltration, the amount of drug infiltrate, the concentration of the agent, the vesicant nature of the agent, and, possibly, the management of the extravasation by the nurse or physician (Clamon, 2001).
3. Antidotes: Animal studies have demonstrated a few effective antidotes for extravasation; however, applicability of these studies to humans is limited (Camp-Sorrell, 1998; Ener, Meglathery, & Styler, 2004) and the use of antidotes continues to be controversial. Ener et al. wrote, "Unfortunately, the lack of large scale comparative trials owing to the infrequent nature of these episodes and the unethical nature of placebo controlled trials make treatment mostly empirical, based on small uncontrolled trials, case reports and animal studies" (p. 860). Currently, sodium thiosulfate is the recommended antidote for mechlorethamine hydrochloride and concentrated solution of cisplatin (0.5 mg/ml) extravasation (Bertelli, 1995; Ener et al.). The topical application of dimethyl sulfoxide (DMSO) on extravasations of anthracyclines shows mixed results, with some authors concluding it is safe and effective as an antidote (Bertelli et al., 1995; St. Germain, Houlihan, & D'Amato, 1994), whereas others show delayed healing (Harwood & Bachur, 1987). However, Clamon (2001) concluded that "the role of antidotes in extravasation injury is not entirely clear" (p. 434).
4. Risk factors for peripheral extravasation include the following (Kassner, 2000; Langhorne & Barton-Burke, 2001; Steele, 2001).
   a) Small, fragile veins
   b) Poor vascular integrity or history of vascular or circulatory disease
   c) History of diabetes, other medical conditions, or previous chemotherapies leading to peripheral neuropathy
   d) Previous multiple venipunctures and IV medications causing decreased vascular integrity

Table 13. Vesicants and Irritants

Vesicants			
Classification	**Medication Name(s)**	**Local Care**	**Nursing Considerations**
Alkylating agent	Cisplatin (Platinol®)	Isotonic sodium thiosulfate may be used as an antidote. Prepare 1/6 molar solution. • If 10% sodium thiosulfate solution: Mix 4 ml with 6 ml sterile water for injection. • If 25% sodium thiosulfate solution: Mix 1.6 ml with 8.4 ml sterile water. Aspirate residual drug. Use 2 ml 10% sodium thiosulfate for each 100 mg cisplatin. Remove needle. Inject into subcutaneous (SQ) tissue.	Vesicant potential is seen when a concentration of more than 20 ml of 0.5 mg/ml extravasates. If less than this, drug is an irritant; no treatment is recommended (Dorr, 1994).
	Mechlorethamine hydrochloride (nitrogen mustard, Mustargen®)	Isotonic sodium thiosulfate may be used as an antidote. Prepare 1/6 molar solution. • If 10% sodium thiosulfate solution: Mix 4 ml with 6 ml sterile water for injection. • If 25% sodium thiosulfate solution: Mix 1.6 ml with 8.4 ml sterile water. Aspirate residual drug. Use 2 ml antidote for every 1 mg drug extravasated. Remove needle. Inject antidote into SQ tissue.	Sodium thiosulfate neutralizes nitrogen mustard, which then is excreted via the kidneys. Time is essential in treating extravasation. Heat and cold have not proven effective (Dorr, 1990, 1994).
Antitumor antibiotic	Doxorubicin (Adriamycin®)	Apply cold pad with circulating ice water, ice pack, or cryogel pack for 15–20 minutes at least four times per day for the first 24–48 hours (Harwood & Govin, 1994). Elevate site for 48 hours, then resume normal activity (Goodman, 2000).	Extravasations of less than 1–2 ml often heal spontaneously. If greater than 3 ml, ulceration often results (Goodman, 2000). Protect area of extravasation from sunlight and heat. Some studies suggest that 99% dimethyl sulfoxide (DMSO) 1–2 ml applied to site every six hours is beneficial (Bertelli, 1995; Olver et al., 1988; St. Germain et al., 1994). Other studies show delayed healing with DMSO (Harwood & Bachur, 1987).
	Daunorubicin (Cerubidine®)	–	Little information is known. In mouse experiments, topical DMSO afforded some benefit (Olver et al., 1988).
	Mitomycin (Mutamycin®)	–	Protect area of extravasation from sunlight. Delayed skin reactions have occurred in areas far from original IV site. Some research studies show benefit with use of 99% DMSO 1–2 ml applied to site every six hours for 14 days. More studies are needed (Alberts & Dorr, 1991).
	Dactinomycin (actinomycin-D, Cosmegen®)	Apply ice to increase comfort at the site. Elevate site for 48 hours, then resume normal activity (Goodman, 2000).	Application of heat may exacerbate tissue damage.
	Epirubicin (Ellence®), idarubicin (Idamycin®)	–	Local care measures are unknown. Cold, DMSO, and corticosteroids were shown to be ineffective in experiments with mice (Soble et al., 1987).

(Continued on next page)

Table 13. Vesicants and Irritants *(Continued)*

Classification	Medication Name(s)	Local Care	Nursing Considerations
Vinca alkaloid or micro-tubular inhibiting agent	Vincristine (Oncovin®)	Apply warm pack for 15–20 minutes at least four times per day for the first 24–48 hours and elevate (Larson, 1985; Rudolph & Larson, 1987).	This method of treatment is very effective for rapid absorption of drug (Bellone, 1981; Dorr, 1994; Goodman, 2000; Laurie et al., 1984).
	Vinblastine (Velban®)	Same as above	Same as above
	Vindesine (Eldisine® [in Canada])	Same as above	Same as above
	Vinorelbine (Navelbine®)	Same as above	Same as above
Taxane	Paclitaxel (Taxol®)	Apply ice pack for 15–20 minutes at least four times a day for the first 24 hours.	Its vesicant potential has been documented (Ajani et al., 1994; Herrington & Figueroa, 1997). Paclitaxel has rare vesicant potential (probably because of dilution in 500 ml diluent) (Dorr et al., 1996). In a review of the literature, Stanford and Hardwicke (2003) concluded that paclitaxel may be a mild vesicant. Ice has been effective in decreasing local tissue damage in a mouse model (Dorr et al., 1996). Conservative management with cold packs may be the most appropriate strategy (Stanford & Hardwicke, 2003).
		Irritants	
Classification	**Medication Name(s)**	**Local Care**	**Nursing Considerations**
Alkylating agent	Carboplatin (Paraplatin®)	–	May cause phlebitis Local care measures are unknown.
	Dacarbazine (DTIC-Dome®)	–	May cause phlebitis Protect dacarbazine from sunlight.
	Ifosfamide (Ifex®)	–	May cause phlebitis Local care measures are unknown.
	Melphalan (Alkeran®)	–	May cause phlebitis Local care measures are unknown.
	Oxaliplatin (Eloxatin®)	–	Vesicant properties have been reported, and the agent is at least an irritant (Ener et al., 2004; Kretzschmar et al., 2003). Extravasation of moderate to high doses led to pronounced symptoms of inflammation but without subsequent necrosis. High-dose dexamethasone should be considered as a therapeutic intervention (Kretzschmar et al., 2003).
Nitrosourea	Carmustine (BiCNU®)	–	May cause phlebitis Local care measures are unknown.
Antitumor antibiotic	Bleomycin (Blenoxane®)	–	May cause irritation to tissue Little information is known.
	Daunorubicin citrate liposomal (DaunoXome®)	–	May cause pain or buring at IV site Little information is known.

(Continued on next page)

Table 13. Vesicants and Irritants *(Continued)*

Classification	Medication Name(s)	Local Care	Nursing Considerations
Antitumor antibiotic *(cont.)*	Doxorubicin liposomal (Doxil®)	–	May produce redness and tissue edema Low ulceration potential If ulceration begins or if pain, redness, or swelling persists, treat like doxorubicin.
	Mitoxantrone (Novantrone®)	–	Administer with caution; may cause tissue damage if extravasation occurs. Local care measures are unknown. Ulceration is rare unless a concentrated dose infiltrates (Dorr, 1990).
Epipodophyllotoxin	Etoposide (VP-16, Etopophos®, VePesid®)	Apply warm pack.	Treatment is necessary only if large amount of a concentrated solution extravasates. In this case, treat like vincristine or vinblastine (Dorr, 1994). May cause phlebitis, urticaria, or redness
	Teniposide (VM-26, Vumon®)	–	Same as above
Taxane	Docetaxel (Taxotere®)	Apply cool or warm cloth to reduce discomfort.	Extravasation reactions are self-limiting. May cause mild symptoms followed by edema, erythema, and occasional pain and blister formation (usually resolving within three weeks) (Ascherman, Knowles, & Attkiss, 2000).

e) Limited vein selection because of lymph node dissection or limb removal

f) Superior vena cava syndrome or other medical conditions causing peripheral edema

g) Use of medications that produce somnolence, altered mental status (i.e., patient cannot communicate discomfort at IV site), excessive movement, vomiting, or coughing

h) Venipuncture technique

i) Drug administration technique

j) Site of venous access (avoid veins in the hand, wrist, and antecubital fossa whenever possible)

k) Device selection (avoid use of steel-tipped, winged infusion [butterfly] needles for infusion) (Clamon, 2001)

5. Extravasation involving a central line: The use of central venous catheters (CVCs) does not preclude extravasation injuries (Clamon, 2001; Ener et al., 2004). Extravasation in the upper torso or neck area may result in serious defects and require extensive reconstructive surgery. It is imperative that the nurse administer vesicant therapy into a central line of any type very carefully. Extravasation may result from any of the following (Ener et al.; Schulmeister & Camp-Sorrell, 2000; Steele, 2001).

a) Backflow secondary to fibrin sheath or thrombosis in CVC

b) Dislodgment of needle from port

c) Catheter damage, breakage, or separation of a vascular access device (VAD)

d) Displacement or migration of the catheter from the vein

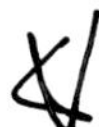

6. Signs, symptoms, and results of extravasation (Langhorne & Barton-Burke, 2001; Otto, 2001): Patients with central VADs also should report any of these symptoms at the site surrounding a central line or across the chest wall. Table 14 distinguishes the manifestations of extravasation from those of vein irritation and flare reaction. See also Appendix 4. The signs, symptoms, and results of extravasation are as follows (Goodman, 2000; Steele, 2001).

a) Swelling (most common)

b) Stinging, burning, or pain at the injection site (not always present)

c) IV flow rate that slows or stops

d) Leaking around catheter or implanted port needle

e) Lack of blood return (not always a sign of extravasation; extravasation can occur with the presence of a blood return)

f) Erythema, inflammation, or blanching at the injection site (not always immediately evident)

g) Induration

h) Vesicle formation

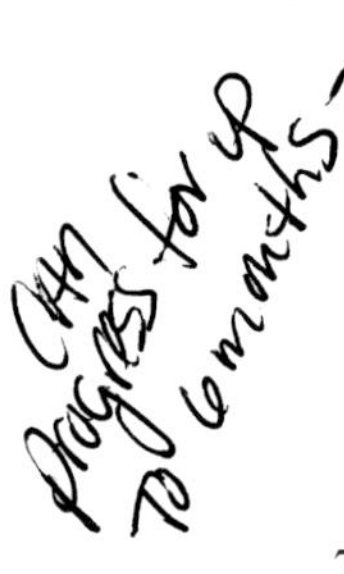

i) Ulceration
j) Necrosis: Tissue damage may progress for six months after the incident. Tissue destruction ultimately may interfere with the affected extremity's function or lead to the loss of a limb or breast (Albanell & Baselga, 2000; Bertelli, 1995).
k) Sloughing
l) Damage to tendons, nerves, and joints (Clamon, 2001)

7. Collaborative management of extravasation: The nurse should be aware of the institution's policies and procedures regarding vesicant extravasation prior to administration of the medication. Document compliance with said policies and procedures.
   a) Initial management of extravasation (Kassner, 2000; Langhorne & Barton-Burke, 2001; Otto, 2001): At the first sign of infiltration,
      (1) Stop administration of vesicant and IV fluids immediately.
      (2) Disconnect the IV tubing from the IV device. Do not remove.
      (3) If the patient has an implanted port, assess the site for proper needle placement.
      (4) Attempt to aspirate the residual drug from the IV device by using a small (1–3 cc) syringe.
      (5) Remove the needle and dress the site; notify the physician.
      (6) Initiate standing orders, if applicable.
      (7) Apply hot or cold compress as directed in Table 13.
   b) Antidote administration: At the time of this publication, controversy continues about the appropriate use of antidotes because of insufficient data and lack of commercial availability (Clamon, 2001; Ener et al., 2004). Therefore, ONS no longer recommends antidotes for extravasation (except sodium thiosulfate). Initiate appropriate nursing management measures according to Table 13 and institutional policies.
   c) Post-extravasation care
      (1) Photograph the initial extravasation site and repeat weekly if appropriate (Goodman, 2000) and if institutional

Table 14. Nursing Assessment of Extravasation Versus Other Reactions

Assessment Parameter	Extravasation		Irritation of the Vein	Flare Reaction
	Immediate Manifestations	Delayed Manifestations		
Pain	Severe pain or burning that lasts minutes or hours and eventually subsides; usually occurs while the drug is being given and around the needle site	Usually occur within 48 hours	Aching and tightness along the vein	No pain
Redness	Blotchy redness around the needle site; not always present at the time of extravasation	Later occurrence	The full length of the vein may be reddened or darkened.	Immediate blotches or streaks along the vein, which usually subside within 30 minutes with or without treatment
Ulceration	Develops insidiously; usually occurs 48–96 hours later	Later occurrence	Not usually	Not usually
Swelling	Severe swelling; usually occurs immediately	Usually occurs within 48 hours	Unlikely	Unlikely; wheals may appear along the vein line.
Blood return	Inability to obtain blood return; good blood return during drug administration	–	Usually	Usually
Other	Change in the quality of infusion	Local tingling and sensory deficits	–	Urticaria

policy requires that the site be photographed.

(2) Instruct the patient to rest and elevate the site for 48 hours and then to resume normal activity. Patients should be given written instructions regarding what symptoms they should report immediately, local care of the site, pain management, and the plan for follow-up (Goodman, 2000; Langhorne & Barton-Burke, 2001). Ensure that no medications are given distally to an extravasation injury (Infusion Nurses Society, 2000).

(3) Evaluate the extent of extravasation and tissue damage. Arrange for a return appointment depending on the type and amount of drug that has extravasated (Goodman, 2000) and the location and the degree of tissue damage.

(4) Consult a plastic surgeon if a large volume was extravasated, if the patient experiences severe pain after the initial injury, or if minimal healing is evident one to three weeks after the initial injury (Bertelli, 1995; Clamon, 2001; Dorr, 1994; Scuderi & Onesti, 1994).

(5) Collaborate with the physician regarding the need for a radiographic flow study to determine the cause of extravasation and future plans for IV access and patient management.

8. Documentation of an extravasation episode: Follow documentation guidelines provided in Figure 15 and/or institutional guidelines.

B. Flare reaction: Flare reaction is distinguishable from extravasation by the lack of pain or swelling and the presence of a good blood return (Goodman, 2000).

1. Flush the vein slowly with saline and watch for resolution of flare.
2. If resolution does not occur, get a physician's order to administer hydrocortisone. For adults, the dose is 25–50 mg IV followed by a saline flush.
3. Once the flare reaction has resolved, slowly resume infusion of the drug (Goodman, 2000).
4. If the drug is to be readministered at a later date, consider premedication with antihistamines and/or corticosteroids. Slowing infusion rates may be helpful (Goodman, 2000; Labovich, 1999).
5. Document the episode, including all treatment and the patient's responses, according to institutional policy.

C. Hypersensitivity and anaphylaxis

1. Pathophysiology: Hypersensitivity and anaphylaxis related to chemotherapy agents are mediated by the immune system—usually by IgE. These reactions may be triggered by the therapeutic agent, the diluent, or the delivery vehicle (solution) (Labovich, 1999; Weiss, 2001). The response may range from itching at the injection site to systemic shock (Shepherd, 2003). The response usually occurs within 5 to 30 minutes of the initiation of chemotherapy (Labovich, 1999).
2. Risk factors for hypersensitivity and anaphylaxis (Labovich, 1999; Langhorne & Barton-Burke, 2001)
   a) A chemotherapy agent known to cause hypersensitivity reactions (see Figure 16)
   b) A history of allergies, particularly a drug allergy
   c) Previous exposure to the agent
   d) Failure to administer known effective prophylactic premedications
3. Preadministration guidelines: Implement the following steps to prevent and manage hypersensitivity reactions (Langhorne & Barton-Burke, 2001; Weiss, 2001).
   a) Obtain and record baseline vital signs.
   b) Review the patient's allergy history.
   c) Administer premedications as ordered. Common premedications include an H_1 blocker (diphenhydramine), H_2 blocker (such as cimetidine), and dexamethasone IV.
   d) Ensure that emergency equipment and medications are readily available. This is especially important if chemotherapy is administered in the patient's home or other non–acute care setting.
   e) Obtain physician's orders for emergency drug procedures before drug administration. Written standing orders for management of hypersensitivity reactions are recommended (Myers & Kearney, 2000; Timoney, Eagan, & Sklarin, 2003).

Figure 15. Chemotherapy Drug Extravasation Record

Patient ______________________________ Date infiltration occured ____________

Drug ______________________ Dilution mg/mL __________ vesicant ______ irritant ________

Amount of drug infiltrated: < 1 mL ______ 1–3 mL ______ 3–5 mL ______ 5 mL ______ > 10 mL ______

Method of drug administration:

______ Two-syringe technique IV push

______ Side-arm with IV freely running

______ Continuous infusion: rate _____ ml/hour
peristaltic pump _____ yes _____ no

______ VAD: _____ port _____ tunneled catheter
type of needle _____

______ Other ________________

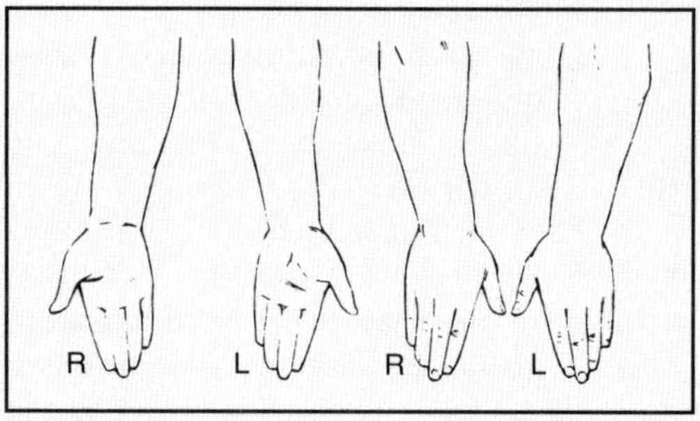

R L R L

right arm

left arm
(attach photograph)

Description of site:
Size ________ Color ________ Texture ________
(Indicate location on diagram)

Process Documentation: Describe the events that occured during the drug administration

S: (Patient's Symptoms) ____

O: (Clinical Symptoms) ____

A: (Assessment) ____________________ suspected extravasation ______ definite extravasation ______

P: (Plan of care) Initial actions: ____

Physicians notified: ________ Instructions ________________________________

Follow-up Instructions: ____

Additional Comments: ____

Consultations: __________ Plastic Surgery __________ Physical Therapy __________ Other __________

Date of referral: __________ Follow-up ________________________________

Return appointment: ________ Written instructions for site care reviewed with patient ______________

(RN Signature ____)

Follow-up visit #1 (date _____) Describe site and care instruction (attach photo) ______________

Follow-up visit #2 (date _____) Describe site and care instruction (attach photo) ______________

Follow-up visit #3 (date _____) Describe site and care instruction (attach photo) ______________

Note. Figure courtesy of Michelle Goodman, RN, MS, Rush College of Nursing, Chicago, IL. Used with permission.

f) Instruct the patient to report hypersensitivity symptoms.

g) Review reports of hypersensitivity before each treatment; hypersensitivity reactions can occur with a patient's repeated exposure to a drug and at any point during the infusion. For example, the incidence of carboplatin hypersensitivity may increase with multiple doses and can occur after 50% of the drug has infused (Rose, Fusco, Smrekar, Mossbruger, & Rodriguez, 2003).

h) Perform a scratch test or intradermal skin test, or administer a test dose before administering the initial dose of the drug to a patient who has a high likelihood of a hypersensitivity reaction. For a patient receiving repeated doses of carboplatin, a skin test is recommended after the seventh dose (Markman et al., 2003).

(1) Observe the patient for any local or systemic reaction for a minimum of 30 minutes. If no sign of hypersensitivity is evident, proceed with the initial dosing.

(2) When administering an IV bolus drug that is associated with hypersensitivity, infuse the drug slowly and continue to observe the patient for signs and symptoms of hypersensitivity.

(a) Any patient who has had a severe anaphylactic reaction with hypotension should not be treated again with that agent unless special circumstances exist (Labovich, 1999; Weiss, 2001).

(b) Avoid administering subsequent doses if a patient is considered sensitized to the drug. If the drug is considered critical to the treatment plan, premedication with antihistamines and/or corticosteroids may prevent a recurrent hypersensitivity reaction (Timoney et al., 2003; Weiss, 2001).

4. Clinical manifestations of hypersensitivity response and anaphylaxis (Labovich, 1999; Langhorne & Barton-Burke, 2001; Shepherd, 2003)

a) Uneasiness or agitation

b) Tightness in the chest

c) Shortness of breath, with or without wheezing

d) Hypotension

e) Urticaria (hives) or rash

f) Localized or generalized itching

g) Periorbital or facial edema

h) Lightheadedness or dizziness

i) Abdominal cramping, diarrhea, nausea, vomiting (less common)

5. Emergency management of anaphylaxis: The need for emergency management usually arises within 30 minutes of initial administration or an increase in the infusion rate (Carr & Burke, 2001; Labovich, 1999; Timoney et al., 2003). Immediate action is imperative.

a) Stop chemotherapy infusion immediately.

b) Maintain an IV line with NS or another appropriate solution.

c) Stay with the patient. Have another staff member notify the physician and emergency team or, if outside a hospital setting, call the local emergency medical service.

d) Place the patient in a supine position if possible.

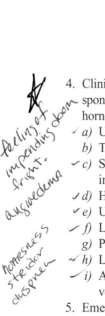

Figure 16. Immediate Hypersensitivity Reactions: Predicted Risk of Chemotherapy

High Risk
- Asparaginase[a, b]
- Docetaxel
- Murine monoclonal antibodies (e.g., rituximab)[c]
- Paclitaxel

Low to Moderate Risk
- Anthracyclines[d]
- Bleomycin[e]
- Carboplatin[f]
- Chimeric and human monoclonal antibodies
- Cisplatin
- Etoposide
- Melphalan[a]
- Methotrexate
- Procarbazine
- Teniposide

Rare Risk
- Cytarabine
- Cyclophosphamide
- Chlorambucil
- Dacarbazine
- 5-fluorouracil
- Ifosfamide
- Interferons
- Interleukins
- Mitoxantrone

[a] Risk is significantly increased with IV route.
[b] There is no reliable way to test for hypersensitivity. Treat each dose of asparaginase as one that could cause a serious reaction (Weiss, 2001).
[c] Reactions are related to cytokine release by malignant lymphocytes. May be minimized by fractionating the dose over several days.
[d] Liposomal versions of these agents may still cause hypersensitivity reactions (Shepherd, 2003; Weiss, 2001).
[e] Occasional and severe reactions to bleomycin have been reported in patients with lymphoma.
[f] Repeated exposure significantly increases chances of reaction. A skin test is recommended after the seventh dose (Markman et al., 2003).

e) Monitor vital signs every 2 minutes until the patient is stable, then every 5 minutes for 30 minutes, then every 15 minutes.
f) Maintain airway, assessing the patient for increasing edema of the respiratory tract. Administer oxygen if needed. Anticipate the need for cardiopulmonary resuscitation (CPR).
g) Administer emergency medications (see Table 15).
h) Provide emotional support to the patient and family.
i) Document all treatments and the patient's response in the medical record.
j) Symptoms of anaphylaxis may recur hours after initial intervention; therefore, patients who have experienced a severe reaction should be hospitalized and monitored closely for 24 hours (Labovich, 1999).

6. Clinical management of localized hypersensitivity (Langhorne & Barton-Burke, 2001)
a) Observe and evaluate symptoms (e.g., urticaria).
b) Administer diphenhydramine, cimetidine, and/or corticosteroids per physician's order or according to protocol.
c) Monitor vital signs at least every 15 minutes for 1 hour or as the patient's condition requires.
d) Document the episode, including all treatments and the patient's response, according to institutional policies.

D. Patient and family education
1. Before cytotoxic therapy, inform the patient and family that extravasation has the potential for immediate complications and instruct them to immediately report signs and symptoms of extravasation, flare, or hypersensitivity reactions.
2. Document all patient teaching. Schulmeister and Camp-Sorrell (2000) stated that "plaintiffs in extravasation lawsuits typically deny being

Table 15. Emergency Drugs and Equipment for Use in Case of Hypersensitivity or Anaphylactic Reaction[a]

Drug	Strength	Usage
Epinephrine	0.1 mg–0.5 mg IV push every 10 minutes as needed Pediatrics: 0.01 mg/kg IV or SQ or 0.1 mg–0.3 mg every 10–15 minutes	Administer by inhalation, SQ, IM, or IV in anaphylaxis or allergic reaction. SQ administration is preferred over IV to minimize adverse cardiac effects (Labovich, 1999).
Antihistamines		
• Diphenhydramine hydrochloride	Adults: 25–50 mg IV Pediatrics: 1 mg/kg (maximum 50 mg)	Administer IV to block further antigen-antibody reaction.
• H_2 blockers		To counteract the multiple effects of histamine release, both H_1 and H_2 blockers should be administered.
- Cimetidine	Adults: 300 mg IV Not used for pediatric patients	
- Ranitidine	Adults: 50 mg IV Not used for pediatric patients	
- Famotidine	Adults: 20 mg IV Not used for pediatric patients	
Aminophylline	Adults: 5 mg/kg Not used for pediatric patients	Administer IV over 30 minutes to enhance bronchodilation.
Dopamine	Adults: 2–20 mcg/kg/minute Not used for pediatric patients	Administer IV to increase cardiac output and blood pressure.
Steroids		All steroids help to prevent a prolonged event or recurrence of symptoms by slowing or halting the inflammatory process (Albanell & Baselga, 2000; Carr & Burke, 2001).
• Methylprednisolone	Adults: 30–50 mg IV Pediatrics: 0.3–0.5 mg/kg	
• Hydrocortisone injection	Adults: 100–500 mg IV Pediatrics: 1–2 mg/kg	Steroids block late allergic symptoms. May repeat in six hours (Albanell & Baselga).
• Dexamethasone	Adults: 10–20 mg IV Pediatrics: 1–2 mg/kg	Administer IV to ease bronchoconstriction and cardiac dysfunction.

[a] Additional emergency medications (e.g., sodium bicarbonate, furosemide, lidocaine, naloxone hydrochloride, sublingual nitroglycerine) and emergency supplies (e.g., oxygen, suction machine with catheters, Ambu® bag [Ambu Inc., Linthicum, MD]) should be available in case of medical emergency.

informed of the risk of extravasation or state that they were led to believe that the risk was minuscule" (p. 532).

3. After therapy, instruct the patient and family about the importance of immediately reporting symptoms of any delayed reaction.

References

Ajani, J.A., Dodd, L.G., Daugherty, K., Warkentin, D., & Ilson, D.H. (1994). Taxol-induced soft-tissue injury secondary to extravasation: Characterization by histopathology and clinical course. *Journal of the National Cancer Institute, 86,* 51–53.

Albanell, J., & Baselga, J. (2000). Systemic therapy emergencies. *Seminars in Oncology, 27,* 347–361.

Alberts, D.S., & Dorr, R.T. (1991). Case report: Topical DMSO for mitomycin-C-induced skin ulceration. *Oncology Nursing Forum, 18,* 693–695.

Ascherman, J.A., Knowles, S.L., & Atkiss, K. (2000). Docetaxel (Taxotere) extravasation: A report of five cases with treatment recommendations. *Annals of Plastic Surgery, 45,* 438–441.

Bellone, J.D. (1981). Treatment of vincristine extravasation [Letter to the editor]. *JAMA, 245,* 343.

Bertelli, G. (1995). Prevention and management of extravasation of cytotoxic drugs. *Drug Safety, 12,* 245–255.

Bertelli, G., Gozzo, A., Forno, G.B., Vidili, M.G., Silvestro, S., Venturini, M., et al. (1995). Topical dimethylsulfoxide for the prevention of soft tissue injury after extravasation of vesicant cytotoxic drugs: A prospective clinical study. *Journal of Clinical Oncology, 13,* 2851–2855.

Camp-Sorrell, D. (1998). Developing extravasation protocols and monitoring outcomes. *Journal of Intravenous Nursing, 21,* 232–239.

Carr, B., & Burke, C. (2001). Outpatient chemotherapy: Hypersensitivity and anaphylaxis—Oncology nurses must know how to respond quickly and correctly. *American Journal of Nursing, 101*(Suppl.), 27–30.

Clamon, G.H. (2001). Extravasation. In M.C. Perry (Ed.), *The chemotherapy source book* (3rd ed., pp. 432–436). Philadelphia: Lippincott Williams & Wilkins.

Dorr, R.T. (1990). Antidotes to vesicant chemotherapy extravasations. *Blood Reviews, 4*(1), 41–60.

Dorr, R.T. (1994). Pharmacologic management of vesicant chemotherapy extravasations. In R.T. Dorr & D.D. Von Hoff (Eds.), *Cancer chemotherapy handbook* (2nd ed., pp. 109–118). Norwalk, CT: Appleton & Lange.

Dorr, R.T., Snead, K., & Liddil, J.D. (1996). Skin ulceration potential of paclitaxel in a mouse skin model in vivo. *Cancer, 78,* 152–156.

Ener, R.A., Meglathery, S.B., & Styler, M. (2004). Extravasation of systemic hemato-oncological therapies. *Annals of Oncology, 15,* 858–862.

Goodman, M. (2000). Chemotherapy: Principles of administration. In C.H. Yarbro, M.H. Frogge, M. Goodman, & S.L. Groenwald (Eds.), *Cancer nursing: Principles and practice* (5th ed., pp. 385–443). Sudbury, MA: Jones and Bartlett.

Harwood, K.V., & Bachur, N. (1987). Evaluation of dimethyl sulfoxide and local cooling as antidotes for doxorubicin extravasation in a pig model. *Oncology Nursing Forum, 14*(1), 39–44.

Harwood, K.V., & Govin, R. (1994). Short-term vs. long-term local cooling after doxorubicin (Dox) extravasation: An Eastern Cooperative Oncology Group (ECOG) study [Abstract]. *Program/Proceedings of the American Society of Clinical Oncology, 13,* 447.

Herrington, J.D., & Figueroa, J.A. (1997). Severe necrosis due to paclitaxel extravasation. *Pharmacology, 17,* 163–165.

Infusion Nurses Society. (2000). Infusion nursing standards of practice. *Journal of Intravenous Nursing, 23*(Suppl. 6), S1–S88.

Kassner, E. (2000). Evaluation and treatment of chemotherapy extravasation injuries. *Journal of Pediatric Oncology Nursing, 17*(3), 135–148.

Kretzschmar, A., Pink, D., Thuss-Patience, P., Dorken, B., Reichart, P., & Eckert R. (2003). Extravasations of oxaliplatin. *Journal of Clinical Oncology, 21,* 4068–4069.

Labovich, T.M. (1999). Acute hypersensitivity reactions to chemotherapy. *Seminars in Oncology Nursing, 15,* 222–231.

Langhorne, M., & Barton-Burke, M. (2001). Chemotherapy administration: General principles for nursing practice. In M. Barton-Burke, G. Wilkes, & K. Ingwersen (Eds.), *Cancer chemotherapy: A nursing process approach* (3rd ed., pp. 608–643). Sudbury, MA: Jones and Bartlett.

Larson, D.K. (1985). What is the appropriate treatment of tissue extravasation by antitumor agents? *Plastic and Reconstructive Surgery, 75,* 397–405.

Laurie, S.W., Wilson, K.L., Kernahan, D.A., Bauer, B.S., & Vistnes, L.M. (1984). Intravenous extravasation injuries: The effectiveness of hyaluronidase in their treatment. *Annals of Plastic Surgery, 13*(3), 191–194.

Markman, M., Zanotti, L., Peterson, G., Kulp, B., Webster, K., & Belinson, J. (2003). Expanded experience with an intradermal skin test to predict for the presence or absence of carboplatin hypersensitivity. *Journal of Clinical Oncology, 21,* 4611–4614.

Mone, A.E., & Summers, M.S. (1998). Immunological disorders. In M.R. Kinney, S.B. Dunbar, J.A. Brooks-Brunn, N. Molter, & J.M. Vitello-Cicciu (Eds.), *AACN's clinical reference for critical care nursing* (4th ed., pp. 947–978). St. Louis, MO: Mosby.

Mosby's medical, nursing and allied health dictionary (6th ed.). (2002). St. Louis, MO: Mosby.

Myers, J.S., & Kearney, K. (2000). Emergency: Chemotherapy-induced hypersensitivity reaction. *American Journal of Nursing, 100*(4), 53–54.

Olver, I.N., Aisner, J., Hament, A., Buchanan, L., Bishop, J.F., & Kaplan, R.S. (1988). A prospective study of topical dimethyl sulfoxide for treating anthracycline extravasation. *Journal of Clinical Oncology, 6,* 1732–1735.

Otto, S.E. (2001). Chemotherapy. In S.E. Otto (Ed.), *Oncology nursing* (4th ed., pp. 638–671). St. Louis, MO: Mosby.

Rose, P.G., Fusco, N., Smrekar, M., Mossbruger, K., & Rodriguez, M. (2003). Successful administration of carboplatin in patients with clinically documented carboplatin hypersensitivity. *Gynecologic Oncology, 89,* 429–433.

Rudolph, R., & Larson, D.L. (1987). Etiology and treatment of chemotherapeutic agent extravasation injuries: A review. *Journal of Clinical Oncology, 5,* 1116–1126.

Schulmeister, L., & Camp-Sorrell, D. (2000). Chemotherapy extravasation from implanted ports. *Oncology Nursing Forum, 27,* 531–538.

Scuderi, N., & Onesti, M.G. (1994). Antitumor agents: Extravasation, management and surgical treatment. *Annals of Plastic Surgery, 32*(1), 39–44.

Sheperd, G.M. (2003). Hypersensitivity reactions to chemotherapeutic drugs. Clinical review in *Allergy and Immunology, 24,* 253–262.

Soble, M.J., Dorr, R.T., Plezia, P., & Breckenridge, S. (1987). Dose-dependent skin ulcers in mice treated with DNA binding antitumor antibiotics. *Cancer Chemotherapy and Pharmacology, 20*(1), 33–36.

St. Germain, B., Houlihan, N., & D'Amato, S. (1994). Dimethyl sulfoxide therapy in the treatment of vesicant extravasation: Two case presentations. *Journal of Intravenous Nursing, 17,* 261–266.

Stanford, B.L., & Hardwicke, F. (2003). A review of clinical experience with paclitaxel extravasations. *Supportive Care in Cancer, 11,* 270–277.

Steele, C.A. (2001). Extravasation. In J.M. Yasko (Ed.), *Nursing management of symptoms associated with chemotherapy* (5th ed., pp. 247–270). West Conshohocken, PA: Meniscus Health Care Communications.

Timoney, J.P., Eagan, M.M., & Sklarin, N.T. (2003). Establishing clinical guidelines for the management of acute hypersensitivity reactions secondary to the administration of chemotherapy/biologic therapy. *Journal of Nursing Care Quality, 18,* 80–86.

Weiss, R.B. (2001). Hypersensitivity reactions. In M.C. Perry (Ed.), *The chemotherapy source book* (3rd ed., pp. 436–452). Philadelphia: Lippincott Williams & Wilkins.

thrombocytopenia - ↓ platelets in bone marrow — tumors - leukemia - aplastic anemia

s/s - petichiae or ecchemosis

blood filled bullae in mouth

- hemorrhage - tachy - SOB LOC,

- electric razor — avoid invasive procedures

soft toothbrush — avoid straining or cough - ↑ICP

VII. Care of the Patient Receiving Cancer Therapy

A. Patient education

1. Patient education, as defined by Bartlett (1985), is "a planned learning experience using a combination of methods such as teaching, counseling, and behavioral modification techniques, which influence patients' knowledge and health behavior" (pp. 323–324).
2. Patient teaching is dependent not only on special expertise in terms of the information to be given but also on understanding the different ways in which individuals learn, the variety of strategies for patient teaching that are available, and how to match appropriate strategies to specific content and specific learners (Blecher, 2004).
3. Outcomes of patient education (Blecher, 2004)
   a) Empower the patient and family to be active participants in health care.
   b) Explain diagnosis and treatment options.
   c) Define signs and symptoms that need to be reported.
   d) Demonstrate the ability to perform self-care and/or adapt to potential limitations.
   e) Promote the ability to cope with the reality of a life-threatening condition.
   f) Make autonomous decisions regarding treatment, including the option to accept no further treatment.
   g) Identify available resources within the community.
4. Barriers to patient education: Barriers to learning should be assessed on an individual basis. Methods of patient teaching should be selected based on patient's preference (e.g., auditory, visual, demonstration). Following are some common barriers to comprehension (JCAHO, 2004).
   a) Lack of knowledge of diagnosis and treatment plan
   b) Expectations regarding treatment
   c) Experience: Patients may have concerns or misconceptions about therapy because of their own prior experience or the experience of a friend or relative. These misconceptions may even prevent the patient from undergoing treatment. Patients should be allowed to express concerns. It is important to correct any misconceptions patients may have concerning treatment, as well as follow-up care.
   d) Language barriers: Access to a translator, either in person or through telecommunications methods, should be available. Family members are not recommended as translators because of role conflicts or their inability to communicate complex medical terminology (Lipson, 1996).
   e) Educational barriers: Teaching should be tailored to the patient's level of understanding. Each patient should be assessed individually, and information should be taught at the patient-appropriate level. Cancer-related literature suitable for patients with low literacy is available through NCI (www.cancer.gov).
   f) Physical barriers: Visual, hearing, and cognitive impairments, as well as the inability to speak, can interfere with patients' comprehension of teaching.

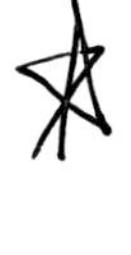

B. Toxicity management

1. General principles of toxicity management
   a) All cancer therapies can cause side effects.
   b) Combined modality therapy has the potential for more side effects than single modality treatment.
   c) Side effects may be exacerbated if the patient
      (1) Has impaired renal or hepatic function
      (2) Has comorbid conditions
      (3) Has protein-calorie malnutrition
      (4) Is younger than one year old or is elderly.
      (5) Has tissues with high growth fractions, which are most affected by cytotoxic therapy. These cells include
         (a) Bone marrow
         (b) Mucosal cells of the GI tract
         (c) Hair follicles and skin
         (d) Organs of the reproductive system.
2. Grading toxicities
   a) The purpose of grading toxicities is to provide an objective assessment.

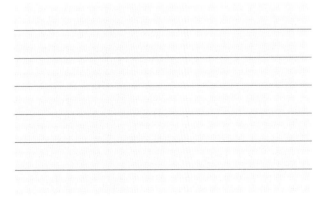

b) Accurate grading of toxicities allows for evaluation of interventions implemented to treat said toxicities.

c) The grade of toxicity is frequently the reason for dosage adjustments or delays.

d) Most toxicity scales range from 0 to 5, with 0 meaning no toxicity and 5 indicating severe or life-threatening toxicity. See Figure 17 for an example of the NCI grading scale for GI symptoms. This scale and others can be accessed via the World Wide Web.

(1) NCI: http://ctep.cancer.gov/forms/CTCAEv3.pdf

(2) WHO Grading of Acute and Subacute Toxicities: http://whqlibdoc.who.int/offset/WHO_OFFSET_48.pdf

Figure 17. National Cancer Institute Common Terminology Criteria for Adverse Events: Selected Gastrointestinal Symptoms

		Grade				
Adverse Event	**Short Name**	**1**	**2**	**3**	**4**	**5**
Diarrhea	Diarrhea	Increase of < 4 stools per day over baseline; mild increase in ostomy output compared to baseline	Increase of 4–6 stools per day over baseline; IV fluids indicated < 24 hrs; moderate increase in ostomy output compared to baseline; not interfering with ADL	Increase of ≥ 7 stools per day over baseline; incontinence; IV fluids ≥ 24 hrs; hospitalization; severe increase in ostomy output compared to baseline; interfering with ADL	Life-threatening consequences (e.g., hemodynamic collapse)	Death
Remark: Diarrhea includes diarrhea of small bowel or colonic origin and/or ostomy diarrhea. Also consider: Dehydration; Hypertension						

		Grade				
Adverse Event	**Short Name**	**1**	**2**	**3**	**4**	**5**
Mucositis/stomatitis (clinical exam) – *Select*: – Anus – Esophagus – Large bowel – Larynx – Oral cavity – Pharynx – Rectum – Small bowel – Stomach – Trachea	Mucositis (clinical exam) – *Select*	Erythema of the mucosa	Patchy ulcerations or pseudomembranes	Confluent ulcerations or pseudomembranes; bleeding with minor trauma	Tissue necrosis; significant spontaneous bleeding; life-threatening consequences	Death
Remark: Mucositis/stomatitis (functional/symptomatic) may be used for mucositis of the upper aero-digestive tract caused by radiation, agents, or GVHD.						

(Continued on next page)

Figure 17. National Cancer Institute Common Terminology Criteria for Adverse Events: Selected Gastrointestinal Symptoms *(Continued)*

		Grade				
Adverse Event	**Short Name**	**1**	**2**	**3**	**4**	**5**
Mucositis/stomatitis (functional/symptomatic) – *Select*: – Anus – Esophagus – Large bowel – Larynx – Rectum – Small Bowel – Stomach – Trachea	Mucositis (functional/symptomatic) – *Select*	Upper aerodigestive tract sites: Minimal symptoms, normal diet; minimal respiratory symptoms but not interfering with function Lower GI sites: Minimal discomfort, intervention not indicated	Upper aerodigestive tract sites: Symptomatic but can eat and swallow modified diet; respiratory symptoms interfering with function but not interfering with ADL Lower GI sites: Symptomatic, medical intervention indicated but not interfering with ADL	Upper aerodigestive tract sites: Symptomatic and unable to adequately aliment or hydrate orally; respiratory symptoms interfering with ADL Lower GI sites: Stool incontinence or other symptoms interfering with ADL	Symptoms associated with life-threatening consequences	Death

		Grade				
Adverse Event	**Short Name**	**1**	**2**	**3**	**4**	**5**
Nausea	Nausea	Loss of appetite without alteration in eating habits	Oral intake decreased without significant weight loss, dehydration or malnutrition; IV fluids indicated < 24 hrs	Inadequate oral caloric or fluid intake; IV fluids, tube feedings, or TPN indicated ≥ 24 hrs	Symptoms associated with life-threatening consequences	Death

		Grade				
Adverse Event	**Short Name**	**1**	**2**	**3**	**4**	**5**
Vomiting	Vomiting	1 episode in 24 hrs	2–5 episodes in 24 hrs; IV fluids indicated < 24 hrs	≥ 6 episodes in 24 hrs; IV fluids, or TPN indicated ≥ 24 hrs	Life-threatening consequences	Death

Note. From *Common Terminology Criteria for Adverse Events* (Version 3.0), by the National Cancer Institute, 2003. Retrieved October 14, 2004, from http://ctep.cancer.gov

(3) Eastern Cooperative Oncology Group (ECOG) Common Toxicity Criteria: http://www.ecog.org/general/common_tox.html

References

Bartlett, E.E. (1985). At last, a definition. *Patient Education Council, 7,* 323–324.

Blecher, C.S. (Ed.). (2004). *Standards of oncology education: Patient/significant other and public* (3rd ed.). Pittsburgh, PA: Oncology Nursing Society.

Joint Commission on Accreditation of Healthcare Organizations. (2004). *Comprehensive accreditation manual for hospitals: The official handbook.* Oakbrook Terrace, IL: Author.

Lipson, J.G. (1996). Culturally competent nursing care. In J.G. Lipson, S. Dibble, & P.A. Minarik (Eds.), *Culture and nursing care: A pocket guide* (pp. 1–6). San Francisco: University of California San Francisco Nursing Press.

RBC count normal M 4.5-5.5 F 4-5

HGB M 12.4-14.9 F 11.7-13.8

HCT normal M 42-52 F 36-48

leukocytosis ↑WBC
leucopenia ↓WBC

$$ANC = WBC \times \left(\frac{Polys + Bands}{100}\right)$$

WBC differential - evaluate distribution + morphology of WBC provides specific info about immune system

neutrophils - 54-75%
eosinophils 1-4%
basophils 0-1%
lymphocytes 25-40%
monocytes 2-8%

components of WBC - polys, bands, basos, Blasts
neutrophils are polys or segs or bands
calculate absolute neutrophyl count ANC
- Convert WBC to total # ex 2.5 x 1000 = 2500
- calculate % of neutrophils - add polys + bands
- multiply WBC by % of neutrophils

BUN - screen for renal damage
☆ creatnine clearance - nonprotein end product of creatnine metabolism / assess glomerular filtration
norm - 0.8-1.2 - hold therapy if 1.5 or greater
uric acid - end metabolite of purine - rapid destruction of neucleic acids -
norm 2.3-6 (3.4-7) impaired renal excretion -

neutropenia - deficiency in # of mature neutrophils - comprimized immune status
<500 severe neutropenia
common infections aerobic gram ⊖ bacilli / RISK for infection
staph aureus
fungal infections - candidasis
aspirgillus

VIII. Side Effects of Cancer Therapy

A. Myelosuppression: Refers to the suppression of bone marrow activity. The results can be a decrease in the number of platelets, red cells, and white cells in the blood. Myelosuppression is the most common dose-limiting toxicity of chemotherapy. It also can be the most lethal (Camp-Sorrell, 2000). Terms used in this discussion include the following.

- *Neutropenia:* The condition in which circulating blood contains an abnormally low number of neutrophils (white blood cells, or WBCs)—in other words, the ANC is $\leq$ 1,000/mm^3. An ANC of < 500/mm^3 defines profound neutropenia (Camp-Sorrell, 2000).
- *Anemia:* The condition in which circulating blood contains an abnormally low number of red blood cells (RBCs) per cubic millimeter, an abnormally small amount of hemoglobin (Hgb) in 100 ml blood, or a volume of RBCs per 100 ml of blood that is less than normal (Camp-Sorrell, 2000).
- *Thrombocytopenia:* The condition in which the number of platelets in circulating blood is abnormally low.
- *Cytopenia:* The lack of cellular elements in circulating blood.
- *Nadir:* After chemotherapy, the point at which the lowest blood cell count is reached. The nadir usually occurs 7–10 days after treatment; the time depends on the chemotherapeutic agent used. Platelet and WBC counts usually are the first to drop (Camp-Sorrell, 2000).
- *Hematopoiesis:* The formation and development of blood cells, a process that involves proliferation, differentiation, and maturation (see Figure 18). In adults, most hematopoiesis occurs in bone marrow, in myeloid tissue.
  - The process begins with a pluripotent stem cell, the most primitive type of blood cell and the source of all hematopoietic cells. A pluripotent stem cell is capable of proliferation, differentiation, and maturation. The forms the cell takes depend on endogenously generated chemical growth factors. Each factor may promote the development of single or multiple cell lines. The process of differentiation involves an intricate and delicate feedback mechanism. The feedback mechanism is affected by stress, infection, hemorrhage, bone marrow depletion, and drug therapy (Amgen Inc., 1999).
  - Life spans of various blood components: The frequency of neutropenia, anemia, and thrombocytopenia is associated with the type of chemotherapy administered. The length and kinetics of the life cycle of each type of blood cell determine when replacement cells will be available (Amgen Inc., 1999). Life spans of blood cells vary greatly (see Table 16). Maturation time will vary depending on the cell line.

1. Neutropenia: Chemotherapy-induced neutropenia (CIN) is the primary dose-limiting toxicity of many chemotherapy agents (Dale, 2003). It has significant negative clinical consequences for patients with cancer, including life-threatening infections, prolonged hospital stays, dose reductions, and dose delays (Crawford, 2004).
   a) Normal physiology of neutrophils (see Figure 18)
      (1) Neutrophils and monocytes stem from the colony-forming unit–granulocyte macrophage (CFU-GM) progenitor cell.
      (2) The earliest identifiable cell of the neutrophil lineage is the myeloblast. Differentiation from myeloblast to segmented neutrophil takes 7–14 days. Normal bone marrow can produce 60–400 x 10^7 neutrophils each day.
   b) Locations of neutrophils (Amgen Inc., 1999)
      (1) A large number of both mature and immature neutrophils, approximately 8.8 x 10^9, are located in the bone marrow of a healthy adult.
      (2) In the bloodstream are 0.8 x 10^9 mature and immature neutrophils. These cells are the body's first line of defense against invading bacteria. Circulating neutrophils have a half-life of six to nine hours.
      (3) Adhering to the walls of blood vessels and stored in tissue are marginated neutrophils, which serve as reserve cells. Neutrophils stored in extravascular tissue can survive for up to two days (Amgen Inc., 1999).
   c) Pathophysiology (Erickson, 2000)

Figure 18. Schema of Hematopoiesis

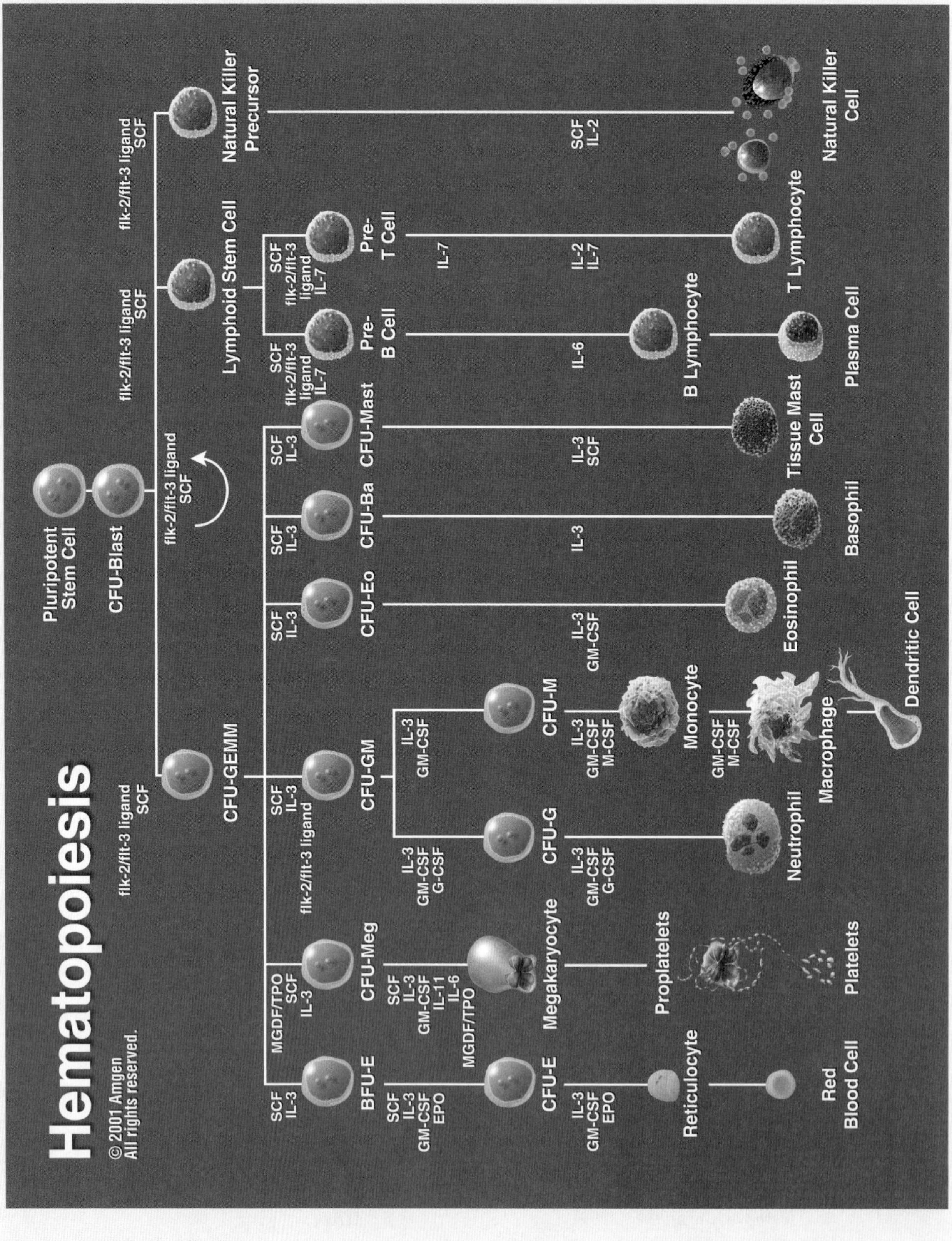

Note. Figure courtesy of Amgen Inc. Used with permission.

(1) The bone marrow must constantly produce neutrophils because the life span of a neutrophil is very short. Chemotherapeutic agents suppress bone marrow activity and damage stem cells; therefore, chemotherapy decreases the neutrophil count as mature neutrophils die and are not replaced.

(2) The WBC nadir depends on the specific drugs and dosages used. A prolonged nadir may occur if the stem cell population fails to repopulate quickly following high-dose chemotherapy (Camp-Sorrell, 2000). The nadir may occur as early as one to two days after treatment if the patient's bone marrow has been damaged as a result of previous chemotherapy or radiation treatments (Schafer, 1998).

(a) Cell-cycle specific agents (e.g., antimetabolites) produce rapid nadirs in 7–14 days, with neutrophil recovery within 7–21 days (Barton-Burke, Wilkes, & Ingwersen, 2001; Scott, 2004).

(b) Cell-cycle nonspecific agents (e.g., antibiotics) cause neutropenia in 10–14 days, with recovery at 21–24 days (Barton-Burke et al., 2001).

(c) Some cell-cycle nonspecific agents (e.g., nitrosoureas) produce a delayed and prolonged neutropenia.

i) For adults, nadir occurs at 26–63 days, with recovery at 35–89 days (Barton-Burke et al., 2001).

ii) For children, nadir occurs at 21–35 days, with recovery at 42–50 days (Scott, 2004).

(d) Agents such as docetaxel can result in an early, short-lasting type of neutropenia at a dose of ≥ 100 mg/m^2 when infused over one hour every three weeks (Camp-Sorrell, 2000).

d) Incidence: The incidence of neutropenia varies according to agents, doses, and administration schedule (Sullivan, 2004).

e) Risk factors for neutropenia

(1) Preexisting neutropenia resulting from disease (Ozer et al., 2000)

(2) Treatment with a highly myelosuppressive chemotherapy regimen

(3) Tumor involvement in the bone marrow (Intragumatornchai, Sutheesophon, Sutcharitchan, & Swasdikul, 2000)

(4) Degeneration of the immune system, resulting in a physiologically elderly patient (Lyman, Balducci, & Agboola, 2001)

(5) Low neutrophil count at the beginning of a chemotherapy cycle

(6) History of neutropenia (current or previous regimens) (Silber et al., 1998; Thomas et al., 2001)

(7) Hepatic or renal dysfunction, which may lead to decreased metabolism and excretion of chemotherapeutic agent (Intragumatornchai et al., 2000)

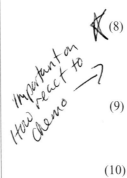

(8) Protein-calorie malnutrition, which decreases the body's ability to manufacture and repair the normal cells destroyed by chemotherapy (Intragumatornchai et al., 2000)

(9) Concurrent use of two or more of the following drugs or types of drugs: antibiotics, antifungals, sulfas, allopurinol, and corticosteroids

(10) Concurrent chemotherapy and radiation therapy to areas with large amounts of bone marrow, especially total body radiation (Silber et al., 1998)

f) Clinical manifestations of infection in patients with neutropenia (Wujcik, 2004)

(1) A fever of ≥ 38°C (100.4°F) is the most reliable, and often the only, sign of infection in patients with neutropenia. Normally, WBCs cause the classic signs of infection (e.g., redness, edema,

Table 16. Life Spans of Blood Components

Blood Component	Typical Life Span
Red blood cell	90–120 days
Platelet	7–8 days
Neutrophil	7–12 hours
Monocyte	3 days
Macrophage	3 days
Eosinophil	3–8 hours
Basophil	7–12 hours
Tissue mast cell	7–12 hours
B lymphocyte	Depends on type and subtype
T lymphocyte	Depends on type and subtype
Natural killer cell	Unknown

pus). Extremely neutropenic patients, however, may not be able to manifest the usual signs—not even a fever.

(2) Common sites of infection and corresponding signs and symptoms of infection in neutropenic patients are the following (Wujcik, 2004).

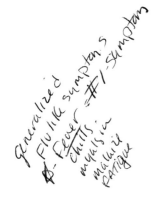

(a) GI tract: Mucositis at any level of the digestive tract or diarrhea

(b) Respiratory tract: Fever, cough, dyspnea on exertion, and adventitious breath sounds

(c) Urinary tract: Fever, dysuria, frequency, hematuria, and cloudy urine

(d) Indwelling devices (e.g., VADs, catheters, ventricular peritoneal [VP] shunts): Fever, erythema, pain or tenderness, edema, drainage, and induration at site

(e) Skin and mucous membranes: Erythema, tenderness, hot skin, and edema (especially in axilla, buttocks, mouth, or perineal or rectal area)

(3) Septic shock associated with neutropenia has a high mortality rate.

g) Assessment: Use laboratory data to assess the presence of neutropenia by calculating ANC. Note that neutropenia can occur when the total WBC count is within a normal range (4,000–10,000/mm^3). Consequently, qualitating the ANC is essential to achieving a correct assessment of neutrophil status (Camp-Sorrell, 2000). To calculate ANC,

(1) Obtain complete WBC count, including differential.

(2) Add neutrophils (polys [segs] and bands).

(3) Convert sum from (2) to percentage.

(4) Multiply total WBC count by total neutrophil percentage (polys + bands). ANC calculation example: WBC count = 1,600, polys = 48, bands = 5.

(a) Add polys and bands: 48 + 5 = 53.

(b) Convert sum to percentage: 53 ÷ 100 = 0.53 = 53%.

(c) Multiply WBC count by percentage to find ANC: 1,600 x 0.53 = 848.

h) Collaborative management

(1) Prevention

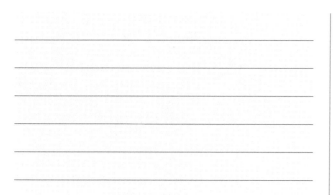

(a) Handwashing is the single most important intervention to prevent infection (Mank & van der Lelie, 2003). Protective isolation has been found to have no effect on the host's endogenous flora and no impact on organisms transmitted by water or food.

(b) Dietary precautions regarding the omission of fresh fruits and vegetables remain unsupported (Wilson, 2002). Recommended restrictions for CIN in adult patients with solid tumors include washing fresh fruits and vegetables with tap water and eliminating raw/unwashed meat, eggs, and fish from the diet.

(c) Treatment with colony-stimulating factors (CSFs): The development of CSFs has had an enormous impact on the incidence of infection related to chemotherapy.

i) Filgrastim (granulocyte-CSF [G-CSF]) and pegfilgrastim are FDA-approved for the prevention of chemotherapy-induced neutropenia.

ii) Sargramostim (granulocyte macrophage–CSF [GM-CSF]) is FDA-approved only for acceleration of bone marrow recovery (recovery of myeloid cells) after autologous or allogeneic BMT.

iii) Both G-CSF and GM-CSF are indicated for use following induction chemotherapy in AML, for mobilization of peripheral blood progenitor cells (PBPCs), following transplantation of autologous PBPCs, and in BMT failure or engraftment delay (Wilkes, Ingwersen, & Barton-Burke, 2003).

iv) The manufacturer recommends initiation of G-CSF no earlier than 24 hours following chemotherapy and continuing daily until the post-nadir ANC > 10,000/mm³ is achieved (Amgen Inc., 2002).

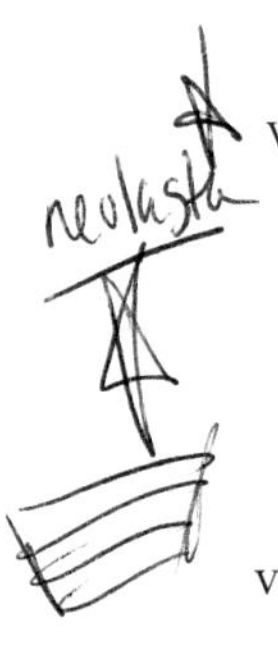

v) Pegfilgrastim is administered as a single 6 mg injection once per chemotherapy cycle and should not be administered in the period between 14 days before and 24 hours after chemotherapy (Amgen Inc., 2004).

vi) Insurance coverage for treatment with all CSFs varies widely.

(d) Prevent trauma to the patient's skin and mucous membranes (Erickson, 2000).

i) Avoid the use of catheters, enemas, nasogastric (NG) tubes, rectal suppositories, and rectal thermometers.

ii) Prevent pressure sores and constipation.

iii) Cleanse and protect wounds as directed.

iv) Use only an electric razor to shave the patient.

v) Consider risk-benefit ratio for invasive procedures (e.g., thoracentesis, paracentesis, percutaneous endoscopic gastrostomy (PEG) tube placement, VAD placement).

(e) Teach neutropenic patients protective measures that they can employ (Camp-Sorrell, 2000).

i) Wash hands frequently with an antimicrobial.

ii) Bathe daily.

iii) Protect skin from cuts and burns.

iv) Wear gloves when working in the garden.

v) Care for the mouth before and after meals or three to four times daily.

vi) Care for the perineal area after voiding and bowel movements.

vii) Use only an electric razor to shave unwanted body hair.

viii) Use a water-soluble lubricant during sexual intercourse, and practice effective postcoital hygiene.

ix) Exercise daily (e.g., walking, running) as tolerated.

x) Do coughing and deep-breathing exercises (e.g., exercises that use an incentive spirometer) to decrease pulmonary stasis, thereby decreasing the potential for respiratory infection.

xi) Avoid exposure to people with colds or contagious illnesses (e.g., chicken pox, herpes zoster, influenza).

xii) Avoid contact with people who were vaccinated with a live vaccine within the past 30 days (CDC, 1993).

xiii) Do not share food utensils.

xiv) Do not provide direct care for pets.

xv) Avoid animal excreta; assign litter box and birdcage cleaning to someone else.

xvi) Do not use tampons, enemas, or rectal suppositories.

xvii) Do not receive live vaccinations (e.g., oral vaccination for polio, varicella, smallpox; nasal flu vaccine).

(2) Management of neutropenic fever: Data regarding the efficacy of CSFs after a patient is diagnosed with febrile neutropenia are inconclusive (Camp-Sorrell, 2000). To manage neutropenic fever, the clinician should (Hughes et al., 1997)

(a) Culture urine, all lumens of CVCs, peripheral blood, and other suspected sources of infection. When dealing with pediatric patients, a peripheral blood culture is indicated only if the patient does not have a CVC.

(b) Perform a physical assessment in an attempt to identify the source of infection.

(c) For all adults, obtain a chest x-ray. For children, obtain a chest x-ray only if the patient's condition warrants.
(d) Administer empiric antibiotics, which should include coverage for gram-positive and gram-negative organisms as ordered until organism source is identified.
(e) Monitor blood culture reports daily.
(3) Patient and family education
(a) Teach patients and significant others to report the following.
i) Temperature elevation ≥ 38°C (100.4°F)
ii) Shaking chills (rigors)
iii) Dysuria
iv) Dyspnea
v) Respiratory congestion or sputum production
vi) Pain
(b) Reinforce the need for meticulous hygiene.
(c) Teach patients and significant others SQ injection technique for G-CSF or GM-CSF administration if applicable.

References

Amgen Inc. (1999). *Neutropenia in malignant diseases: An independent study program for pharmacists and nurses.* Thousand Oaks, CA: Author.

Amgen Inc. (2002). Neupogen [Package insert]. Thousand Oaks, CA: Author.

Amgen Inc. (2004). Neulasta [Package insert]. Thousand Oaks, CA: Author.

Barton-Burke, M., Wilkes, G.M., & Ingwersen, K.C. (2001). *Cancer chemotherapy: A nursing process approach* (3rd ed.). Sudbury, MA: Jones and Bartlett.

Camp-Sorrell, D. (2000). Chemotherapy: Toxicity management. In C.H. Yarbro, M.H. Frogge, M. Goodman, & S.L. Groenwald (Eds.), *Cancer nursing: Principles and practice* (5th ed., pp. 444–486). Sudbury, MA: Jones and Bartlett.

Centers for Disease Control and Prevention. (1993). *Recommendations of the Advisory Committee on Immunization Practices (ACIP): Use of vaccines and immune globulins in persons with altered immunocompetence.* Retrieved March 10, 2004, from http://www.cdc.gov/mmwr/preview/mmwrhtml/00023141.htm

Crawford, J. (2004). Improving management of chemotherapy-induced neutropenia. *Journal of Supportive Oncology, 2*(Suppl. 2), 36–69.

Dale, D. (2003). Optimizing the management of chemotherapy-induced neutropenia. *Clinical Advances in Hematology and Oncology, 1,* 675–680.

Erickson, J. (2000). Myelosuppression. In B.M. Nevidjon & K. Sowers (Eds.), *A nurse's guide to cancer care* (pp. 384–392). Philadelphia: Lippincott Williams & Wilkins.

Hughes, W.T., Armstrong, D., Bodey, G.P., Brown, A.E., Edwards, J.E., & Feld, R. (1997). 1997 guidelines for the use of antimicrobial agents in neutropenic patients with unexplained fever. Infectious Diseases Society of America. *Clinical Infectious Diseases, 25,* 551–573.

Intragumatornchai, T., Sutheesophon, J., Sutcharitchan, P., & Swasdikul, D. (2000). A predictive model for life-threatening neutropenia and febrile neutropenia after the first course of CHOP chemotherapy in patients with aggressive non-Hodgkin's lymphoma. *Leukemia and Lymphoma, 37,* 351–360.

Lyman, G.H., Balducci, L., & Agboola, Y. (2001). Use of colony-stimulating factors in the elderly cancer patient. *Oncology Spectrums, 2,* 414–421.

Mank, A., & van der Lelie, H. (2003). Is there still an indication for nursing patients with prolonged neutropenia in protective isolation? An evidenced-based nursing and medical study of 4 years experience for nursing patients with neutropenia without isolation. *European Journal of Oncology Nursing, 7*(1), 17–23.

Ozer, H., Armitage, J.O., Bennett, C.L., Crawford, J., Demetri, G.D., & Pizzo, P.A. (2000). 2000 update of recommendations for the use of hematopoietic colony-stimulating factors: Evidence-based, clinical practice guidelines. American Society of Clinical Oncology Growth Factors Expert Panel. *Journal of Clinical Oncology, 18,* 3558–3585.

Schafer, S.L. (1998). Infection due to leukopenia. In J.M. Yasko (Ed.), *Nursing management of symptoms associated with chemotherapy* (pp. 135–161). Bala Cynwyd, PA: Meniscus Health Care Communications.

Scott, T.E. (2004). Neutropenia. In N.E. Kline (Ed.), *Essentials of pediatric oncology nursing: A core curriculum* (2nd ed., pp. 67–69). Glenview, IL: Association of Pediatric Oncology Nurses.

Silber, J.H., Fridman, M., Dipaola, R.S., Erder, M.H., Pauly, M.V., & Fox, K.R. (1998). First cycle blood counts and subsequent neutropenia, dose reduction, or delay in early-stage breast cancer therapy. *Journal of Clinical Oncology, 7,* 2392–2400.

Sullivan, C. (2004). Chemotherapy. In N.E. Kline (Ed.), *Essentials of pediatric oncology nursing: A core curriculum* (2nd ed., pp. 81–96). Glenview, IL: Association of Pediatric Oncology Nurses.

Thomas, E.S., Rivera, E., Erder, M.H., Fridman, M., Frye, D., & Hortobagyi, G.N. (2001). Using first cycle nadir absolute neutrophil count as a risk factor for neutropenic events: A validation study [Abstract]. *Proceedings for the American Society of Clinical Oncology, 20,* 37a.

Wilkes, G.M., Ingwersen, K., & Barton-Burke, M. (2003). *2003 oncology nursing drug handbook.* Sudbury, MA: Jones and Bartlett.

Wilson, B.J. (2002). Dietary recommendations for neutropenic patients. *Seminars in Oncology Nursing, 18,* 44–49.

Wujcik, D. (2004). Infection. In C.H. Yarbro, M.H. Frogge, & M. Goodman (Eds.), *Cancer symptom management* (3rd ed., pp. 252–267). Sudbury, MA: Jones and Bartlett.

2. Anemia
a) Normal production and role of RBCs
(1) RBCs are produced in the bone marrow and then reside in the sternum, ribs, vertebrae, pelvis, and proximal end of the femur and humerus. The Hgb

molecule transports oxygen from the lungs to body tissue(s). Carbon dioxide is then returned from the tissues to the lungs.

(2) Decreased oxygen tension initiates a feedback mechanism by which an increased release of erythropoietin (EPO) from the kidney stimulates production of RBCs (Lynch, 2000).

b) Iron is necessary for the normal production of RBCs. It is carried to the precursor cells by transferrin, where it is then incorporated into a heme molecule and stored as ferritin in various tissues. Daily dietary sources of iron are needed to maintain iron stores (Loney & Chernecky, 2000). The major steps of erythropoiesis follow (see Figure 18).

(1) A pluripotent stem develops into a progenitor cell committed to the development of RBCs.

(2) The stem cell divides and matures to form a reticulocyte.

(3) Hgb synthesis begins at the erythroblast stage. RBCs develop increased amounts of Hgb as they mature in the bone marrow. Approximately 25% of Hgb is synthesized after reticulocytes leave the marrow (Bron, Meuleman, & Mascaux, 2001; Dessypris, 1999).

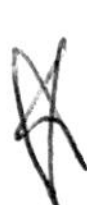

c) The role of EPO in erythropoiesis: EPO is a glycoprotein that acts much like a hormone and is produced or suppressed based on the feedback mechanism in the kidney. More than 90% of EPO is produced in the kidney, with a very small amount produced in the liver. When EPO is secreted into the plasma, erythrocyte precursor cells in the bone marrow are stimulated and RBC production and maturation are accelerated (Loney & Chernecky, 2000). Although erythropoiesis was originally thought to be the sole physiologic function of EPO, it is now known EPO receptors in tissue are not limited to hematopoietic cells. Active EPO receptors also have been identified on endothelial, renal, neuronal, and cardiac cells in vitro (Smith, 2004). This fact helps to explain many of the neuropathic toxicities experienced by patients with anemia. EPO stimulates increased production of RBCs by

(1) Increasing the number of stem cells committed to the red cell line

(2) Shortening the time a stem cell takes to become a mature RBC (Erickson, 1996).

d) RBC mass and volume: EPO production and erythropoiesis usually are orderly and continuous processes that result in a constant circulating RBC mass for each individual, but this volume may vary by more than 10% in people of the same age and gender (Loney & Chernecky, 2000).

e) RBC life span: A typical RBC can survive 90–120 days. This span, longer than that of a neutrophil or platelet, is the primary reason anemia occurs later after chemotherapy than do neutropenia and thrombocytopenia.

f) Pathophysiology

(1) Isolating the cause of anemia to a single factor in the patient with cancer often is difficult. Various mechanisms that interfere with bone marrow functioning, erythropoiesis, RBC destruction, and maintenance of a stable blood volume often are involved (Loney & Chernecky, 2000).

(2) Chemotherapy not only suppresses bone marrow functioning and erythropoiesis, but it also may cause poor dietary intake of iron, RBC lysis, and microangiopathic bleeding (Loney & Chernecky, 2000).

(3) Chemotherapy-induced anemia is associated with bone marrow suppression resulting in decreased RBCs. Cytotoxic chemotherapeutic agents prohibit stem cells from developing into erythrocytes. RBCs have a longer life than WBCs or platelets. As a result, the RBC depression may not be evident for up to six weeks following the treatment (Loney & Chernecky, 2000).

g) Alteration in erythroblast development

(1) DNA cell-cycle specific agents inhibit the overall production of DNA, resulting in the alteration of erythrocyte development.

(2) Cytoplasmic maturation exceeds nuclear maturation (Hoagland, 1992).

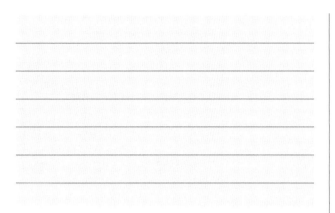

h) Peripheral macrocytosis: An increase in the size of erythrocytes. This results from megaloblastic changes in the bone marrow following chemotherapy, particularly chemotherapy involving methotrexate, which causes folic acid depletion (Hoagland, 1992).

i) Because the kidneys produce more than 90% of EPO, any nephrotoxic agent has the potential to deplete EPO levels. The usual constant level of EPO in circulation is lost, and a greater degree of hypoxia is needed to stimulate the EPO response (Loney & Chernecky, 2000).

j) Increased RBC destruction can occur as a result of the following mechanisms.

(1) Antimetabolites triggering mechanical RBC lysis (e.g., 5-FU, hydroxyurea, methotrexate, gemcitabine, capecitabine)

(2) Enzyme deficiency: People with a hereditary glucose-6-phosphate-dehydrogenase deficiency lack an enzyme needed for antioxidant protection of RBCs. Without the enzyme, exposure to oxidizing agents (e.g., chemotherapy) and viral or bacterial infections can damage RBC, Hgb, and cell membranes (Loney & Chernecky, 2000).

(3) Anemia of chronic disease is an understudied phenomenon that occurs in patients with cancer and is mediated by inflammatory cytokines. These patients will have low serum iron levels, but the iron in their bone marrow will be normal, suggesting a utilization defect versus iron depletion and has been termed "functional iron deficiency" (National Comprehensive Cancer Network [NCCN], 2004).

k) Incidence

(1) The degree of anemia is related to drug, dose, and frequency of treatment regimens. Severe anemia rarely occurs from standard-dose chemotherapy alone.

(2) Macrocytosis is common with long-term hydroxyurea and usually is evidenced by mean corpuscular volumes of > 115 mm^3 (Burns, Reed, & Weng, 1986).

l) Risk factors

(1) Drugs that cause hypoproliferation (i.e., decreased RBC production related to either bone marrow suppression or impaired EPO response) (Loney & Chernecky, 2000)

(a) Platinum drugs or platinum-based regimens (explains the frequency of anemia in patients with ovarian and lung cancer) (Gordon, 2002)

(b) Combination therapy with cyclophosphamide, methotrexate, and 5-FU (a combination known to result in anemia as long as five years after initial treatment)

(c) Biotherapy using an interleukin (IL) or interferon

(d) High-dose methotrexate, ifosfamide, or streptozocin

(2) Tumor infiltration of bone marrow, resulting in decreased RBC precursors

(3) Prior or concomitant radiation exposure to bone marrow, with associated fibrosis. In adults, fibrosis in the sternum, long bones, or sacrum is a risk factor. In children, fibrosis in the spine or pelvis is a risk factor.

(4) Acute bleeding or hemorrhaging, which may cause a rapid drop in Hgb and progressive hypoxia

(5) Age

(a) Patients younger than age five are more tolerant of chemotherapy because their marrow contains more hematopoietic cells and a lower percentage of fat than does the marrow of older patients (Hoagland, 1992).

(b) The influence of age on the risk of chemotherapy-induced anemia has received little attention, despite the prevalence of this condition in older patients with cancer (Repetto, 2003). The prevalence of anemia increases markedly after age 60; therefore, anemia is likely to be a comorbid condition prior to the initiation of any therapy in an elderly patient (Balducci, 2003).

(6) Poor nutrition: Poor dietary intake related to the toxicities associated

with chemotherapy can greatly alter the reabsorption of iron and diminish available iron stores. Patients with a negative nitrogen balance and associated weight loss are unable to repair cells damaged by chemotherapy (Loney & Chernecky, 2000).

(7) Abnormal metabolism: Renal and hepatic dysfunction may result in prolonged blood levels of drug and increased marrow toxicity (Scott, 1998).

(8) Use of certain drugs (Worrall, Tompkins, & Rust, 1999)

(a) Alcohol

(b) Aspirin and nonsteroidal anti-inflammatory drugs (NSAIDs)

(c) Anticonvulsants (e.g., phenytoin sodium, primidone, carbamazepine)

(d) Oral contraceptives

(e) Oral hypoglycemics

(f) Antibiotics

(g) Tranquilizers

(h) Antimicrobials

m) Clinical manifestations: See Table 17.

n) Collaborative management

(1) Patients with cancer have rated fatigue as the leading complaint, superseding

Table 17. Clinical Manifestations of Anemia

Manifestation	Mild Anemia[a]	Severe Anemia
Hemoglobin Normal ranges: • Adults: Males, 14–18 g/dl; females, 12–16 g/dl • Children: 11.5–13.5 g/dl	Adults (males and females): 8–12 g/dl Children: 7–10 g/dl	Adults (males and females): < 8 g/dl Children: < 7 g/dl
Hematocrit Normal ranges: • Adults: Males, 42%–52%; females, 37%–47% • Children: 34%–40%	Adults (males and females): 31%–37% Children: 34%	Adults (males and females): < 25% Children: < 20%
Associated symptoms	Pallor Fatigue Slight dyspnea Palpitations Sweating on exertion	Headache Dizziness Irritability Dyspnea on exertion and at rest Angina Compensatory tachycardia Tachypnea
General	Fatigue	Fatigue Exercise intolerance
Central nervous system	Dizziness Headaches Irritability	Difficulty sleeping Difficulty concentrating
Cardiovascular	Tachycardia Palpitations with exertion	Tachycardia Palpitations at rest Systolic ejection murmur S_3 (extra heart sound)
Pulmonary	Dyspnea with exertion	Dyspnea at rest
Gastrointestinal	–	Anorexia Indigestion
Genitourinary	–	Menstrual problems Male impotence
Skin	Pallor	Pallor Sensitivity to cold

[a] Mild anemia often is asymptomatic.

Note. From "A New Approach to Managing Chemotherapy-Related Anemia: Nursing Implications of Epoetin Alfa," by P.T. Rieger and D. Haeuber, 1995, *Oncology Nursing Forum, 22,* p. 73. Copyright 1995 by the Oncology Nursing Society. Adapted with permission. Also based on information from "Side Effects of Treatment" (pp. 120–154) by K. Wilson in M. Hockenberry-Eaton (Ed.), *Essentials of Pediatric Oncology Nursing,* 1998, Glenview, IL: Association of Pediatric Oncology Nurses; and *Childhood Leukemia,* 1997, by N. Keene, Sebastopol, CA: O'Reilly and Associates.

nausea and vomiting and having the greatest impact on their energy and activity levels. Fatigue may be the first indication of anemia. Quality-of-life issues become paramount. However, until recently, the symptom of fatigue often has been inadequately assessed (Gillespie, 2003; Tchekmedyian, 2002).

(2) Identify the underlying cause of the anemia.

(3) Implement iron supplementation only for patients with anemia related to iron deficiency. In general, serum ferritin levels less than 100 or transferrin saturation levels less than 20% are taken as evidence of functional iron deficiency, and oral supplementation may be warranted (NCCN, 2004).

(4) Address symptoms related to hypoxia. Improved Hgb and, thus, oxygen levels, have been shown to have a positive impact on treatment—both chemotherapy and radiation. Anoxic tumor cells are two to three times more resistant to radiation therapy than are normally oxygenated cells (Weiss, 2003).

(a) Encourage adult patients to rest to conserve energy. This recommendation only is made if the patient is hypoxic and benefits from the use of oxygen. The new paradigm regarding exercise versus rest has been greatly influenced by recent studies that have identified the positive influence of exercise on the quality of life of patients receiving treatment (Mock, 2003). Children with anemia will set their own limits on activity. They may nap more often or not want to participate in favorite activities.

(b) Encourage the use of or administer oxygen if oxygen saturation is less than 90%.

(5) Compare lab results with important lab indices. Table 18 presents results that are considered in the normal range for healthy men and women. If a patient's results are abnormal, take appropriate action.

(6) Administer recombinant human (rHu) EPO-alfa as ordered. Know the differences between the types of rHu EPO currently available—epoetin alfa and darbepoetin alfa—their recommended administration as well as dosing schedules and their mechanisms of action (Capo & Waltzman, 2004). The traditional definitions of "clinically significant anemia" have been reconsidered in clinical studies, and anemia of lesser grades may be more important than previously suspected (NCCN, 2004). Note: The FDA has not approved the use of rHu EPO for children.

(a) Patient selection and target Hgb: An increase in EPO production occurs as Hgb levels fall below 12 g/dl, and the best treatment outcomes in the retrospective radiation and anemia data appear to occur around relatively normal

Table 18. Laboratory Assessment of Anemia: Normal Values (Adults)

Laboratory Test	Normal Value
Red blood cell count	Male: 4.7–6 m/µl; female: 4.2–5.4 m/µl
Hemoglobin	Male: 13.5–18 g/dl; female: 12–16 g/dl
Hematocrit	Male: 42%–52%; female: 37%–47%
Mean corpuscular volume (MCV)	78–100 fl
Mean corpuscular hemoglobin (MCH)	27–31 pg/cell
Red cell distribution width (RDW)	11.5%–14%
Reticulocyte count	0.5%–1.85% of erythrocytes
Ferritin	Male: 20–300 ng/ml; female: 15–120 ng/ml
Serum iron	Male: 75–175 µg/dl; female: 65–165 µg/dl
Total iron binding capacity (TIBC)	250–450 µg/dl
Serum erythropoietin level	Male: 17.2 mIU/ml; female: 18.8 mIU/ml
Coomb's test (direct and indirect)	Negative
Serum B_{12}	190–900 mg/ml
Serum folate	> 3.5 µg/l

Note. From "Anemia of Chronic Disease" (p. 659) by M.P. Lynch in D. Camp-Sorrell and R.A. Hawkins (Eds.), *Clinical Manual for the Oncology Advanced Practice Nurse,* 2000, Pittsburgh, PA: Oncology Nursing Society. Copyright 2000 by the Oncology Nursing Society. Reprinted with permission.

Hgb values; therefore, is it essential to define the "end point" of intervention (Ades et al., 2003). The quality-of-life data support that optimal improvement occurs by moving Hgb into the 11–12 g/dl range (Crawford, Cella, & Cleeland, 2002). Based on large community studies, the most recent NCCN panel recommended using 11 g/dl as the level to begin intervention when improvement in patient function is the goal (Ades et al.). Other factors that need to be considered when deciding to initiate the use of epoetin alfa or darbepoetin are

i) Radiation and/or chemotherapy
ii) Bone marrow infiltrated by tumor
iii) Myelodysplastic syndrome
iv) Transferrin saturation of at least 20%
v) Serum ferritin level > 100 ng/ml.

(b) Dosing criteria (Amgen Inc., 2002; Ortho Biotech, 2004; Weiss, 2003): The recommended starting dose for rHu EPO alfa is 150 U/kg SQ administered three times a week. If no response is seen after eight weeks, increase dose by 50–100 U/kg three times a week. Epoetin alfa 40,000 U weekly has been shown to be clinically effective in healthy subjects and commonly is used in the clinical setting (Capo & Waltzman, 2004). Darbepoetin's potential benefit is that it may be able to be administered once every two to three weeks.

i) Although darbepoetin alfa is closely related to epoetin alfa, it has three N-linked carbohydrate chains, which gives it a much heavier molecular weight and confers a half-life of 33–48 hours, versus 16–19 hours for epoetin alfa. It may, thus, be administered less frequently, sparing the patient from multiple needle sticks (Capo & Waltzman, 2004).
ii) A commonly used starting dose is 3 mcg/kg SQ q two weeks and increased to 5 mcg/kg q two weeks if no response. The "fixed" dose would be 200 mcg q two weeks or 300 mcg q two weeks (Ades et al., 2003).
iii) A study of q-three-week darbepoetin administered for chemotherapy-induced anemia was presented as an abstract at the 2003 American Society of Hematology meeting (Rearden et al., 2003).
   - The authors found that q-three-week dosing was effective in treating both mild and moderate anemia caused by chemotherapy.
   - It also can simplify the management of anemia in that many chemotherapy regimens are administered on a q-three-week basis and could, therefore, be administered when the patient comes for treatment.

(c) Monitoring (NCCN, 2004)

i) After initiation of rHu EPO alfa therapy, monitor Hgb at least weekly until it reaches 12 g/dl.
ii) Once the target Hgb had been achieved, monitor Hgb at least monthly. Therapy should be held until Hgb is < 12 g/dl.
iii) If hematocrit (HCT) drops below 25%, Hgb drops below 8g/dl, or cardiopulmonary symptoms develop, administer 1–2 units packed RBCs over 2–3 hours.
iv) If the patient has a history of hypersensitivity, premedicate 30 minutes before transfusion with acetaminophen 650 mg po and diphenhydramine

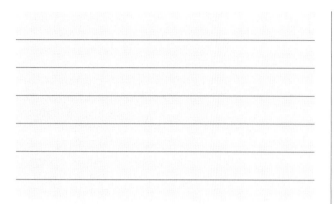

25–50 mg po or IV. Use a leukocyte filter during administration, or administer leukocyte-depleted packed RBCs.

v) If the patient is immunocompromised, administer irradiated packed RBCs (Aledort & Mohandas, 1996) using a leukocyte filter. One unit of packed RBCs can raise HCT by 3% and Hgb by 1 g/dl (Van Gulick, 1998). Monitor tolerance to fluids; if the patient retains fluids, administer furosemide 10–40 mg IV, per physician's order, after the first unit infuses. Repeat after 2–3 hours if needed. Monitor for transfusion reaction (see Labovich, 1997, for a detailed discussion).

o) Patient and family education

(1) Encourage patients to set short-term goals for activities of daily living to conserve energy (Loney & Chernecky, 2000).

(2) Encourage patients to change positions slowly to prevent dizziness secondary to postural hypotension.

(3) Acknowledge patients' reports of symptoms, such as fatigue, as real, even if stated in vague terminology (Loney & Chernecky, 2000).

(4) Discuss the potential for anemia and the signs and symptoms of anemia when teaching patients about the side effects of chemotherapy and/or radiation.

(5) Help patients and caregivers develop mechanisms for managing persistent symptoms of anemia (e.g., fatigue, shortness of breath, decreased stamina).

(6) Provide instruction regarding the self-administration of EPO, including written materials, if applicable.

(7) When applicable, encourage the patients to maintain an optimum level of physical activity and consider referral to physical therapy, physical medicine, or rehabilitation therapy for deconditioned patients (Mock, 2003).

(8) Consult with a registered dietitian regarding an iron-rich diet for the patient and the relation between diet and RBC production (Van Gulick, 1998).

(9) Teach patients and caregivers about the hazards, risks, and benefits of blood transfusions.

3. Thrombocytopenia (Camp-Sorrell, 2000; Shuey, 1996)

a) Normal physiology of platelets: See Figure 18.

(1) Platelets, or thrombocytes, are fragments of bone marrow cells known as megakaryocytes.

(2) A megakaryocyte develops from a pluripotent stem cell. In its final phase of development, it sheds platelets.

(3) A normal platelet count is 150,000–400,000 cells/mm^3. The average life span of a platelet is 7–10 days. Platelets are not stored in bone marrow.

(4) Following an initial insult to a blood vessel, platelets adhere to collagen along the subendothelial surface and release several compounds, including serotonin and adenosine diphosphate (ADP). All these compounds cause the recruitment of more platelets, which adhere to collagen and stick together. This leads to the formation of a clot, a large platelet aggregate, or a hemostatic plug. The entire process should occur within three to five minutes.

(5) When factors VII and XII are activated, as a result of proteins on the platelet surface coming into contact with the damaged endothelial cells, secondary hemostasis occurs.

(6) When the extrinsic and intrinsic pathways are activated, they converge at the common pathway, producing activated factor that converts prothrombin to thrombin. Thrombin converts fibrinogen to fibrin, leading to a stable clot.

(7) Fibrinolysis is the mechanism by which clots are broken down. The factors responsible for fibrinolysis (plasminogen activators) are present in most body

fluids and normal and neoplastic tissue (Gobel, 2000).

b) Pathophysiology (Camp-Sorrell, 2000)
   (1) Bone marrow suppression caused by acute or delayed effects of chemotherapy decreases platelet production.
   (2) Thrombocytopenia usually occurs with neutropenia.
   (3) Indices vary by institution and protocol, but a general rule of thumb for solid tumors is to hold chemotherapy if the platelet count is < 100,000/mm³ (Camp-Sorrell, 2000). Check with the patient's physician before holding chemotherapy. Treatment may be administered with much lower counts, and the physician then may decide to support the patient with platelet transfusions if it becomes necessary. Thrombocytopenia in a child receiving chemotherapy may necessitate dosing changes and a delay in treatment (Felgenhauer et al., 2000).
   (4) The following drugs are known to cause thrombocytopenia as a dose-limiting toxicity (Wilkes, Ingwersen, & Barton-Burke, 2003).
      (a) Platinums (carboplatin and cisplatin)
      (b) Dacarbazine
      (c) Daunorubicin
      (d) Docetaxel
      (e) Doxorubicin
      (f) Gemcitabine
      (g) Lomustine
      (h) Mitomycin
      (i) Thiotepa
      (j) Trimetrexate
      (k) Taxanes
   (5) A cumulative and delayed onset of thrombocytopenia has been observed with the following (Wilkes et al., 2003).
      (a) Carmustine
      (b) Dactinomycin
      (c) Fludarabine
      (d) Lomustine
      (e) Mitomycin
      (f) Paclitaxel
      (g) Streptozocin
      (h) Thiotepa
      (i) 6-thioguanine

c) Incidence
   (1) Chemotherapy commonly causes thrombocytopenia. With the recent increase in the use of growth factors (e.g., G-CSF), which allow higher doses of chemotherapeutic drugs, the incidence of dose-limiting thrombocytopenia has increased.
   (2) Incidence varies depending on the agent used.

d) Risk factors (Gobel, 2000; Lynch, 2000)
   (1) Myelosuppressive chemotherapy, chemotherapy and radiation, or radiation therapy alone
   (2) Disease infiltration of bone marrow
   (3) Disseminated intravascular coagulation (DIC)
   (4) Elevated temperature leading to destruction of platelets (Fuller, 1990)
   (5) Concomitant diseases (Gobel, 2000; Lynch, 2000)
      (a) Cirrhosis or metastasis to the liver
      (b) Diabetes mellitus
      (c) Infection, sepsis, human immunodeficiency virus (HIV)
      (d) Scleroderma, systemic lupus erythematosus, sarcoidosis
      (e) Aplastic anemia
   (6) Nutritional deficiencies (vitamin B_{12}, folate)
   (7) Drug therapy known to affect platelet production or function (Wilkes et al., 2003)
      (a) Antibiotics
      (b) Anticoagulants
      (c) Antidepressants
      (d) Aspirin
      (e) Codeine
      (f) Ethanol
      (g) Indomethacin
      (h) NSAIDs (The effect of an NSAID is temporary; an NSAID prolongs clotting time as long as the drug is in the system.)
      (i) Sulfa drugs
      (j) In children, amphotericin B

e) Clinical manifestations (Camp-Sorrell, 2000; Gobel, 2000; Petursson, 1998; Shelton, 1998)

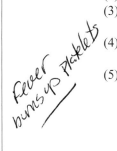

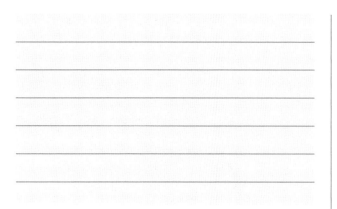

(1) Petechiae (tiny purplish red dots) and ecchymoses (purplish bruises) indicate capillary microvascular bleeding in the soft tissue.
(2) Overt bleeding (e.g., nosebleeds; bleeding from gums, wounds, body orifices, or around existing tubes). Mucous membranes (i.e., nasopharynx, oral mucosa, GI and urinary tracts, upper airways) have capillaries close to the surface, so they bleed easily.
(3) Enlarged and tender liver or spleen indicates that the organ may be capturing enlarged or fragmented cells.
(4) Occult or overt blood in stool or urine
(5) Headaches (may indicate an intracranial bleed)
(6) Hypotension or tachycardia in adults; hypotension and tachycardia do not occur in cases of thrombocytopenia in children.
(7) Prolonged menstruation and amount of pad saturation during menses

f) Laboratory indicators
(1) Platelet count and risk of bleeding
(a) ≤ 50,000/mm³: A moderate risk of bleeding exists.
(b) ≤ 15,000/mm³: A severe risk exists for spontaneous hemorrhage (Gobel, 2000).
(2) Hgb and HCT: Monitor for signs of blood loss in thrombocytopenic patients.
(3) Assessment of coagulation tests (e.g., prothrombin time, activated partial thromboplastin time, thrombin time, platelet aggregation) to determine if patient has DIC.
(4) Occult blood in the urine, stool, or emesis. The stool of patients taking iron supplements may test false guaiac-positive.

g) Collaborative management
(1) Maintain and reinforce bleeding precautions when the platelet count is ≤ 50,000/mm³.
(2) Decrease patients' activity to prevent injury (e.g., falls, bumping into objects). Discourage activities that pose a high risk of injury (e.g., bicycle riding, contact sports).
(3) Maintain a safe environment (e.g., use nonskid rugs in the home).
(4) Maintain the integrity of skin.
(a) Use electric versus straight-edged razors.
(b) Use an emery board versus metal file for nail care, or use metal nail clippers.
(c) Ensure that the patient knows to avoid wearing restrictive clothing (especially restrictive undergarments).
(d) Do not use tourniquets.
(e) Minimize invasive procedures (e.g., needle sticks, injections [especially IM injections]).
(5) Maintain integrity of mucous membranes (Gobel, 2000; Petursson, 1998; Shelton, 1998).
(a) Encourage patients to
i) Blow their nose gently.
ii) Use a water-based lubricant before sexual intercourse.
iii) Use only a soft toothbrush or sponge-tipped applicator, and rinse the mouth with a mild saltwater solution.
(b) Discourage patients from
i) Having dental care until platelets normalize
ii) Using dental floss or oral irrigation tools
iii) Having sexual intercourse if the platelet count is ≤ 50,000/mm³
iv) Using tampons
v) Having anal intercourse.
(6) Maintain the integrity of the genitourinary tract (Gobel, 2000; Petursson, 1998; Shelton, 1998).
(a) Increase patients' hydration and avoid the use of indwelling catheters whenever possible. If catheterization becomes necessary, use only a small-lumen catheter and ample lubrication.
(b) Encourage patients to drink more fluids; they should drink two to three liters per day.

(7) Maintain the integrity of the GI tract (Gobel, 2000; Petursson, 1998; Shelton, 1998).
   (a) Encourage patients to take steroids with food, if steroids are ordered.
   (b) Use prophylactic stool softeners and stimulants to avoid constipation; avoid using enemas, suppositories, harsh laxatives, or rectal thermometers.
(8) Maintain optimal nutritional status (Gobel, 2000; Petursson, 1998; Shelton, 1998).
   (a) Encourage consumption of protein-containing foods; protein is needed for megakaryocyte production.
   (b) Encourage patients to consume a soft diet and avoid foods that are irritating (e.g., hot foods, acidic foods, spicy foods).
   (c) Discourage alcohol use.
(9) Avoid all medications that have the potential to induce bleeding. The anti-inflammatory choline magnesium trisalicylate is platelet sparing.
(10) Administer appropriate medications and treatments.
   (a) Administer platelets prophylactically to adults when the platelet count is 10,000–20,000/mm^3 or when the patient is symptomatic (bleeding), based on institutional guidelines or protocol. (Patients with brain tumors usually receive platelet transfusions if the count drops below 50,000/mm^3). The general rule of thumb is to hold transfusions until the platelet count drops to $\leq$ 10,000/mm^3 (Rebulla et al., 1997).
   (b) Administer stool softeners or laxatives to avoid constipation.
   (c) Consider administering IL 11, also known as oprelvekin, to minimize chemotherapy-induced thrombocytopenia. The FDA has approved IL 11 as a growth factor for megakaryocytes in nonmyeloid malignancies and nonmyeloblative chemotherapy regimens (Camp-Sorrell, 2000). IL 11 presently is not used in pediatrics.
      i) Be cautious when administering IL 11 to patients with a history of fluid retention, congestive heart failure (CHF), atrial arrhythmias, or coronary artery disease; patients who are at risk for developing any of the preceding symptoms, such as the elderly; or patients who are heavily pretreated with anthracyclines (Camp-Sorrell, 2000; Rust, Wood, & Battiato, 1999).
      ii) If IL 11 is ordered, administer the dosage subcutaneously on a daily basis at 50 mcg/kg per day, beginning 6–24 hours after completion of chemotherapy. The manufacturer recommends that the drug be discontinued when the post-nadir platelet count reaches 50,000/mm^3 (Rust et al., 1999). Monitor patients closely (preferably daily) for dyspnea, pleural effusion, and edema. These side effects are thought to result from an increase in renal sodium retention and plasma volume expansion, which cause an increase in intravascular fluid.

h) Patient and family education (Camp-Sorrell, 2000; Shelton, 1998)
   (1) Tell patients and significant others to immediately notify the nurse or physician of symptoms of bleeding.
   (2) Instruct patients about the signs of transfusion reaction.
   (3) Provide reassurance by discussing the fact that chemotherapy-related platelet disorder is generally short-lived. Share the prediction for nadir and outline the patient's specific regimen.

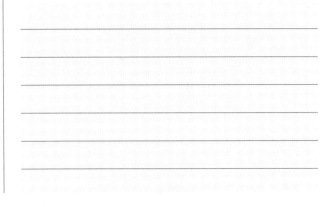

(4) Reinforce the need to avoid injuries; list the activities that patients should avoid to prevent injury.
(5) Provide instruction regarding self-administration of IL 11, if applicable.
(6) Provide instruction on interventions to manage bleeding.
(7) Provide healthcare providers' names and telephone numbers, and instruct patients to call if any of the following occur.
(a) Bleeding from any body orifice
(b) New petechiae or bruising
(c) Change in level of consciousness
(8) Provide an inclusive list of medications that may interfere with megakaryocyte production.

References

Ades, T., Alteri, R., Esclante, C., Johnson, E., McClure, J., Mock, V., et al. (2003). *Cancer-related fatigue and anemia: Treatment guidelines for patients.* Retrieved February 9, 2005, from http://www.cancer.org/downloads/CRI/944601%20-%20Fatigue%20and%20Anemia%20(En).pdf

Aledort, L.M., & Mohandas, K. (1996). Transfusion requirements in patients with malignancy. *Seminars in Hematology, 33,* 6–9.

Amgen Inc. (2002). Aranesp [Package insert]. Thousand Oaks, CA: Author.

Balducci, L. (2003). Anemia, cancer and aging. *Cancer Control, 10,* 478–486.

Bron, D., Meuleman, N., & Mascaux, C. (2001). Biological basis of anemia. *Seminars in Oncology, 28*(2 Suppl. 8), 1–6.

Burns, E.R., Reed, L.J., & Weng, B. (1986). Volumetric erythrocyte macrocytosis is induced by hydroxyurea. *American Journal of Clinical Pathology, 3,* 413.

Camp-Sorrell, D. (2000). Chemotherapy: Toxicity management. In C.H. Yarbro, M.H. Frogge, M. Goodman, & S.L. Groenwald (Eds.), *Cancer nursing: Principles and practice* (5th ed., pp. 444–486). Sudbury, MA: Jones and Bartlett.

Capo, G., & Waltzman, R. (2004). Managing hematologic toxicities. *Journal of Supportive Oncology, 2,* 65–78.

Crawford, J., Cella, D., & Cleeland, C. (2002). Relationship between changes in hemoglobin level and quality of life during chemotherapy in anemic cancer patients receiving epoetin alfa therapy. *Cancer, 95,* 888–895.

Dessypris, E.N. (1999). Erythropoiesis. In G.R.M. Lee, J. Foester, J. Lukens, F. Paraskevas, J.P. Greer, & G.M. Rodgers (Eds.), *Wintrobe's clinical hematology* (10th ed., pp. 169–192). Baltimore: Williams & Wilkins.

Erickson, J.M. (1996). Anemia. *Seminars in Oncology Nursing, 12,* 2–14.

Felgenhauer, J., Hawkins, D., Pendergrass, T., Lindsley, K., Conrad, E.U., III, & Miser, J.S. (2000). Very intensive, short-term chemotherapy for children and adolescents with metastatic sarcomas. *Medical and Pediatric Oncology, 34*(1), 29–38.

Fuller, A.K. (1990). Platelet transfusion therapy for thrombocytopenia. *Seminars in Oncology Nursing, 6,* 123–128.

Gillespie, T.W. (2003). Anemia in cancer: Therapeutic implications and interventions. *Cancer Nursing, 26,* 119–128.

Gobel, B.H. (2000). Bleeding. In C.H. Yarbro, M.H. Frogge, M. Goodman, & S.L. Groenwald (Eds.), *Cancer nursing: Principles and practice* (5th ed., pp. 709–736). Sudbury, MA: Jones and Bartlett.

Gordon, M.S. (2002). Managing anemia in the cancer patient: Old problems, future solutions. *Oncologist, 7,* 331–341.

Hoagland, H.C. (1992). Hematologic complications of cancer chemotherapy. In M.C. Perry (Ed.), *The chemotherapy source book* (2nd ed., pp. 498–507). Baltimore: Williams & Wilkins.

Labovich, T. (1997). Transfusion therapy: Nursing implications. *Clinical Journal of Oncology Nursing, 1,* 61–72.

Loney, J., & Chernecky, C. (2000). Anemia. *Oncology Nursing Forum, 27,* 951–964.

Lynch, M.P. (2000). Overview of anemia. In D. Camp-Sorrell & R.A. Hawkins (Eds.), *Clinical manual for the oncology advanced practice nurse* (pp. 665–678). Pittsburgh, PA: Oncology Nursing Society.

Mock, V. (2003). Clinical excellence through evidence-based practice: Fatigue management as a model. *Oncology Nursing Forum, 30,* 787–796.

National Comprehensive Cancer Network. (2004). *Cancer and Treatment-Related Anemia, 1,* MS1–MS9.

Ortho Biotech. (2004). Procrit (epoetin alfa) [Package insert]. Bridgewater, NJ: Author.

Petursson, C.T. (1998). Bleeding due to thrombocytopenia. In J.M. Yasko (Ed.), *Nursing management of symptoms associated with chemotherapy* (4th ed., pp. 127–134). Bala Cynwyd, PA: Meniscus Health Care Communications.

Rearden, T., Charu, V., Saidman, B., Ben-Jacob, A., Justice, G.R., Manaim, A.S., et al. (2003). Results of a randomized study of every three-week dosing of darbepoetin alfa for chemotherapy-induced anemia (CIA). *Blood, 102*(11), 20B.

Rebulla, P., Finazzi, G., Marangoni, F., Avvisati, G., Gugliotta, L., Tognoni, G., et al. (1997). The threshold for prophylactic platelet transfusions in adults with acute myeloid leukemia. Gruppo Italiano Malattie Ematologiche Maligne dell'Adulto. *New England Journal of Medicine, 337,* 1870–1875.

Repetto, L. (2003). Greater risks of chemotherapy toxicity in elderly patients with cancer. *Journal of Supportive Oncology, 1*(2), 18–24.

Rust, D.M., Wood, L.S., & Battiato, L.A. (1999). Oprelvekin: An alternative treatment for thrombocytopenia. *Clinical Journal of Oncology Nursing, 3,* 57–62.

Scott, T.E. (1998). Anemia. In M.J. Hockenberry-Eaton (Ed.), *Essentials of pediatric oncology nursing: A core curriculum*. Glenview, IL: Association of Pediatric Oncology Nurses.

Shelton, B.K. (1998). Bleeding disorders. In C.R. Ziegfeld, B.G. Lubejko, & B.K. Shelton (Eds.), *Oncology fact finder* (pp. 244–261). Philadelphia: Lippincott.

Shuey, K.M. (1996). Platelet-associated bleeding disorders. *Seminars in Oncology Nursing, 12,* 15–27.

Smith, R.E., Jr. (2004). Erythropoietic agents in the management of cancer patients. Part 2: Studies on their role in neuroprotection. *Journal of Supportive Oncology, 2,* 39–49.

Tchekmedyian, M.S. (2002). Anemia in cancer patients: Significance, epidemiology, and current therapy. *Oncology, 16*(9 Suppl. 10), 17–24.

Van Gulick, A.J. (1998). Anemia. In J.M. Yasko (Ed.), *Nursing management of symptoms associated with chemotherapy* (pp.

115–125). Bala Cynwyd, PA: Meniscus Health Care Communications.

Weiss, M.J. (2003). New insights into erythropoietin and epoetin alfa: Mechanisms of action, target tissues, and clinical applications. *Oncologist, 8*(Suppl. 3), 18–29.

Wilkes, G.M., Ingwersen, K., & Barton-Burke, M. (2003). *2003 oncology nursing drug handbook.* Sudbury, MA: Jones and Bartlett.

Worrall, L.M., Tompkins, C.A., & Rust, D.M. (1999). Recognizing and managing anemia. *Clinical Journal of Oncology Nursing, 3,* 153–160.

B. Gastrointestinal and mucosal side effects

1. Nausea and vomiting: Studies suggest that healthcare providers perceive that patients have less acute and delayed chemotherapy-induced nausea and vomiting (CINV) than they actually do and that patients do not receive adequate preventive antiemetics (Fabi et al., 2003; Grunberg, Hansen, Deuson, & Mavros, 2002). Oncology nurses must be knowledgeable about and proactive in the treatment of CINV. Terms used in this discussion include the following.
   - *Nausea:* Nausea is an unpleasant subjective experience that is described as a "wavelike" feeling occurring in the stomach and/or the back of the throat that may be accompanied by vomiting (NCI, 2004). Nausea is mediated by the autonomic nervous system and accompanied by symptoms such as tachycardia, perspiration, lightheadedness, dizziness, pallor, excess salivation, and weakness (Camp-Sorrell, 2000).
   - *Retching:* A rhythmic and spasmodic movement involving the diaphragm and abdominal muscles, controlled by the respiratory center in the brain stem, near the vomiting center (Camp-Sorrell, 2000). Retching also is known as the dry heaves.
   - *Vomiting:* The forceful expulsion of gastric, duodenum, or jejunum contents through the mouth (NCI, 2004).

   a) Pathophysiology (NCCN, 2005)

      (1) Mechanisms of emesis (see Figure 19): Nausea, retching, and vomiting are independent phenomena that can occur sequentially or as separate entities. The subjective nature of nausea prevents a clear understanding of it; however, mechanisms of vomiting

Figure 19. Mechanics of Emesis

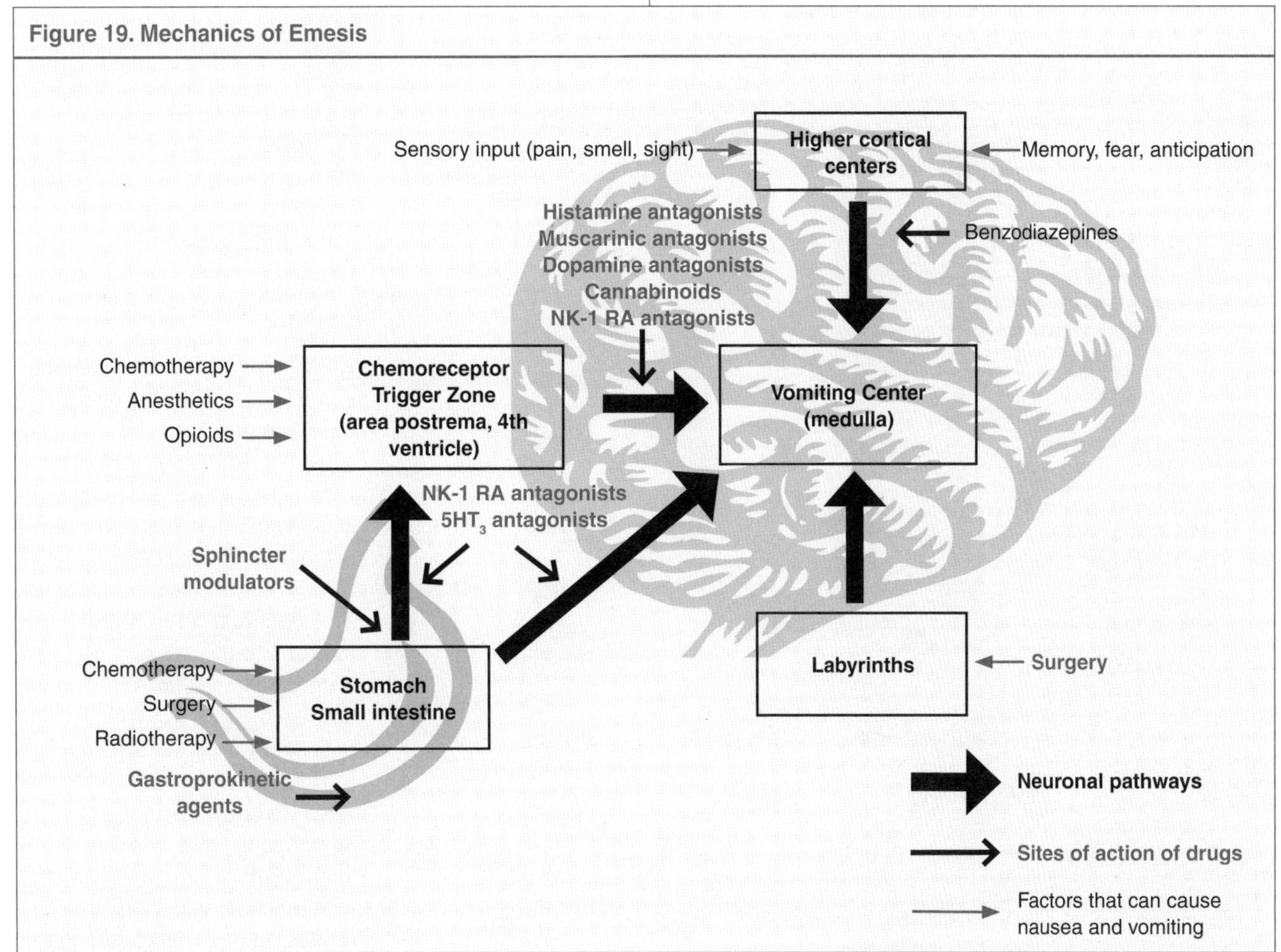

related to chemotherapy administration are becoming better understood.

(a) Vomiting results from the stimulation of a complex process that involves the activation of various pathways and neurotransmitter receptors (see Figures 19 and 20).

(b) Vomiting occurs when certain neurons in the brain stem, collectively called the vomiting center (VC), are stimulated (Wickham, 1997). The VC is activated by the visceral and vagal afferent pathways from the GI tract, the chemoreceptor trigger zone (CTZ), the vestibular apparatus (VA), and the cerebral cortex (Camp-Sorrell, 2000).

(c) Chemotherapy and radiation to the gut stimulate enterochromaffin cells, causing them to release serotonin ($5HT_3$). The vagus nerve plays a key role in emesis caused by chemotherapy, radiation therapy to the epigastrium, and abdominal distention or obstruction. Serotonin release causes the activation of the vagus nerve, which stimulates vomiting through either the CTZ or the VC (O'Bryant, Gonzales, & Bestul, 2004).

(d) The CTZ, a highly vascular area, lies at the surface of the fourth ventricle, close to the VC. The CTZ is not confined within the blood-brain barrier. Therefore, it can detect chemical stimuli in the cerebrospinal fluid and the blood. The CTZ plays a role in nausea and vomiting associated with chemotherapy as well as in emesis associated with other causes such as anesthetics and opioids.

(e) Substance P is found in vagal afferent neurons and binds to NK-1 receptors, causing vomiting. The study of this specific mechanism of vomiting has led to the development of a new class of antiemetics, NK-1 receptor antagonists (Campos et al., 2001; Hesketh, 2001).

(f) Motion sickness and labyrinthitis are the most common stimuli to the VA of the inner ear that induce nausea and vomiting. The VA may play a minor role in CINV. Surgery also can induce vomiting through stimulation at the vestibular system. Drugs that are ototoxic, such as cisplatin, may secondarily induce nausea and vomiting via the VA (Wickham, 1997).

(g) Memory, fear, anticipation, pain, and a distasteful smell can trigger nausea and vomiting at the cerebral cortex.

(h) Factors that can cause nausea and vomiting include chemotherapy, biotherapy, radiation therapy, surgery, opioids, and other medications.

(2) Patterns of therapy-related emesis (NCCN, 2005)

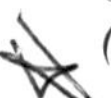

(a) Anticipatory nausea and vomiting: A conditioned response that occurs most commonly before treatment and can be triggered by a particular smell, taste, or sight. Anticipatory nausea and vomiting also can occur during treatment and may even last one to two days after therapy. This usually is a result of a previous unpleasant experience(s) with uncontrolled nausea and vomiting and may be worse in patients with high levels of anxiety. Anticipatory nausea usually occurs after two or three cycles of chemotherapy. To minimize the risk of this side effect, adequate antiemetic control with initial treatments is essential. Infants and young children usu-

Figure 20. Neurotransmitter Receptors

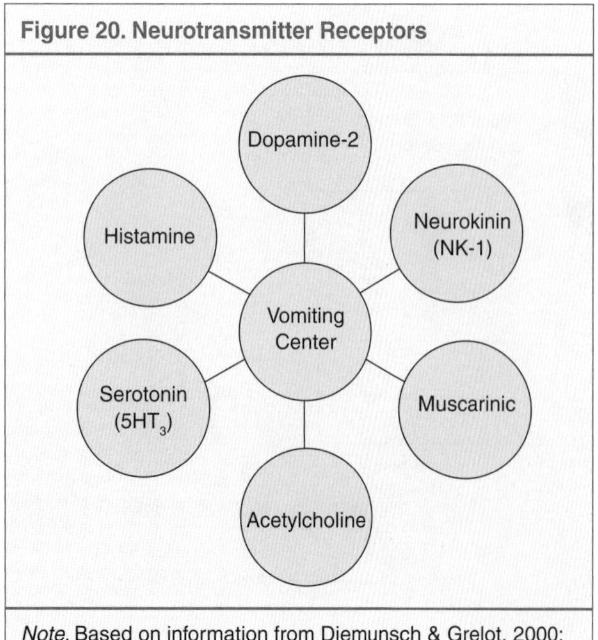

Note. Based on information from Diemunsch & Grelot, 2000; Hornby, 2001.

ally do not experience anticipatory nausea and vomiting.

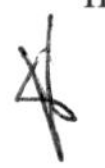

i) Incidence: Anticipatory nausea and vomiting occurs in 25% of patients as a result of classical conditioning from stimuli associated with chemotherapy (e.g., odors, tastes of drugs, visual cues) (Camp-Sorrell, 2000).

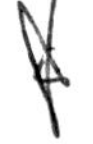

ii) Risk factors: The factors that follow may increase susceptibility to anticipatory nausea and vomiting (NCI, 2004).

- Being young or middle-aged: Patients younger than age 50 are at increased risk for anticipatory nausea and vomiting.
- High levels of anxiety prior to and during treatment
- Feeling warm or hot after chemotherapy
- Having a susceptibility to motion sickness
- Feeling generalized weakness after chemotherapy

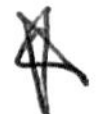

(b) Acute nausea and vomiting: Starts within minutes to hours after chemotherapy administration and may last 24 hours, depending on the agent (NCCN, 2005). The type of chemotherapy, dose, and administration schedule influence the severity and risk of acute nausea and vomiting.

i) Incidence: Determined by the emetogenicity of the chemotherapy agents (see Table 19) and whether pretreated with an antiemetic agent (Camp-Sorrell, 2000)

ii) Risk factors: The following factors increase susceptibility to acute nausea and vomiting (Doherty, 1999; Osoba et al., 1997).

Table 19. Emetogenic Potential of Various Chemotherapeutic Drugs

Incidence	Level	Agent	Onset (hours)	Duration (hours)
Very high (> 90%)	5	Cisplatin (> 50 mg/m^2)	1–6	24–48+
		Dacarbazine	1–3	1–12
		Mechlorethamine	0.5–2	8–24
		Melphalan – high dose	0.3–6	6–12
		Streptozocin	1–6	12–24
		Cytarabine – high dose (> 1 g/m^2)	1–4	12–48
High (60%–90%)	4	Carmustine	2–4	4–24
		Cyclophosphamide	4–12	12–24
		Procarbazine	24–72	variable
		Etoposide – high dose	4–6	24+
		Semustine	1–5	12–24
		Lomustine	4–6	12–24
		Dactinomycin	2–5	24
		Methotrexate – high dose	1–12	24–72
		Actinomycin-D	1–12	24–48
		Cytarabine (500 mg/m^2)	1–12	24–48
		Epirubicin/Idarubicin	6–12	24+

(Continued on next page)

Table 19. Emetogenic Potential of Various Chemotherapeutic Drugs *(Continued)*

Incidence	Level	Agent	Onset (hours)	Duration (hours)
Moderate (30%–60%)	3	Doxorubicin	4–6	6+
		Mitoxantrone	4–6	6+
		5-fluorouracil	3–6	24+
		Mitomycin C	1–4	48–72
		Carboplatin	4–6	12–24
		Daunorubicin (> 50 mg/m^2)	2–6	24
		L-asparaginase	1–4	2–12
		Topotecan	6–12	24–72
		Ifosfamide	3–6	24–72
		Irinotecan	6–12	24+
		Epirubicin	–	–
		Idarubicin	–	–
Low (10%–30%)	2	Bleomycin	3–6	–
		Cytarabine	6–12	3–12
		Etoposide	3–8	–
		Melphalan	6–12	–
		6-mercaptopurine	4–8	–
		Methotrexate (< 100 mg/m^2)	4–12	3–12
		Vinblastine	4–8	–
		Hydroxyurea	–	–
		Teniposide	–	–
		Gemcitabine	–	–
		Vinorelbine	–	–
		Fludarabine	–	–
		Topotecan	–	–
		Capecitabine	–	–
		Trimetrexate	–	–
Very low (< 10%)	1	Vincristine	4–8	–
		Chlorambucil	48–72	–
		Busulfan	–	–
		Thioguanine	–	–
		Hormones	–	–
		Paclitaxel	4–8	–
		Docetaxel	–	–
		Thiotepa	–	–

Note. From "Chemotherapy: Toxicity Management" (p. 458), by D. Camp-Sorrell in C.H. Yarbro, M.H. Frogge, M. Goodman, and S.L. Groenwald (Eds.), *Cancer Nursing: Principles and Practice* (5th ed.), 2000, Sudbury, MA: Jones and Bartlett. Copyright 2000 by Jones and Bartlett. Reprinted with permission.

- Gender: Menstruating women experience more acute nausea and vomiting than do men.
- Age: Patients older than 50 years experience less nausea and vomiting than patients younger than 50.
- Alcohol use: Patients with a history of chronic or high alcohol intake generally have less severe nausea than do those without such a history.
- Advanced-stage disease
- Fatigue
- Pain
- Tumor burden
- Concomitant medical conditions (e.g., obstruction, pancreatitis, hepatic metastases)
- Presence of strong taste disturbances during chemotherapy
- A high level of pretreatment anxiety
- Susceptibility to GI distress
- Poor performance status
- A history of hyperemesis during pregnancy or morning sickness throughout pregnancy

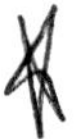

(c) Delayed nausea and vomiting: Occurs at least 24 hours after chemotherapy administration and may last up to six days (O'Bryant et al., 2004). Nausea often is worse for patients than vomiting. Delayed nausea and vomiting may be caused by the ongoing effect that the metabolites of chemotherapy continue to exert on the CNS or GI tract (Camp-Sorrell, 2000). Cisplatin is associated with the highest incidence of delayed nausea and vomiting. Roila et al. (1991) found that patients who were suboptimally treated for acute nausea and vomiting with cisplatin had higher levels of delayed and anticipatory nausea and vomiting. In a multisite, longitudinal, descriptive study of patients with breast cancer by Dibble, Isreal, Nussey, Casey, and Luce (2003), younger, heavier women experienced delayed nausea more frequently than other women. In addition, this study found that women who had a history of experiencing nausea with stressful situations were more likely to have delayed nausea after receiving cyclophosphamide.

b) Risk factors: See the preceding section, which relates risk factors to specific types of nausea and vomiting. See also Table 19, which cites the emetogenic potential of various chemotherapeutic agents.

c) Assessment: Determine the potential causes of nausea and vomiting and the level of emetogenicity (Potter & Schafer, 1999).

(1) Chemotherapy: Utilizing the emetogenic levels as described by Hesketh (1997), the emetogenic potential of a particular regimen can be estimated.

(a) Begin with the most highly emetogenic agent in the regimen and then add levels based on the other agents in the regimen.

(b) In general, *level 1* agents do not add to the emetogenicity of a regimen.

(c) As one or more *level 2* chemotherapy agents are added to a regimen, the emetogenicity of the regimen should be increased by one level.

(d) Each *level 3 or 4* agent added to the regimen increases the emetogenicity of the regimen by one level per agent.

(2) Biotherapy (interferon or IL-2): Patients receiving biologic agents may experience nausea and/or vomiting as part of a flu-like syndrome. Biotherapy involving the infusion of monoclonal antibodies may be associated with nausea and/or vomiting during the infusion; the cause seems related to the infusion process, not the antibodies.

When nausea or vomiting occurs, it usually does so during the first infusion (e.g., an infusion with rituximab) (Kosits & Callaghan, 2000).

(3) Physical causes: Tumor obstruction, constipation, increased intracranial pressure, brain metastasis, vestibular dysfunction, uncontrolled pain

(4) Metabolic causes: Hypercalcemia, hyponatremia, hyperglycemia, uremia, increased creatinine

(5) Other medications (e.g., opioids, antibiotics)

(6) Psychological causes: Anxiety, fear, emotional distress.

d) Potential complications of nausea and vomiting

(1) Discomfort

(2) Delay of treatment

(3) Interference with quality of life (e.g., impaired mobility, fatigue)

(4) Dehydration

(5) Metabolic disturbances

(6) Anorexia and weight loss

(7) Physical debilitation from malnutrition

(8) Straining of abdominal muscles

(9) Danger of aspiration

e) Collaborative management—Pharmacologic actions: See Table 20. Prevention of nausea and vomiting is the primary goal. Choose antiemetics appropriate to the chemotherapeutic regimen. Consider level of emetogenicity based on route of administration and dose administered. Consider cumulative chemotherapy emetogenicity. Administer antiemetics to cover the expected emetogenic period of the chemotherapy agent, considering duration and pattern of emesis. Note: Steroids often are contraindicated for patients receiving biotherapy agents because of their immunosuppressive effects.

(1) To manage acute nausea and vomiting (NCCN, 2005)

(a) For patients at high risk (Level 5): Use a combination of a $5HT_3$ antagonist, NK-1 antagonist, plus a corticosteroid before chemotherapy. Lorazepam also may be used in combination with the above antiemetics to improve control in high-risk regimens. The administration of a corticosteroid with a $5HT_3$ antagonist has been found to improve the control of nausea and vomiting when compared to a $5HT_3$ antagonist alone (Perez et al., 1998).

(b) For patients at moderate risk (Level 3–4): Use a combination of a corticosteroid and a $5HT_3$ antagonist. The addition of lorazepam and/or an NK-1 antagonist may be considered in select patients.

(c) For patients at low risk (Level 2): Use a single agent or a combination of a corticosteroid, metoclopramide, and/or phenothiazine. Lorazepam also may be added.

(d) For patients at minimal risk (Level 1): No routine prophylaxis. Ongoing assessment for the occurrence of nausea and/or vomiting should be performed.

(e) For patients undergoing multiple consecutive days of chemotherapy: Each day, use antiemetics appropriate to the risk category of the chemotherapy to be administered that day.

(2) To manage delayed nausea and vomiting (NCCN, 2005)

(a) For patients at risk for delayed nausea and vomiting (e.g., patients receiving cisplatin): Use a single agent such as a corticosteroid, a $5HT_3$ antagonist, or metoclopramide. Use a combination of the previously listed antiemetics based on patient-specific needs, or consider utilizing an NK-1 antagonist on days two and three for delayed nausea and vomiting in combination with a corticosteroid. Metoclopramide is rarely used for pediatric patients.

(b) Delayed nausea and vomiting is a significant problem for the patients with cancer who are receiving chemotherapy. New approaches such as NK-1 antagonists and lon-

ger-acting $5HT_3$ antagonists have been investigated in an attempt to improve nausea and vomiting in this setting (Massaro & Lenz, 2005).

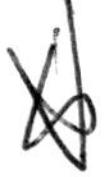

(3) To manage anticipatory nausea and vomiting: Use the most active antiemetic regimens appropriate to the chemotherapy being given. Such regimens must be used with the initial chemotherapy rather than after assessment of the patient's emetic response to less-effective treatment. Benzodiaz-

Table 20. Antiemetic Therapy: Select Pharmacologic Agents for the Control of Chemotherapy-Induced Nausea and Vomiting

Category	Medication Name	Dose and Schedule	Indications	Comments	Side Effects
Serotonin antagonist	Ondansetron	8–32 mg IV once; infuse over 15 minutes; give 30 minutes before chemotherapy. Oral doses vary, ranging from 8–24 mg/day With moderately emetogenic therapy; administer 8 mg bid 30 minutes before chemotherapy and continuing for 1–2 days after chemotherapy. With highly emetogenic chemotherapy, administer 24 mg po 30 minutes before chemotherapy. Orally disintegrating tablet formulation: 8 mg	Prevention of nausea and vomiting associated with single-day highly emetogenic chemotherapy in adults	Ondansetron and dexamethasone can be combined.	Headache, diarrhea, fever, constipation, transient increase in serum SGOT, SGPT, hypotension
	Granisetron	2 mg po up to 1 hour before chemotherapy; 1 mg po or 0.01 mg/kg IV 30 minutes before chemotherapy	Prevention of nausea and vomiting during chemotherapy at initial and repeated cycles Approved for use with high-dose cisplatin	Granisetron can be administered by rapid bolus.	Headache, asthenia, diarrhea, constipation, fever, somnolence
	Dolasetron	100 mg po, or 100 mg IV, 30 minutes before chemotherapy	Prevention of chemotherapy-induced nausea and vomiting	Dolasetron will precipitate with dexamethasone in D5W.	Headache, diarrhea, dizziness, fatigue, abnormal liver function
	Palonosetron	0.25 mg fixed IV dose; infuse over 30 seconds. Give 30 minutes prior to chemotherapy.	Prevention of acute nausea and vomiting associated with initial and repeated courses of moderately and highly emetogenic chemotherapy and the prevention of delayed nausea and vomiting associated with initial and repeat courses of moderately emetogenic chemotherapy	Mean terminal elimination half-life is approximately 40 hours. First $5HT_3$ to be approved for delayed nausea and vomiting Repeat dosing within a seven-day interval is not recommended until further evaluated. Not currently used for pediatric patients	Headache, constipation

(Continued on next page)

Table 20. Antiemetic Therapy: Select Pharmacologic Agents for the Control of Chemotherapy-Induced Nausea and Vomiting *(Continued)*

Category	Medication Name	Dose and Schedule	Indications	Comments	Side Effects
NK-1 antagonist	Aprepitant	Capsules: 125 mg po day one of chemotherapy and then 80 mg po days two and three	Prevention of acute and delayed chemotherapy-induced nausea and vomiting in combination with other antiemetics Approved for initial and repeated courses of highly emetogenic chemotherapy	Drug is given in combination with corticosteroid and $5HT_3$ antagonists on day one and a corticosteroid on days two and three. Use with caution in patients receiving chemotherapy that is primarily metabolized through CYP3A4. The efficacy of oral contraceptives during administration of aprepitant may be compromised. Co-administration of aprepitant and warfarin may decrease INR; monitor closely.	Constipation, hiccups, loss of appetite, diarrhea, fatigue
Corticosteroid	Dexamethasone	Doses vary: 20 mg IV or po before chemotherapy; 4 mg po bid or tid for 2–4 days	Prevention of nausea and vomiting caused by moderately emetogenic chemotherapy Prevention of delayed nausea or vomiting	Adding a corticosteroid increases the efficacy of antiemetic regimens by 15%–25%. Add dexamethasone to $5HT_3$ regimens. Use is contraindicated with most biotherapy agents.	Administer slowly over at least 10 minutes to prevent perianal burning or itching. Insomnia, anxiety, acne
Dopamine antagonists	Metoclopramide	20–40 mg po q 4–6 hours 10 mg IV q 4 hours; IV dose can be given up to 2 mg/kg q 4 hours	Prevention of nausea and vomiting caused by moderately emetogenic chemotherapy Prevention of delayed nausea or vomiting	Incidence of drowsiness is greater with high doses. May cause diarrhea	Sedation, extrapyramidal symptoms, dystonia, dizziness, orthostasis
	Prochlorperazine	Doses vary: 10 mg IV q 4 hours; 10–20 mg po q 4 hours	Prevention of nausea and vomiting caused by moderately emetogenic chemotherapy Prevention of delayed nausea or vomiting	Not used for pediatric patients Highly sedating	
	Haloperidol	1–4 mg IV/po or IM q 2–6 hours	Prevention of acute or delayed nausea or vomiting	Administering haloperidol with diphenhydramine 25–50 mg po or IV prevents extrapyramidal symptoms; more common in younger patients; highly sedating	
Cannabinoid	Dronabinol	5 mg po tid or qid	Prevention of nausea and vomiting caused by moderately emetogenic chemotherapy	Incidence of paranoid reactions or abnormal thinking increases with maximum doses.	Sedation, euphoria, dysphoria, dry mouth, orthostasis
Anxiolytic	Lorazepam	1–3 mg po or sublingual; 0.5–2 mg IV q 4–6 hours	Prevention of anticipatory nausea and vomiting In combination with other antiemetics as needed for acute or delayed nausea and vomiting	Use with caution in elderly patients or those with hepatic or renal dysfunction.	Sedation

Note. From "Serotonin Antagonists: State of the Art Management of Chemotherapy-Induced Emesis," by L.B. Cleri, 1995, *Oncology Nursing Updates: Patient Treatment and Support, 2*(1), pp. 6–7. Copyright 1995 by Lippincott Williams and Wilkins. Adapted with permission. Also based on information from Massaro & Lenz, 2005.

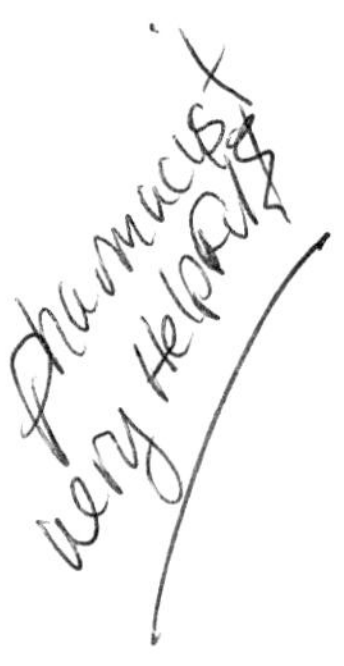

epines (alprazolam or lorazepam) are the primary drugs used for the treatment of anticipatory nausea and vomiting (Aapro, Molassiotis, & Olver, 2004).

(4) For patients experiencing refractory nausea and vomiting despite optimal prophylaxis in current or prior cycles (breakthrough nausea and vomiting): Ascertain that the best regimen is being given based on the emetogenic potential of the regimen (NCCN, 2005).

(a) Conduct a careful evaluation of risk, antiemetic agents, type of disease, concurrent conditions, and medication factors.

(b) Consider adding an antianxiety agent to the regimen.

(c) Consider adding a dopamine receptor antagonist, such as metoclopramide.

(d) Multiple agents used in combination may be required to gain control over nausea and vomiting.

(e) Around-the-clock scheduling is suggested.

f) Collaborative management—Nonpharmacologic interventions should be used in conjunction with antiemetics.

(1) In a randomized study of 33 BMT recipients receiving high-dose chemotherapy, music therapy was found to significantly reduce the incidence of nausea and vomiting. Music therapy is the controlled use of music to influence physiologic, psychological, and emotional responses. Music therapy often is used with other techniques. It also decreases the perceptions of the degree of vomiting (Ezzone, Baker, & Terrepka, 1998).

(2) Moderate aerobic exercise has been demonstrated to provide relief of nausea (Potter & Schafer, 1999).

(3) Acupressure wristbands have been used with some success. Acupressure is a form of massage in which the practitioner uses energy channels, called meridians, to increase energy flow and affect emotions (King, 1997).

(4) In a review of the experimental literature related to the effects of acupuncture treatment for CINV, Mayer (2000) found evidence that acupuncture is effective.

(5) Behavioral interventions—such as self-hypnosis, progressive muscle relaxation, biofeedback, guided imagery, cognitive distraction, and systemic desensitization—have been used either alone or in combination with pharmacologic agents to prevent or control CINV. These behavioral methods are similar in that their use is an attempt to induce relaxation as a learned response. Each method induces relaxation in a different manner (King, 1997).

(6) Dietary interventions

(a) Encourage patients to eat small, frequent meals.

(b) Medicate patients prior to meals so that the antiemetic effect is active during and immediately after eating.

(c) Encourage patients to avoid fatty, spicy, and highly salted foods and foods with strong odors.

(d) Determine and repeat past measures that have been effective in controlling nausea and vomiting (Ropka, 1998).

(e) Encourage patients to eat cold or room-temperature foods because these give off fewer odors than do hot foods.

(f) Suggest that patients cook meals between chemotherapy regimens, when they are not nauseated, and freeze the meals for later use, or suggest that another family member cook meals.

(g) Encourage patients to avoid favorite foods on the day of chemotherapy and while nausea and vomiting persist so that aversions to the foods do not develop (Wickham, 1997).

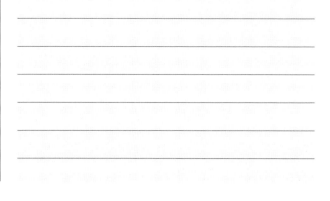

(h) Suggest that the patients try foods containing ginger when feeling nauseated. In folk medicine, ginger is known as an agent that decreases

nausea and vomiting (Wickham, 1997).

g) Patient and family education

(1) Instruct adult patients to notify the staff if nausea and vomiting persist for more than 24 hours or if they are unable to maintain fluid intake. Ensure that parents of pediatric patients know to notify staff after a few hours of vomiting. In children, just a few hours of vomiting can cause dehydration.

(2) Remind patients as necessary to take antiemetics before arriving for treatment. Ensure that antiemetics have been taken prior to administration of chemotherapy (Potter & Schafer, 1999).

(3) Follow up 24–48 hours after outpatient treatment to ensure adherence to or effectiveness of the antiemetic regimen is essential (Camp-Sorrell, 2000).

References

Aapro, M.S., Molassiotis, A., & Olver, I. (2004). Anticipatory nausea and vomiting. *Supportive Care in Cancer.* Retrieved January 10, 2005, from http://www.springerlink.com/app/home/contribution.asp?wasp=524c86wymq2xnh95yj2q&referrer=parent&backto=issue,20,54;journal,1,66;linkingpublicationresults,1:101182,1

Campos, D., Pereira, J.R., Reinhardt, R.R., Carracedo, C., Poli, S., Vogel, C., et al. (2001). Prevention of cisplatin-induced emesis by the oral neurokinin-1 antagonist, MK-869, in combination with granisetron and dexamethasone or with dexamethasone alone. *Journal of Clinical Oncology, 19,* 1759–1767.

Camp-Sorrell, D. (2000). Chemotherapy: Toxicity management. In C.H. Yarbro, M.H. Frogge, M. Goodman, & S.L. Groenwald (Eds.), *Cancer nursing: Principles and practice* (5th ed., pp. 444–486). Sudbury, MA: Jones and Bartlett.

Dibble, S.L., Isreal, J., Nussey, B., Casey, K., & Luce, J. (2003). Delayed chemotherapy-induced nausea in women treated for breast cancer [Online exclusive]. *Oncology Nursing Forum, 30,* E40–E47.

Diemunsch, P., & Grelot, L. (2000). Potential of substance P antagonists as antiemetics. *Drugs, 60,* 533–546.

Doherty, K.M. (1999). Closing the gap in prophylactic antiemetic therapy: Patient factors in calculating the emetogenic potential of chemotherapy. *Clinical Journal of Oncology Nursing, 3,* 113–119.

Ezzone, S., Baker, R., & Terrepka, E. (1998). Music as an adjunct to antiemetic therapy. *Oncology Nursing Forum, 25,* 1551–1556.

Fabi, A., Barduagni, M., Lauro, S., Portalone, L., Mauri, M., Marinis, F., et al. (2003). Is delayed chemotherapy-induced emesis well managed in oncological clinical practice? An observational study. *Supportive Care in Cancer, 11,* 156–161.

Grunberg, S.M., Hansen, M., Deuson, R., & Mavros, P. (2002). Incidence and impact of nausea/vomiting with modern antiemetics: Perception vs. reality [Abstract 996]. *Proceedings of the American Society of Clinical Oncology, 21,* 250a.

Hesketh, P.J. (1997). Proposal for classifying the acute emetogenicity of cancer chemotherapy. *Journal of Clinical Oncology, 15,* 103–109.

Hesketh, P.J. (2001). Potential role of NK1 receptor antagonists in chemotherapy-induced nausea and vomiting. *Supportive Care in Cancer, 9,* 350–354.

Hornby, P.J. (2001). Receptors and transmission in the brain-gut axis: II. Excitatory amino acid receptors in the brain-gut axis. *American Journal of Physiology—Gastrointestinal and Liver Physiology, 280,* 1055–1060.

King, C. (1997). Nonpharmacologic management of chemotherapy-induced nausea and vomiting. *Oncology Nursing Forum, 24*(Suppl. 7), 41–47.

Kosits, C., & Callaghan, M. (2000). Rituximab: A new monoclonal antibody therapy for non-Hodgkin's lymphoma. *Oncology Nursing Forum, 27,* 51–59.

Massaro, A.M., & Lenz, K.L. (2005). Aprepitant: A novel antiemetic for chemotherapy-induced nausea and vomiting. *Annals of Pharmacotherapy, 39,* 77–85.

Mayer, D.J. (2000). Acupuncture: An evidence-based review of the clinical literature. *Annual Review of Medicine, 51,* 49–63.

National Cancer Institute. (2004). *Nausea and vomiting.* Retrieved April 20, 2004, from http://www.nci.nih.gov/cancerinfo/pdq/supportivecare/nausea/healthprofessional#Section_3

National Comprehensive Cancer Network. (2005). *NCCN clinical practice guidelines in oncology, v.1.2005: Antiemesis.* Jenkintown, PA: Author.

O'Bryant, C.L., Gonzales, J.A., & Bestul, D. (2004). Guide to the prevention and management of nausea and vomiting in the oncology setting. The Annual Clinical Reference. *Multinational Association of Supportive Care in Cancer, 7,* 67–74.

Osoba, D., Zee, B., Pater, J., Warr, D., Latreille, J., & Kaizer, L. (1999). Determinants of postchemotherapy nausea and vomiting in patients with cancer. Quality of Life and Symptom Control Committees of the National Cancer Institute of Canada Clinical Trials Group. *Journal of Clinical Oncology, 15,* 116–123.

Perez, E.A., Hesketh, P., Sandbach, J., Reeves, J., Chawla, S., Markman, M., et al. (1998). Comparison of single-dose oral granisetron versus intravenous ondansetron in the prevention of nausea and vomiting induced by moderately emetogenic chemotherapy: A multicenter, double-blind, randomized parallel study. *Journal of Clinical Oncology, 16,* 754–760.

Potter, K., & Schafer, S. (1999). Nausea and vomiting. *American Journal of Nursing, 99*(Suppl. H), 2–4.

Roila, F., Boschetti, E., Tonato, M., Basurto, C., Bracarda, S., Picciafuoco, M., et al. (1991). Predictive factors of delayed emesis in cisplatin-treated patients and antiemetic activity and tolerability of metoclopramide or dexamethasone. A randomized single-blind study. *American Journal of Clinical Oncology, 14,* 238–242.

Ropka, M. (1998). Nutrition. In B. Johnson & J. Gross (Eds.), *Handbook of oncology nursing* (3rd ed., pp. 377–416). Sudbury, MA: Jones and Bartlett.

Wickham, R. (1997). Nausea and vomiting: Are they still a problem? In R. Gates & R. Fink (Eds.), *Oncology nursing secrets* (pp. 250–261). Philadelphia: Hanley & Belfus, Inc.

2. Diarrhea

a) Pathophysiology

(1) Diarrhea is defined as loose or watery stools. Diarrhea resulting from administration of chemotherapy or specific biotherapy agents is a frequent problem. Left untreated or inadequately treated, diarrhea can lead to severe dehydration, hospitalizations, che-

motherapy delays, dose reductions, and even death (Arbuckle, Huber, & Zacher, 2000).

(2) The pathophysiology and etiology of diarrhea in patients with cancer can be multifaceted. All possible causes of diarrhea need to be considered to treat the patient appropriately. The most common mechanisms of chemotherapy-induced diarrhea are osmotic, secretory, and exudative (Martz, 2002).

(a) Osmotic diarrhea: Osmotic diarrhea usually is related to injury to the gut, dietary factors, or problems with digestion. Unabsorbable substances draw water into the intestinal lumen by osmosis, resulting in increased stool volume and weight (Field, 2003). Lactose intolerance is an example of this type of diarrhea, which can occur in patients undergoing cancer treatment (Roy, 2003). Osmotic diarrhea is associated with large stool volumes and sometimes is improved with fasting or elimination of the causative factor (e.g., lactose, glucose) (Vogel, Viele, & Stern, 2004).

(b) Secretory diarrhea: The small and large intestines secrete more fluids and electrolytes than can be absorbed. Infection and inflammation of the gut; damage to the gut caused by chemotherapy, radiation, or graft-versus-host disease (GVHD); and certain endocrine tumors can cause secretory diarrhea. The imbalance between absorption and secretion leads to the production of a large volume of fluid and electrolytes in the small bowel. The fluid can overwhelm the absorptive capacity of the colon, resulting in chemotherapy-induced diarrhea (Wadler et al., 1998). This type of diarrhea is associated with large volumes and usually is not improved with fasting.

(c) Exudative diarrhea: Caused by alterations in mucosal integrity, epithelial loss, and enzyme destruction. Alterations in mucosal integrity coupled with the destruction of enzymes essential to carbohydrate and protein digestion combine to produce moderate to severe levels of diarrhea immediately following, and up to 14 days after, chemotherapy (Engelking, 1998). Mucosal inflammation and ulceration caused by inflammatory diseases, cancers, and cancer treatment may result in the outpouring of plasma, proteins, mucus, and blood into the stool, all of which can result in exudative diarrhea (Field, 2003).

b) Chemotherapy agents presenting the highest risk of diarrhea (Weaver & Buckner, 2004)

(1) Topoisomerase inhibitors

(a) Irinotecan

(b) Topotecan

(2) 5-FU

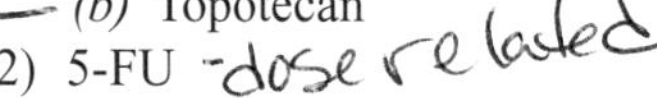

(3) Paclitaxel

(4) Dactinomycin

(5) Dacarbazine

c) Biotherapy agents that may cause diarrhea

(1) IL-2

(2) Interferons

(3) Monoclonal antibodies

d) Other agents that may cause diarrhea

(1) Fludarabine

(2) Cytarabine

(3) Idarubicin

(4) Mitoxantrone

(5) Pentostatin

(6) Floxuridine

(7) Capecitabine

(8) Cisplatin

(9) Oxaliplatin

(10) Docetaxel

(11) Pemetrexed

e) Incidence of diarrhea following cytotoxic therapy

(1) Up to 90% of patients undergoing chemotherapy and/or radiation therapy may experience diarrhea (Tuchmann &

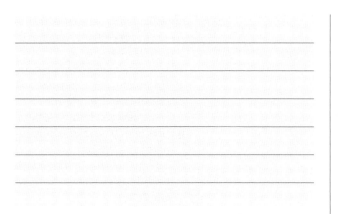

Engelking, 2001). Of patients receiving chemotherapy only, 10%–30% experience chemotherapy-induced diarrhea (Prudden, 2000).

(2) The specific agent, dose, schedule, and combination with other anticancer therapies all influence the severity of chemotherapy-induced diarrhea.

f) Clinical manifestations and consequences: If manifestations are severe, the course of action may be to modify or hold the chemotherapeutic agent, which could compromise the benefit of the regimen. The clinical manifestations of diarrhea include the following (Vogel et al., 2004).

(1) Dehydration: Diarrhea dehydrates pediatric patients very quickly.

(2) Life-threatening hypokalemia, metabolic acidosis, hypercalcemia, malnutrition

(3) Cardiovascular compromise

(4) Impaired immune function following frequent episodes of chemotherapy-induced diarrhea

(5) Reduced absorption of oral medications

(6) Pain

(7) Anxiety

(8) Exhaustion and decreased quality of life

g) Risk factors (Hogan, 1998)

(1) Radiation therapy to the pelvis, abdomen, or lower thoracic and lumbar spine. This can lead to destruction of the cells of the lumen of the bowel.

(2) 5-FU in combination with high-dose leucovorin (500 mg/m^2) or 5-FU administered as a weekly bolus (versus continuous infusion) (Goldberg et al., 2004). Irinotecan can be associated with both acute and delayed diarrhea.

(3) Immunosuppression

(4) Intestinal resection or gastrectomy

(5) Manipulation of bowel during surgery, which may cause diarrhea or ileus

(6) Intestinal infection secondary to mucositis and neutropenia (e.g., infection with *Rotavirus, Escherichia coli, Shigella, Salmonella, Giardia,* or *Clostridium difficile*)

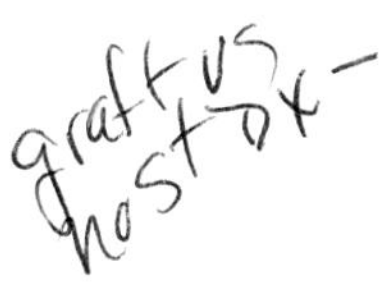

(7) GVHD

(8) Dietary causes (e.g., lactose intolerance; ingestion of caffeine, alcohol, or spicy or fatty foods; use of hyperosmotic dietary supplements)

(9) Inflammatory conditions, such as diverticulitis, irritable bowel syndrome, or ulcerative colitis

(10) Malabsorption with partial bowel obstruction, bowel edema, motility disruption

(11) Anxiety and stress

h) Assessment: Accurate assessment is vital in determining the cause and type of diarrhea; knowing the cause and type can be crucial to proper treatment (e.g., mistakenly using an antidiarrheal to treat diarrhea caused by infection can intensify diarrhea severity and infectious complications). Likewise, irinotecan causes two distinct forms of diarrhea (early onset and late onset), and each requires a different management strategy (Pfizer Oncology, 2004).

(1) Assess stools.

(a) Assess the pattern of elimination and stool character in relation to treatments (i.e., onset, duration, frequency, consistency, amount, odor, color). Chemotherapy-induced diarrhea usually consists of frequent, watery to semisolid stools with an onset 24–96 hours after chemotherapy administration (Engelking, 2003).

(b) Grade the diarrhea according to NCI criteria.

(c) Watch for the presence of blood or mucus in the stools.

(d) Monitor the patient for incontinence.

(2) Conduct a physical examination: The presence of fever, blood in the stool, abdominal pain, weakness, or dizziness warrant medical attention to rule out infection, bowel obstruction, or dehydration (Wadler, 2004). The steps of a physical examination follow.

(a) Auscultate for bowel sounds.

(b) Palpate and assess the abdomen.
(c) Assess for fecal impaction. Use caution with thrombocytopenic and/or neutropenic patients.
(d) Look for signs of malnutrition, dehydration, electrolyte imbalance, and infectious process.
(e) Ask about the experience of pain.
(f) Assess for fever, weakness, and dizziness.
(g) Determine if blood has been present in the stool.

(3) Take a diet history (Tuchmann & Engelking, 2001).
(a) Determine if dietary habits have changed. Be especially aware of clues that indicate that the amount of fiber in the diet has increased rapidly.
(b) Assess for intake that could contribute to diarrhea (e.g., irritating foods, alcohol, coffee, fiber, fruit, sorbitol-based gum).
(c) Assess for food or lactose intolerances or allergies.

(4) Take a medication history: Assess for use of the following (Tuchmann & Engelking, 2001).
(a) Antacids (especially magnesium-containing compounds)
(b) Antibiotics
(c) Antihypertensives
(d) Potassium supplements
(e) Diuretics
(f) Caffeine
(g) Theophylline
(h) NSAIDs
(i) Antiarrhythmic drugs
(j) Overuse of laxatives or stool softeners
(k) Promotility agents (metoclopramide)
(l) Magnesium oxide
(m) Opioid withdrawal

(5) Assess other factors: As recommended by Hogan (1998), ask about
(a) Travel history (such as to other countries).
(b) Use of alternative therapies (e.g., dietary supplements, herbal remedies).

(6) Take objective measurements (Engelking, 2003).
(a) Monitor intake and output.
(b) Monitor weight.
(c) Monitor laboratory data.
i) Check stool culture results to determine the presence of infection.
ii) Check serum chemistries to determine if electrolyte imbalance, specifically the levels of potassium, and protein-calorie malnutrition (hypoalbuminemia) play roles.
iii) Assess complete blood count (CBC) to determine if infection is present.
(d) Check skin turgor.
(e) Check vital signs.

i) Collaborative management
(1) Monitor number, amount, and consistency of bowel movements. For patients with colostomies, an increase in the number of loose stools daily should be monitored to assess for chemotherapy-induced diarrhea.
(2) Replace fluid and electrolytes, including potassium.
(3) Administer antidiarrheal medication as appropriate to reduce stool frequency, volume, and peristalsis. Reassess the severity of chemotherapy-induced diarrhea at the appropriate interval after antidiarrheal medication. Table 21 lists antidiarrheal medications.

j) Patient and family education: Instruct patients to
(1) Know when to start antidiarrheal medications (e.g., with certain chemotherapeutic agents, antidiarrheal medication should be provided so that patients can self-administer at the onset of diarrhea).
(2) Eat foods containing pectin, such as bananas, avocados, and asparagus tips (all three also are high in potassium); beets; unspiced applesauce; and peeled apples (Hogan, 1998).

Table 21. Common Antidiarrheal Medications

Agent	Dose and Mechanism of Action*	Contraindications*
	Antimotility agents	
Diphenoxylate HCl with atropine sulfate (Lomotil®)	Adults: Individualize dosage. Initial dose is 5 mg 4 times a day. Slows gut and promotes reabsorption of water; antiperistaltic	Invasive bacterial diarrhea, pseudomembranous colitis Patients with advanced liver disease Should not be used in children younger than age two
Loperamide (Imodium® AD, Kaopectate® II, Maalox® Antidiarrheal)	Adults: 4 mg initially, followed by 2 mg after each unformed stool; do not exceed 16 mg/day (see product information); doses are higher for irinotecan-induced diarrhea prophylaxis. Slows the gut and promotes reabsorption of water; antiperistaltic	Invasive bacterial diarrhea Should not be used in children younger than age two
	Absorbent agents	
Attapulgite, activated (Kaopectate®)	Adults: 1,200 mg after each bowel movement, up to 7 doses per day. Binds to bacteria and prevents water loss	Patients with blood or mucus in stool May interfere with absorption of some medications
Calcium polycarbophil (FiberCon®, Equalactin®)	Adults: 1 g 1–4 times daily or as needed; do not exceed 6 g in 24 hours. Binds to bacteria and prevents water loss	Patients with blood or mucus in stool May interfere with absorption of some medications
	Antisecretory agents	
Bismuth subsalicylate (Pepto-Bismol®)	Adults: 2 tablets or 30 ml every 30 minutes to 1 hour, as needed, up to 8 doses in 24 hours	Interacts with warfarin and tetracycline Caution with concomitant aspirin/salicylates Can darken stool and tongue
Octreotide (Sandostatin®)	Adults: IV/IM and SQ doses for chemotherapy-induced diarrhea vary. Studies are under way to determine the therapeutic dose and efficacy for long-acting Sandostatin. Slows the gut and promotes reabsorption and decreases secretion of fluids	May interact with insulin, oral hypoglycemic medications, beta blockers, calcium channel blockers May decrease levels of cyclosporine when given concurrently May increase risk of gallstones
	Anticholinergics	
Atropine	Adults: Used for early onset cholinergic diarrhea (e.g., irinotecan-induced) 0.25–1 mg IV or SQ	Dry mouth, blurred vision, photophobia
Belladonna	Consult product information.	Dry mouth, blurred vision, photophobia Many formulations exist.
Scopolamine (transdermal scopolamine patch)	1.5 mg patch lasts 72 hours.	Dry mouth, blurred vision, photophobia Do not apply to irritated skin. Wash hands after applying and removing patch.

*Consult product information for complete list of contraindications, drug interactions, and dosage ranges.

Note. Based on information from Rosenoff, 2004; Wadler, 2004.

(3) Drink ginger tea, which has a high pectin level (Hogan, 1998).
(4) Eliminate from the diet foods that are stimulating or irritating to the GI tract (e.g., whole-grain products, nuts, seeds, popcorn, pickles, relishes, rich pastries, raw vegetables).
(5) Eat a low-residue, low-roughage, low-fat diet that includes potassium-rich foods, such as the BRAT diet (bananas, rice, apples [peeled], and toast [dry]).
(6) Avoid alcohol, caffeine-containing products, and tobacco.

(7) Avoid greasy foods, spicy foods (curry, chili powder, garlic), and fried foods.
(8) Maintain fluid intake by drinking 8–10 large glasses each day of clear fluids (e.g., bouillon; weak, tepid tea; gelatin; sports drinks). Water alone lacks the needed electrolytes and vitamins. Carbonated and caffeinated drinks contain relatively few electrolyes and may worsen diarrhea. Fluids with glucose are useful because glucose absorption drives sodium and water back into the body (Tuchmann & Engelking, 2001).
(9) Avoid prune juice and orange juice.
(10) Eat food at room temperature. Hot and cold foods may aggravate diarrhea.
(11) Avoid milk and dairy products.
(12) Avoid hyperosmotic supplements (e.g., Ensure® [Ross Products, Columbus, OH]), which can contribute to the production of loose, high-volume stools (Wadler, 2004).
(13) Clean the rectal area with mild soap and water after each bowel movement, rinse well, and pat dry with a soft towel. Cleaning decreases the risk of infection and skin irritation. Moisture-barrier ointment may provide additional protection.
(14) Take warm sitz baths to relieve pain related to perianal inflammation. Corticosteroid creams or sprays also may help to relieve pain related to inflammation (Tuchmann & Engelking, 2001).
(15) Understand when diarrhea can be self-managed and when to seek help.
(16) Report excessive thirst, fever, dizziness or lightheadedness, palpitations, rectal spasms, excessive cramping, watery or bloody stools, and continued diarrhea in spite of antidiarrheal treatment. These symptoms can be life-threatening.

References

Arbuckle, R.B., Huber, S.L., & Zacher, C. (2000). The consequences of diarrhea occurring during chemotherapy for colorectal cancer: A retrospective analysis. *Oncologist, 5,* 250–259.

Engelking, C. (1998). Cancer-treatment-related diarrhea: Challenges and barriers to clinical practice. *Oncology Nursing Updates: Patient Treatment and Support, 5*(2), 1–16.

Engelking, C. (2003). Diarrhea. In C.H. Yarbro, M.H. Frogge, & M. Goodman (Eds.), *Cancer symptom management* (3rd ed.). Sudbury, MA: Jones and Bartlett.

Field, M. (2003). Intestinal ion transport and the pathophysiology of diarrhea. *Journal of Clinical Investigation, 111,* 931–943.

Goldberg, R.M., Sargent, D.J., Morton, R.F., Fuchs, C.S., Ramanathan, R.K., Williamson, S.K., et al. (2004). A randomized controlled trial of fluorouracil plus leucovorin, irinotecan, and oxaliplatin combinations in patients with previously untreated and metastatic colorectal cancer. *Journal of Clinical Oncology, 22,* 23–30.

Hogan, C. (1998). The nurse's role in diarrhea management. *Oncology Nursing Forum, 25,* 879–886.

Martz, C. (2002). *Diarrhea in cancer symptom management* (2nd ed.). Retrieved January 10, 2005, from http://www.cancersource.com

Pfizer Oncology. (2004). *Camptosar: Side effects.* Retrieved December 6, 2004, from http://www.camptosar.com/camptosarEffects1.asp

Prudden, J. (2000). Clinical consequences and prophylaxis of chemotherapy-induced diarrhea. *Oncology Special Edition, 3.* New York: McMahon Publishing Group.

Rosenoff, S.H. (2004). Octreotide LAR resolves severe chemotherapy-induced diarrhea (CID) and allows continuation of full-dose therapy. *European Journal of Cancer Care, 13,* 380–383.

Roy, P. (2003). *Lactose intolerance.* Retrieved January 10, 2005, from http://www.emedicine.com

Tuchmann, L., & Engelking, C. (2001). Cancer-related diarrhea. In R.A. Gates & R.M. Fink (Eds.), *Oncology nursing secrets* (2nd ed., pp. 310–322). Philadelphia: Hanley & Belfus, Inc.

Vogel, W., Viele, C., & Stern, J. (2004, April). *Cancer treatment-induced diarrhea: Interventions to minimize the roller coaster ride* [Continuing education program]. Ancillary event presented at the Oncology Nursing Society 29th Annual Congress, Anaheim, CA.

Wadler, S. (2004). Treatment guidelines for chemotherapy-induced diarrhea. *Oncology Special Edition, 7,* 83–87.

Wadler, S., Benson, A., Engelking, C., Catalano, R., Field, M., Kornblau, S., et al. (1998). Recommended guidelines for the treatment of chemotherapy-induced diarrhea. *Journal of Clinical Oncology, 16,* 3169–3178.

Weaver, C., & Buckner, C.D. (2004). *Managing side effects treatment and prevention: Chemotherapy-induced diarrhea.* Retrieved January 10, 2005, from http://patient.cancerconsultants.com/supportive_treatment.aspx?id=1002

3. Mucositis: Mucositis is a common complication of both systemic cytotoxic therapy and radiation therapy. It can be a dose-limiting toxicity of hyperfractionated radiotherapy and concurrent chemotherapy and radiation (NCI, 2004; Rubenstein et al., 2004). Terms used in this discussion include the following.
   - *Mucositis:* A general term referring to an inflammation of the mucosa, including inflammation of the oral cavity
   - *Stomatitis* or *oral mucositis:* Inflammation of the oral cavity

   a) Pathophysiology: Oral mucositis traditionally has been attributed to the direct effects of cytotoxic drugs or radiation on the epithelial stem cells. More recently, evidence has suggested that microvascular injury and connective tissue damage in the submucosa precede epithelial damage. Oral mucositis is now described as having five phases (Sonis, 2004; Sonis et al., 2004).

(1) Initiation: Stomatotoxic drugs or radiation therapy generate reactive oxygen species that damage DNA, resulting in cell, tissue, and blood vessel damage in the mucosa.

(2) Upregulation and generation of messenger signals: Nuclear factor-κB (NF-κB) is activated by chemotherapy or radiation therapy. This results in the upregulation of a large number of genes and the release of pro-inflammatory cytokines, such as tumor necrosis factor-alpha (TNF-α), IL-1 beta (IL-1β), and IL-6. These and other cytokines are responsible for tissue injury and apoptosis.

(3) Signaling and amplification: In addition to direct tissue damage caused by the pro-inflammatory cytokines, these activate the further production of tissue-damaging TNF-α, IL-1β, and IL-6, and other cytokines that alter the tissues in the mucosa.

(4) Ulceration: Tissue injury in the oral mucosa appears as ulcers that penetrate through the epithelium to the submucosa. Bacteria penetrate the submucosa and stimulate macrophage activity, which further increases the release of pro-inflammatory cytokines. Angiogenesis also is stimulated.

(5) Healing: Signals from the extracellular tissues stimulate epithelial proliferation until the mucosa returns to its normal thickness. Tissues do not return completely to normal, however, placing them at increased risk for future injury.

b) Incidence: Oral mucositis occurs in

(1) 30%–40% of patients receiving standard-dose chemotherapy (Goldberg, Chiang, Selina, & Hamarman, 2004; NCI, 2004; Rubenstein et al., 2004)

(2) 80% of stem cell transplant recipients (NCI, 2004)

(3) Up to 100% of patients undergoing head and neck radiation therapy (NCI, 2004).

c) Risk factors

(1) Chemotherapeutic agents that affect DNA synthesis are the most stomatotoxic (Dodd, 2004), but the drug class alone does not predict mucositis risk (NCI, 2004). The following classes of chemotherapy agents have been associated with mucositis.

(a) Antimetabolites

(b) Antitumor antibiotics

(c) Alkylating agents

(d) Plant alkaloids

(2) Biotherapeutic agents, particularly IL-2, lymphokine-activated killers (LAKs), TNF, and interferons (Madeya, 1996a)

(3) Drugs or therapies that alter mucous membranes (Beck, 2004)

(a) Oxygen therapy: Dries out the mucosal lining

(b) Anticholinergics: Decrease salivary flow

(c) Phenytoin: Causes gingival hyperplasia

(d) Steroids: Can result in fungal overgrowth

(4) Total body irradiation or radiation therapy to the head or neck

(5) Dental disease and poor oral hygiene (Beck, 2004)

(6) Ill-fitting dentures: Ill-fitting dentures irritate the mucosa and break integrity (Beck, 2004).

(7) Advanced age and youth: Elderly patients and children have a higher risk of mucositis than do others (Beck, 2004).

(a) Elderly patients are at risk because of degenerative changes, decreased salivary flow, diminished keratinization of mucosa, and increased prevalence of gingivitis.

(b) Children are at risk because of immature immune response, increased cellular proliferation, and higher prevalence of hematologic malignancies.

(8) History of alcohol and/or tobacco use: Alcohol and tobacco irritate the mucosa (Beck, 2004).

(9) Poor nutrition

(a) Reduced nutritional intake delays healing.

(b) A diet high in refined sugars promotes dental decay (Beck, 2004).

(10) Consumption of irritating foods: Acidic or spicy foods inflame and traumatize mucosa (Beck, 2004).

(11) Dehydration: Dehydration alters mucosal integrity.

(12) Head and neck cancer: Patients with head and neck cancer are at especially high risk if they have surgery followed by radiation therapy.

(13) Leukemia, lymphoma, stem cell transplant: These conditions put patients at risk because their treatment involves drugs with a great potential to produce oral mucositis and cause prolonged neutropenia. They also predispose patients to secondary opportunistic infections (Kemp & Brackett, 1997).

(14) Hepatic or renal impairment: These can result in inadequate metabolism or excretion of certain chemotherapeutic agents (Daeffler, 1998).

(15) Multimodal therapies that traumatize the mucosa (Beck, 2004)

d) Clinical manifestations: The pattern of mucositis varies both by drug regimen and by individual. Intensity and duration vary by type of drug and by dose and frequency of administration. Visible signs of oral mucositis are evident four to five days following standard-dose chemotherapy. Stem cell transplant recipients experience mucositis three to five days following the conditioning regimen. In patients receiving head and neck radiation therapy, mucositis is clinically evident during week two of therapy. Intensity increases with higher doses of cytotoxic drugs. Even drugs that are not usually stomatotoxic (e.g., cyclophosphamide) can cause cellular damage to the mucosa at high doses. The duration of mucositis may be prolonged with frequent administration because there is no time for cellular recovery and healing (Beck, 2004). Signs and symptoms include

(1) Changes in taste and ability to swallow

(2) Hoarseness or decreased voice strength

(3) Pain when swallowing or talking

(4) Changes in the color of the oral mucosa (e.g., pallor, erythema of varying degrees, white patches, discolored lesions or ulcers) (Beck, 2004)

(5) Changes in oral moisture (e.g., amount of saliva, quality of secretions)

(6) Edema of oral mucosa and tongue

(7) Mucosal ulcerations.

e) Assessment

(1) Use a standardized assessment tool when performing a physical examination. Scales designed for clinical use take into account symptoms, signs, and functional disturbances associated with oral mucositis and assign an overall score. Three common tools are

(a) Oral Assessment Guide: This tool contains eight categories that reflect oral health and function (see Table 22).

(b) Oral Cavity Assessment: This tool uses a numeric rating, 1–4, in each of five categories (lips, gingival/oral mucosa, tongue, teeth, and saliva). The total score represents the level of dysfunction: mild (6–10), moderate (11–15), or severe (16–20) (Beck, 2004).

(c) Common Terminology Criteria for Adverse Events: The NCI tool consists of a 0–4 grading index that is associated with descriptions of mucosal changes (NCI, 2003).

(2) Examine the lips, tongue, and oral mucosa after removing dental appliances, for color, moisture, integrity, and cleanliness (Beck, 2004).

(3) Assess the patient for changes in taste, voice, ability to swallow, and comfort during swallowing (Beck, 2004).

(4) Examine the saliva for amount and quality (Beck, 2004).

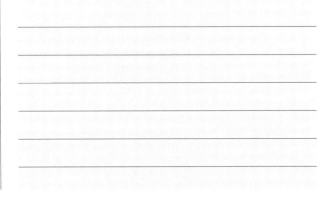

f) Collaborative management: Currently no standard of care exists for the prevention and treatment of oral mucositis. The Multinational Association for Supportive Care in Cancer (MASCC), in collaboration

Table 22. Oral Assessment Guide

Category	Tools for Assessment	Methods of Measurement	Numeric and Descriptive Ratings		
			1	2	3
Voice	Sense of hearing	Converse with patient.	Normal	Deeper than normal or raspy	Difficulty talking or painful to talk
Swallowing	Tongue blade and vision	Ask patient to swallow. To test gag reflex, gently place blade on back of tongue and depress. Observe result.	Normal	Some pain on swallowing	Unable to swallow
Lips	Vision and/or palpation	Observe and feel tissue.	Smooth, pink, and moist	Dry or cracked	Ulcerated or bleeding
Tongue	Vision and/or palpation	Observe and feel tissue.	Pink, moist; papillae present	Coated with a shiny appearance and few papillae, with or without redness	Blistered or cracked
Saliva	Tongue blade and vision	Insert blade into the patient's mouth, touching the center of the tongue and the floor of the mouth. Assess the saliva.	Watery	Thick or ropey	Absent
Mucous membranes	Vision	Observe the tissue.	Pink and moist	Reddened or coated (increased whiteness without ulcerations)	Ulcerations with or without bleeding
Gingiva	Tongue blade and vision	Gently press tissue with tip of blade. Observe the gingiva.	Pink, stippled, and firm	Edematous with or without redness	Spontaneous bleeding or bleeding with pressure
Teeth or dentures (or denture-bearing area)	Vision	Observe the teeth or denture-bearing area.	Clean; no debris	–	Plaque or debris generalized along gum line or denture-bearing area

Note. Table courtesy of June Eilers, PhD, APRN, BC, The Nebraska Health System in Omaha. Used with permission.

with the International Society for Oral Oncology, issued clinical practice guidelines in 2004 with several suggestions and a few recommendations based on literature published between 1966 and 2001. These include the following.

(1) Oral care protocols, including patient education, should be instituted in an attempt to reduce the severity of oral mucositis from chemotherapy and radiation therapy (Rubenstein et al., 2004).

(a) Provide patient education, which is essential in promoting good oral hygiene (Dodd, 2004).

(b) Conduct a pretreatment dental evaluation with attention to potentially irritating teeth surfaces, underlying gingivitis, periodontal infection, and ill-fitting dentures (Dodd, 2004). Crucial dental work should be done before chemotherapy begins. Once therapy begins, neutropenia and throm-

bocytopenia contraindicate corrective dental work (Beck, 2004). Removing braces may be necessary in pediatric patients if they are to undergo transplantation or if prolonged periods of neutropenia are anticipated.

(c) Emphasize intake of high-protein foods and plenty of fluids (> 1,500 ml/day) to encourage oral mucous membrane regeneration (Kemp & Brackett, 1997).

(2) Prevention of oral mucositis (Rubenstein et al., 2004)

(a) Oral cryotherapy (ice chewing) is recommended for patients receiving bolus 5-FU.

(b) Chlorhexidine and acyclovir should not be used to prevent oral mucositis resulting from head and neck radiation or chemotherapy.

(3) Prevention of GI mucositis (Rubenstein et al., 2004)

(a) Either ranitidine or omeprazole is recommended for the prevention of epigastric pain after treatment with cyclophosphamide, methotrexate and 5-FU, or 5-FU with or without folinic acid.

(b) Amifostine is suggested for reducing the severity of esophagitis caused by the combination of chemotherapy and radiation therapy for non-small cell lung cancer.

(4) Treatment: Currently, there are no evidence-based recommendations for the treatment of established oral mucositis. Interventions are aimed at symptom relief and preventing further tissue damage. These interventions may include the following.

(a) Encourage the use of oral agents to promote cleansing, prevent infection, moisturize the oral cavity, maintain mucosal integrity, and promote healing (see Table 23).

(b) Administer systemic pain medications for mucositis pain. The MASCC guidelines recommend the use of patient-controlled analgesia in stem cell transplant recipients experiencing oral mucositis pain (Rubenstein et al., 2004).

(c) Culture mucosal lesions so that appropriate antimicrobial agents can be prescribed (Daeffler, 1998). Candidal lesions look like whitish plaques on the mucosa and often are treated while cultures are pending.

g) Patient and family education: Stress the goals of keeping the oral cavity clean, moist, and intact to prevent further damage to the mucosa during stomatotoxic therapy (Daeffler, 1998). To do this, patients should

(1) Perform a daily oral self-exam and report signs and symptoms of mucositis.

(2) Comply with an oral hygiene program: When mild to moderate dysfunction is present, the frequency of oral hygiene should be increased to every two hours. If the condition progresses to a more severe dysfunction, hourly care may be indicated (Beck & Yasko, 1993). The program should include the following.

(a) Flossing the teeth daily with nontraumatic dental tape (if not contraindicated)

(b) Brushing the teeth with a soft toothbrush or, during periods of neutropenia or thrombocytopenia, a sponge swab

(c) Cleansing the oral cavity after meals, at bedtime, and at other times by vigorously swishing the mouth with an appropriate cleansing agent (see Table 23). Oral rinsing should be done to remove excess debris before applying local anesthetic agents (Kemp & Brackett, 1997).

(d) Avoiding use of oral irrigators, which may force microorganisms into ulcerated and compromised gingival tissue, leading to bacteremia (Madeya, 1996b)

(e) Avoiding irritating agents: Such agents include commercial mouth-

Table 23. Treatment for Oral Mucositis: Available Agents

Agent	Efficacy	Comments
Bland rinses		
0.9% saline solution	Formal evaluation is lacking.	Relatively innocuous and economical
Sodium bicarbonate	Formal evaluation is lacking.	Creates an alkaline environment that promotes bacterial microflora Unpleasant taste may affect adherence. Recommended by NCI
0.9% saline/sodium bicarbonate	Formal evaluation is lacking.	Recommended by NCI
Rinse, multiagent	Data demonstrating efficacy are lacking.	Limited rationale for use Alcohol-based elixirs should be avoided.
Cryotherapy (ice chips)	Demonstrates consistent reduction in incidence and severity of oral mucositis among patients receiving bolus chemotherapy infusion	Impractical for certain patient groups
Coating agents, mucosal protectants		
Sucralfate suspension	Most data demonstrate no statistically significant difference in oral mucositis severity, pain intensity scores, and other subjective symptoms (e.g., taste alteration, dry mouth).	May offer little or no benefit compared to oral hygiene and symptomatic treatment
Prostaglandin E_2	Studies have produced controversial results. Pilot trials have demonstrated significant reductions in pain and mucositis severity compared to placebo, whereas a smaller randomized clinical trial showed no benefit and higher incidence of herpes simplex virus and severe mucositis. Other treatment-associated adverse effects include vomiting, diarrhea, and fever.	Evidence base is insufficient. Further study is needed.
Hydroxypropyl cellulose film	Initial studies are mostly open-label. Certain products may provide some relief for at least three hours. Facilitates ability to cover affected areas over long time periods.	Further study is needed. Protective film must remain intact for effectiveness.
Polyvinylpyrrolidone/sodium hyaluronate	Early data demonstrate statistically significant declines in pain scores and improvement in oral mucositis with short onset times.	Further study is needed. Identified as a class 1 medical device. Provides an occlusive dressing for oral lesions.
Amifostine	Data suggest marked or significant reductions in mucositis severity compared to placebo or no treatment. Adverse events, including nausea and hypotension, appear to be more pronounced at higher doses.	Optimal dose and route of administration remain to be clarified.
Antiseptic agents		
Chlorhexidine	Overall, data demonstrate no significant change in oral mucositis severity or suppression of any type of oral microflora.	Reports of rinse-induced discomfort, taste alteration, and teeth staining
Hydrogen peroxide	Mixed results: Linked to exacerbation or dryness, stinging, pain, and nausea; some reports of intensification of symptoms as a result of glossodynia	Long-term use is discouraged. At full potency, it may break down new granulation tissue and disrupt normal oral flora.

(Continued on next page)

Table 23. Treatment for Oral Mucositis: Available Agents *(Continued)*

Agent	Efficacy	Comments
Povidone-iodine	Possesses antiviral, antibacterial, and antifungal efficacy; well tolerated	Potency limits use in patients with new granulation tissue. Swallowing is contraindicated. Further study is needed.
Anti-inflammatory agents		
Kamillosan liquidum rinse	Unfavorable results in clinical trials	Most patients appear to develop mucositis despite treatment.
Chamomile	Lacks data demonstrating its efficacy	Inexpensive, readily available, and innocuous
Oral corticosteroids	No significant difference in degree of mucositis compared to placebo	Data are limited; definitive conclusions cannot be drawn.
Topical analgesics		
Lidocaine	Limited data; may provide significant relief of limited duration	Requires frequent application; may lead to decreased sensitivity and additional trauma, and may impair taste perception Prophylaxis is not recommended.
Capsaicin	Pilot data demonstrated marked reduction in oral pain.	Clinical potential possibility linked to re-epithelization and elevation of pain threshold. Further study is warranted.
Topical morphine	May have limited utility. Data suggest reduction in pain severity and duration of pain.	Alcohol-based formulations may cause burning.
Antiproliferative, mucosal protectant, cytokine-like agents and growth factors		
Granulocyte macrophage–colony-stimulating factor	Some data indicate reduction in oral mucositis severity and pain; others do not.	May prove especially beneficial for patients receiving chemotherapy or radiation therapy High drug discontinuation because of intolerable side effects, including local skin reaction, fever, bone pain, and nausea when administered subcutaneously
Granulocyte–colony-stimulating factor	Limited data; some indication of significant reductions of oral mucositis severity in bone marrow transplant recipients and oral mucositis occurrence in patients undergoing radiation therapy when used prophylactically	Further study is needed to draw any conclusion.
Transforming growth factor-β3	Limited data, mixed outcome; animal data demonstrate favorable results, but clinical data fail to demonstrate any significant advantage compared to placebo.	Further study is warranted.
Epidermal growth factor	Limited data, animal studies only; in hamsters, linked to worsening of severity and duration of mucositis	Utility in treatment of mucositis appears to be limited.

Note. Based on information from Cerchietti et al., 2002; Clarkson et al., 2003; Foncuberta et al., 2001; Knox et al., 2000; Kostler et al., 2001; Mantovani et al., 2003; Miller & Kearney, 2001; NCI, 2004; Redding & Haveman, 1999; Saarilahti et al., 2002; Shih et al., 2002; Smith, 2001; Sprinzl et al., 2001; Valcarcel et al., 2002. From "Nursing Interventions and Supportive Care for the Prevention and Treatment of Oral Mucositis Associated With Cancer Treatment," by J. Eilers, *Oncology Nursing Forum, 31*(Suppl. 4), pp. 19–20. Copyright 2004 by the Oncology Nursing Society. Reprinted with permission.

washes containing phenol, astringents, or alcohol; highly abrasive toothpastes; hot or spicy foods and beverages; alcohol; tobacco; poorly fitting dentures; braces; and lemon-glycerin swabs and solutions.

References

Beck, S. (2004). Mucositis. In C.H. Yarbro, M.H. Frogge, & M. Goodman (Eds.), *Cancer symptom management* (3rd ed., pp. 276–287). Sudbury, MA: Jones and Bartlett.

Beck, S., & Yasko, J. (1993). *Guidelines for oral care* (2nd ed.). Crystal Lake, IL: Sage Products, Inc.

Cerchietti, L.C., Navigante, A.H., Bonomi, M.R., Zaderajko, M.A., Menendez, P.R., Pogany, C.E., et al. (2002). Effect of topical morphine for mucositis-associated pain following concomitant chemoradiotherapy for head and neck carcinoma. *Cancer, 95,* 2230–2236.

Clarkson, J.E., Worthington, H.V., & Eden, O.B. (2003). Interventions for preventing oral mucositis for patients with cancer receiving treatment. *Cochrane Database System Review, 3,* CD000978.

Daeffler, R. (1998). Protective mechanisms: Mucous membranes. In B. Johnson & J. Gross (Eds.), *Handbook of oncology nursing* (3rd ed., pp. 440–459). Sudbury, MA: Jones and Bartlett.

Dodd, M.J. (2004). The pathogenesis and characterization of oral mucositis associated with cancer therapy. *Oncology Nursing Forum, 31*(Suppl. 4), 5–23.

Foncuberta, M.C., Cagnoni, P.J., Brandts, C.H., Mandanas, R., Fields, K., Derigs, H.G., et al. (2001). Topical transforming growth factor-b3 in the prevention or alleviation of chemotherapy-induced oral mucositis in patients with lymphomas or solid tumors. *Journal of Immunotherapy, 24,* 384–388.

Goldberg, S.L., Chiang, L., Selina, N., & Hamarman, S. (2004). Patient perceptions about chemotherapy-induced oral mucositis: Implications for primary/secondary prophylaxis strategies. *Supportive Care in Cancer, 12,* 526–530.

Kemp, J., & Brackett, H. (1997). Mucositis. In R. Gates & R. Fink (Eds.), *Oncology nursing secrets* (pp. 245–249). Philadelphia: Hanley & Belfus.

Knox, J.J., Puodziunas, A.L.V., & Feld, R. (2000). Chemotherapy-induced oral mucositis. Prevention and management. *Drugs and Aging, 17,* 257–267.

Kostler, W.J., Hejna, M., Wenzel, C., & Zielinski, C.C. (2001). Oral mucositis complicating chemotherapy and/or radiotherapy: Options for prevention and treatment. *CA: A Cancer Journal for Clinicians, 51,* 290–315.

Madeya, M. (1996a). Oral complications from cancer therapy: Part 1—Pathophysiology and secondary complications. *Oncology Nursing Forum, 23,* 801–807.

Madeya, M. (1996b). Oral complications from cancer therapy: Part 2—Nursing implications for assessment and treatment. *Oncology Nursing Forum, 23,* 808–819.

Mantovani, G., Massa, E., Astara, G., Murgia, V., Gramignano, G., Lusso, M.R., et al. (2003). Phase II clinical trial of local use of GM-CSF for prevention and treatment of chemotherapy- and concomitant chemoradiotherapy-induced severe oral mucositis in advanced head and neck cancer patients: An evaluation of effectiveness, safety and costs. *Oncology Reports, 10,* 197–206.

Miller, M., & Kearney, N. (2001). Oral care for patients with cancer: A review of the literature. *Cancer Nursing, 24,* 241–254.

National Cancer Institute. (2003). *Common terminology criteria for adverse events v.3.0.* Retrieved October 16, 2004, from http://ctep.cancer.gov/forms/CTCAEv3.pdf

National Cancer Institute. (2004). *Oral complications of chemotherapy and head/neck radiation.* Retrieved October 16, 2004, from http://www.cancer.gov/cancertopics/pdq/supportivecare/oralcomplications/HealthProfessional

Redding, S.W., & Haveman, C.W. (1999). Treating the discomfort of oral ulceration resulting from cancer chemotherapy. *Compendium of Continuing Education in Dentistry, 20,* 389–392, 394, 396.

Rubenstein, E.B., Peterson, D.E., Schubert, M., Keefe, D., McGuire, D., Epstein, J., et al. (2004). Clinical practice guidelines for the prevention and treatment of cancer therapy-induced oral and gastrointestinal mucositis. *Cancer, 100*(Suppl. 9), 2026–2046.

Saarilahti, K., Kajanti, M., Joensuu, T., Kouri, M., & Joensuu, H. (2002). Comparison of granulocyte-macrophage colony-stimulating factor and sucralfate mouthwashes in the prevention of radiation-induced mucositis: A double-blind prospective randomized phase III study. *International Journal of Radiation Oncology, Biology, Physics, 54,* 479–485.

Shih, A., Miaskowski, C., Dodd, M.J., Stotts, N.A., & MacPhail, L. (2002). A research review of the current treatments for radiation-induced oral mucositis in patients with head and neck cancer. *Oncology Nursing Forum, 29,* 1063–1080.

Smith, T. (2001). Gelclair: Managing the symptoms of oral mucositis. *Hospital Medicine, 62,* 623–626.

Sonis, S.T. (2004). A biological approach to mucositis. *Journal of Supportive Oncology, 2,* 21–36.

Sonis, S.T., Elting, L.S., Keefe, D., Peterson, D.E., Schubert, M., Hauer-Jensen, M., et al. (2004). Perspectives on cancer therapy-induced mucosal injury. *Cancer, 100*(Suppl. 9), 1995–2011.

Sprinzl, G.M., Galvan, O., de Vries, A., Ulmer, H., Gunkel, A.R., Lukas, P., et al. (2001). Local application of granulocyte-macrophage colony stimulating factor (GM-CSF) for the treatment of oral mucositis. *European Journal of Cancer, 37,* 2003–2009.

Valcarcel, D., Sanz, M.A., Jr., Sureda, A., Sala, M., Munoz, L., Subirá, M., et al. (2002). Mouth-washings with recombinant human granulocyte-macrophage colony stimulating factor (rhGM-CSF) do not improve grade III-IV oropharyngeal mucositis (OM) in patients with hematological malignancies undergoing stem cell transplantation. Results of a randomized double-blind placebo-controlled study. *Bone Marrow Transplantation, 29,* 783–787.

4. Anorexia
   a) Pathophysiology: *Anorexia* refers to a loss of appetite and subsequent reduction in food intake that results from a complicated process involving numerous physiologic and psychological factors.
      (1) Alterations in the sense of taste
         (a) These may result as a direct effect of the tumor itself, from oral infections (e.g., *Candida* infections), or from the effect of various treatments (e.g., chemotherapy, radiation therapy, surgery, antibiotic treatment) (Capra, Ferguson, & Ried, 2001).

(b) Patients receiving biotherapeutic agents commonly report changes in the sense of taste (Rieger, 1999).

(c) Taste abnormalities may resolve shortly after treatment or may persist, leading to food aversions and slowed digestion caused by decreases in digestive enzymes (Cunningham, 2004).

(d) Altered sense of taste is referred to as *dysgeusia.*

(e) Diminished sense of taste is called *hypogeusia.*

(f) Common taste alterations include the following (Cunningham, 2004).

i) A decreased threshold for bitter tastes, causing a dislike of or an aversion to beef, pork, chocolate, coffee, or tomatoes

ii) An increased threshold for sweet tastes, leading patients to add sugar to many foods

iii) A decreased threshold for sweet tastes

iv) An increased desire for salt on foods

v) A decreased threshold for sour foods

vi) A metallic or medicinal taste

(2) Alterations in GI function: Chemotherapy can be toxic to normal cells found along the GI mucosa, affecting the digestion and absorption of nutrients (Capra et al., 2001).

(a) Ulceration of the mucous membranes may produce mucositis or diarrhea, which can interfere with ingestion, digestion, or absorption.

(b) Nausea and vomiting may decrease appetite and create food aversions.

(c) Early satiety may be related to GI tumors, ascites, hepatomegaly, or splenomegaly.

(3) Metabolic abnormalities

(a) Abnormalities in glucose metabolism may lead to elevated blood glucose levels, which may suppress appetite (Cunningham, 2004).

(b) Increases in circulating amino acids or lactic acid may cause early satiety (Cunningham, 2004).

(c) Increases in free fatty acids may cause early satiety (Cunningham, 2004).

(d) Increases in levels of serotonin or tryptophan in the brain affect CNS control over appetite (Tisdale, 2001).

(e) Electrolyte abnormalities as seen in TLS, including hypercalcemia, hypokalemia, uremia, and hyponatremia (Richerson, 2004)

(4) Psychological changes (Finley, 2003)

(a) Depression

(b) Grief

(c) Anxiety

(d) Pain

(e) Fatigue

(5) GI abnormalities: Anorexia is one of the most common neurologic side effects of cytokine immunotherapy. It can be accompanied by other GI manifestations, such as nausea, vomiting, or taste aversion (Plata-Salaman, 1998).

(6) Social or cultural food preferences or dining behaviors

(7) Effects of the tumor (Inui, 2002)

(a) Tumors can secrete substances (e.g., cytokines, IL-1) that circulate and affect various regulatory mechanisms involving hunger, satiety, and metabolism.

(b) Malignant cells may produce peptides that cause satiety.

(c) Malignant processes might cause abnormal neuronal or hormonal signals from the GI tract that directly influence the hypothalamic appetite centers.

b) Incidence (Haapoja, 2000)

(1) Anorexia may occur with any type of cancer.

(2) Although difficult to determine, the incidence of anorexia and cachexia in

the oncologic population is estimated to occur in 60%–70% of patients with advanced malignant disease.

(3) Anorexia-cachexia can occur at any time during the disease process and usually is related to a high tumor burden.

(4) Anorexia frequently is one of the earliest manifestations of cancer. It has been shown to improve with successful anticancer treatment, which supports the idea that it is a paraneoplastic process.

c) Clinical consequences (Finley, 2003)

(1) Decreases in digestive enzymes, which may yield a delay in digestion

(2) Progressive deterioration of nutrition resulting in cachexia, which is characterized by weight loss, skeletal muscle atrophy, and asthenia

(3) Compromise of other bodily functions (e.g., weakness, fatigue)

(4) Lower resistance to infection

(5) Slow healing

d) Risk factors (Cunningham, 2004)

(1) Advanced age

(2) Health problems that can affect nutrition, such as diabetes, renal disease, and thyroid disorders

(3) Type of therapy used: Multimodality therapy may increase risk of nutritional complications.

(4) Uncontrolled pain

(5) Psychological factors (e.g., patients' body image, factors relating to the home environment)

e) Assessment: Nutritional screening is helpful to identify patients at risk for malnutrition due to the disease or treatment process (Cunningham, 2004).

(1) Assess factors related to food.

(a) Obtain a diet history.

(b) Ask about food preferences, food intolerances, food aversions, and food allergies.

(c) Encourage patients to use a food diary to record the amount and types of food and beverages consumed. This usually is done over three consecutive 24-hour periods. Other means of documenting intake include a food frequency questionnaire, direct observation and recording, and evaluation of nutrient intake according to standard nutrition criteria (such as the Recommended Dietary Allowances) (Cunningham, 2004).

(d) Assess education needs regarding diet and nutrition and psychosocial factors (e.g., family support, religious and cultural factors) that affect eating.

(e) Determine patients' ability to obtain, purchase, and prepare food.

(2) Perform a physical examination.

(a) Monitor patients' height and weight. Weigh patients on the same scale each day/visit. Compare current measurements with pretreatment measurements. An unintentional weight loss of 10% or more of body weight within the previous six months or more than 5% in one month signifies a substantial nutrition deficit (Cunningham, 2004).

(b) Assess skin, hair, mouth, teeth, and general muscle tone for signs of nutrition deficiencies. (Look for dry, flaky skin; muscle wasting; pale skin or sclera; unhealed wounds.)

(c) Take anthropometric measurements, which quantify body compartments and correlate them with values from age- and sex-matched normal populations. Mid-arm muscle circumference provides a measure of muscle mass. Measurements of subscapular and triceps skinfolds represent an index of body fat (Cunningham, 2004).

(3) Evaluate laboratory results. (Be aware of the fact that biotherapy, which usually involves an increase in interferon alpha, IL-1, TNF, and other cytokines, increases the rate of lipolysis, decreases lipoprotein lipase activity, increases fatty-acid synthesis, decreases insulin receptor tyrosine kinase activity, and increases serum triglyceride levels.

These effects may be evident in the lab results of patients with anorexia who are undergoing biotherapy.) In regard to patients undergoing biotherapy and chemotherapy, monitor the levels of the following (Foltz, 2000).

(a) Serum transferrin: The level of serum transferrin reflects the body's ability to make serum proteins. A value < 200 mg/dl reflects acute changes in visceral protein (Bender et al., 2002).

(b) Serum albumin: Measurements of serum albumin are used to estimate visceral protein levels. A value < 3.5 g/dl indicates protein depletion (Bender et al., 2002). Albumin levels may be influenced by body stresses (e.g., trauma, infection), changes in hydration status, and alteration in liver and renal functions.

(c) Serum prealbumin: The level of serum prealbumin is a sensitive indicator of changes in nutrition status. A level < 15 mg/dl indicates protein depletion (Bender et al., 2002).

(d) Lymphocyte count: A depleted lymphocyte count indicates decreased immunocompetence.

(e) Electrolytes, minerals, trace elements, and vitamins: Levels of these components can help to confirm or dispute physical observations. Zinc deficiency can cause taste and smell alterations. A deficiency of magnesium, potassium, or calcium can cause muscle twitching. Pallor can indicate an iron deficiency (Wilson, 2000).

f) Collaborative management: The extent of nutritional intervention depends on the cause of weight loss and the overall goals of the patient and healthcare team. Treatment includes steps to improve patients' nutritional intake while changing the metabolic environment to inhibit muscle and fat wasting (Inui, 2002).

(1) Consult a dietitian for help in diet planning. Patients need to maintain access to the dietitian, especially during chemotherapy (McGrath, 2002).

(2) Administer high-calorie, high-protein dietary supplements if indicated.

(3) Administer megestrol acetate if appropriate. Megestrol acetate has been shown to increase appetite, caloric intake, and body weight and provides a sensation of well-being. The recommended dose is 800 mg/day (Inui, 2002).

(4) Glucocorticoids may be used to decrease nausea and improve appetite when used for a limited time (Inui, 2002).

(5) Administer dronabinol if appropriate. Dronabinol has been found to stimulate appetite and improve mood for selected patients (Inui, 2002).

(6) Administer enteral nutrition if the patient cannot meet caloric requirements by oral intake. Enteral nutrition helps to maintain normal gut floral and prevents atrophy of the microvilli lining the intestinal wall (Cunningham, 2004).

(7) Administer total parenteral nutrition (TPN) in patients with altered or absent GI function or those who are intolerant of enteral therapy.

(8) Alert patients to community resources (e.g., Meals on Wheels, or the Special Supplemental Nutrition Program for Women, Infants, and Children [known as WIC]) to assist with nutrition.

g) Patient and family education: Patients and families need well-written, informative material addressing nutritional issues (McGrath, 2002). Teach patients and significant others techniques to help to increase intake and optimize nutritional health (Cunningham, 2004; Sherry, 2002).

(1) Monitor weight weekly, using the same scale at the same time of day.

(2) Eat small, frequent meals.

(3) Incorporate high-protein foods into the diet. Marinate meats to enhance or disguise flavor. Substitute other high-protein foods (e.g., cheese, milk, eggs, beans, nuts, yogurt, puddings, wheat germ) for meat.

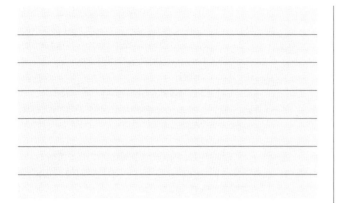

(4) Avoid filling and gas-forming foods (e.g., broccoli, cabbage, fruits, carbonated beverages).
(5) Drink fluids with meals to rinse away bad tastes. Fruit-flavored drinks tend to be well tolerated; coffee and tea frequently are not.
(6) Avoid drinking large quantities of liquids, which may reduce the intake of solid foods.
(7) Eat slowly to allow the stomach to empty while eating.
(8) Take medication for pain or nausea to minimize discomfort, if indicated.
(9) Minimize odors that can affect taste by drinking fluids cold and with a straw and by choosing cold foods such as cheese, milkshakes, cold cuts, and tuna and egg salad.
(10) Use hard candies and fresh fruit, if possible, to eliminate bad tastes in the mouth and leave a more pleasant taste.
(11) Plan daily food-preparation activities to conserve energy.
(12) Experiment with approaches to eating and food preparation.
    (a) Ordering takeout
    (b) Preparing large quantities and freezing smaller portions for later
    (c) Purchasing frozen dinners
    (d) Varying the surroundings (e.g., dining out)
    (e) Using distractions (e.g., radio, TV)
    (f) Trying new foods and recipes
    (g) Arriving at the table immediately before meals to minimize the effect of food odor on appetite
(13) Use gravies or sauces on foods to help spread taste through the mouth and add calories.
(14) Use tart foods to help to overcome metallic tastes.
(15) Use plastic eating utensils and glass or plastic cooking containers if a metallic taste is noted while eating.
(16) In the absence of a sodium restriction, use salt to decrease the excessive sweetness of sugary foods.
(17) Add a small amount of seasoning (e.g., oregano, basil, cinnamon, ginger) to food to enhance food flavor. Strongly seasoned foods (e.g., Italian, Mexican, curried, barbequed dishes) may satisfy the patient who has a diminished sense of taste.
(18) Brush the teeth or rinse the mouth before and after meals to keep the mouth clean and reduce bad tastes. If mucositis is a problem, rinse the mouth with a solution of salt, baking soda, and warm water before eating; the rinse will help eliminate bad tastes.
(19) Avoid cigarette smoke or smoking, which can affect the sense of smell, which affects the sense of taste.
(20) Perform mild exercise for about 20 minutes per day to stimulate muscles and increase strength.
(21) Report symptoms associated with anorexia to the healthcare team.
(22) Report physical changes (e.g., fatigue, anemia, mouth sores) that decrease appetite and require management.

References

Bender, C.M., McDaniel, R.W., Murphy-Ende, K., Pickett, M., Rittenberg, C.N., Rogers, M.P., et al. (2002). Chemotherapy-induced nausea and vomiting. *Clinical Journal of Oncology Nursing, 6,* 94–101.

Capra, S., Ferguson, M., & Ried, K. (2001). Cancer: Impact of nutrition intervention outcome—nutrition issues for patients. *Nutrition, 17,* 769–772.

Cunningham, R.S. (2004). The anorexia-cachexia syndrome. In C.H. Yarbro, M.H. Frogge, & M. Goodman (Eds.), *Cancer symptom management* (3rd ed., pp. 137–167). Sudbury, MA: Jones and Bartlett.

Finley, J. (2003). Detection and management of cachexia in cancer patients. *Advanced Studies in Nursing, 1*(1), 8–12.

Foltz, A.T. (2000). Nutritional disturbances. In C.H. Yarbro, M.H. Frogge, M. Goodman, & S.L. Groenwald (Eds.), *Cancer nursing: Principles and practice* (5th ed., pp. 754–775). Sudbury, MA: Jones and Bartlett.

Haapoja, I.S. (2000). Paraneoplastic syndromes. In C.H. Yarbro, M.H. Frogge, M. Goodman, & S.L. Groenwald (Eds.), *Cancer nursing: Principles and practice* (5th ed., pp. 792–812). Sudbury, MA: Jones and Bartlett.

Inui, A. (2002). Cancer anorexia-cachexia syndrome: Current issues in research and management. *CA: A Cancer Journal for Clinicians, 52,* 72–91.

McGrath, P. (2002). Reflections on nutritional issues associated with cancer therapy. *Cancer Practice, 10,* 94–101.

Plata-Salaman, C. (1998). Cytokines and anorexia: A brief overview. *Seminars in Oncology, 25,* 64–72.

Richerson, M.T. (2004). Electrolyte imbalances. In C.H. Yarbro, M.H. Frogge, & M. Goodman (Eds.), *Cancer symptom management* (3rd ed., pp. 440–453). Sudbury, MA: Jones and Bartlett.

Rieger, P.T. (1999). *Clinical handbook for biotherapy.* Sudbury, MA: Jones and Bartlett.

Sherry, V.W. (2002). Taste alterations among patients with cancer. *Clinical Journal of Oncology Nursing, 6,* 73–76.

Tisdale, M.J. (2001). Cancer anorexia and cachexia. *Nutrition, 17,* 438–442.

Wilson, R. (2000). Optimizing nutrition for patients with cancer. *Clinical Journal of Oncology Nursing, 4,* 23–27.

5. Constipation: Constipation may be a presenting symptom of the cancer diagnosis, a side effect of therapy, or the result of tumor progression. It may be unrelated to the cancer or the therapy (Massey, Haylock, & Curtiss, 2004). Depression and anxiety caused by cancer treatment or pain can lead to constipation, either alone or with other functional and physiologic disorders. The most common causes are inadequate fluid intake and pain medications (NCI, 2004).
   a) Pathophysiology: Decreased motility of the large intestine is the primary cause of constipation. Mechanisms of constipation include altered strength of contractions within the intestines, poor muscle tone within the colon, and sensory changes relating to the rectum and anus (Pace, 1999).
      (1) Agents that decrease motility
         (a) Vinca alkaloids: May cause autonomic nerve dysfunction manifested as colicky abdominal pain and ileus. Specifically, rectal emptying is diminished because nonfunctional afferent and efferent pathways from the sacral cord are interrupted (Camp-Sorrell, 2000).
            i) Vincristine and vinblastine may cause neurotoxicity that affects the smooth muscles of the GI tract, leading to decreased peristalsis or paralytic ileus.
            ii) Vincristine may damage the myenteric plexus of the colon.
            iii) Vinorelbine
      (2) Certain chemotherapy agents that cause nausea and vomiting may contribute to constipation in that they cause the patient to decrease oral intake, slowing peristaltic push-down in the GI tract. When a patient does not eat, less stool is produced, the transit time increases, and the stool becomes hard and difficult to eliminate (Bisanz, 1997).
      (3) Opioids profoundly impact the bowel's ability to maintain appropriate motility. They are the primary cause of medication-induced constipation (Robinson et al., 2000).
   b) Incidence
      (1) Clinically, constipation is a common problem for patients with cancer, especially in advanced stages, and its occurrence has been reported in 40% of individuals with cancer referred to a palliative care service (Massey et al., 2004). Severe constipation may occur in up to 35% of patients receiving chemotherapy. It is more common in elderly patients than in others and may lead to bowel obstruction (Tuchmann, 2001).
      (2) Constipation has been reported in 20% of patients receiving vinblastine, especially in high doses or after prolonged treatment (Clinical Pharmacology, 2004c).
      (3) Constipation, abdominal pain, and paralytic ileus are common side effects of vincristine (Chu & DeVita, 2004).
      (4) Vinorelbine may cause severe (grade III–IV) constipation, with an overall incidence of all grades of 35% (GlaxoSmithKline, 2003).
      (5) Constipation occurs in 3%–30% of patients receiving thalidomide, with an increased incidence at doses > 400 mg/day (Clinical Pharmacology, 2004b).
      (6) Bortezomib causes constipation in 43% of patients (Clinical Pharmacology, 2004a).

c) Clinical consequences
   (1) Discomfort or pain
   (2) Nausea and/or vomiting
   (3) Impaction
   (4) Ileus
   (5) Ruptured bowel and life-threatening sepsis

d) Risk factors (Bisanz, 1997)
   (1) Mechanical pressure on the bowel (e.g., bowel obstruction secondary to tumor in the GI tract, pressure from ascites) (Massey et al., 2004)
   (2) Damage to the spinal cord from T8 to L3, which causes compression of nerves that innervate the bowel
   (3) Decreased mobility
   (4) Dehydration
   (5) Low dietary fiber intake
   (6) Metabolic and endocrine disorders (NCI, 2004; Wright & Thomas, 1995)
      (a) Hypercalcemia
      (b) Addison's disease
      (c) Hypothyroidism and hyperthyroidism
      (d) Cushing's syndrome
      (e) Hypokalemia
      (f) Diabetes mellitus
   (7) Use of certain medications (Massey et al., 2004)
      (a) Neurotoxic chemotherapy drugs
      (b) Anticholinergic medications
      (c) Diuretics
      (d) Opioids
      (e) Aluminum- and calcium-based antacids
      (f) Calcium and iron supplements
      (g) Tricyclic antidepressants
      (h) Antihypertensives
      (i) Anxiolytics
      (j) $5HT_3$ antagonists
      (k) NSAIDs
   (8) Overuse of laxatives

e) Assessment
   (1) Assess patterns of elimination, including the amount and frequency of elimination and the urge to defecate, character of the stool, volume of stool, chronic use of laxatives or softeners, other measures to enhance bowel function (Pace, 1999).
   (2) Assess patients' usual dietary patterns, focusing on fluid and fiber intake.
   (3) Assess mobility, activity level, and functional status.
   (4) Assess abdominal pain or cramping.
   (5) Determine facts about the patient's last bowel movement (e.g., when, amount, consistency, color, presence of blood).
   (6) Determine current medication usage.
   (7) Use laboratory results to assist in metabolic evaluation.
   (8) Perform abdominal palpation and rectal examination. A rectal examination is not routinely performed in pediatric patients.
   (9) Use radiographs to differentiate between mechanical obstruction and decreased motility from an ileus (Tuchmann, 2001).

f) Collaborative management
   (1) Administer laxatives as ordered. Use laxatives from the following groups (Massey et al., 2004).
      (a) Bulk-forming laxatives (e.g., methylcellulose, psyllium): Cause water to be retained in the stool; of limited use for patients who cannot tolerate at least three liters of fluid each day
      (b) Lubricants and emollients (e.g., mineral oil): Coat and soften the stool; excessive doses can lead to rectal seepage and perianal irritation.
      (c) Saline laxatives (magnesium salts, sodium phosphate): Contain magnesium or sulfate ions; act by drawing water into the gut; of little use in a daily prevention program; used most often for acute evacuation of the bowel
      (d) Osmotic laxatives (e.g., lactulose, sorbitol): These attract and retain water in the bowel, resulting in softer stool; effective onset usually is within 24–72 hours after the drug has reached the colon; adverse reactions include abdominal pain, gas, and abdominal distention (Avila, 2004).

(e) Detergent laxatives (e.g., docusate sodium): Have a direct action on the intestines by allowing water and fats to penetrate into dry stool; decrease electrolyte and water absorption from the colon; appropriate for short-term use when straining is to be avoided

(f) Stimulant laxatives: Act directly on the colon to stimulate motility and are activated by bacterial degradation in the intestine; the most commonly used in a prophylactic plan

(g) Suppositories: Stimulate the intestinal nerve plexus and cause rectal emptying. Not indicated for long-term bowel management.

(h) Prokinetic agents (e.g., metoclopramide): Effective for delayed gastric emptying; the appropriate dose is taken prior to meals and at bedtime; the onset of action is within 60 minutes of the oral dose (Avila, 2004).

(2) Use a combination laxative-stool softener prophylactically for patients receiving vinca alkaloids (Tuchmann, 2001).

(3) Include an increase in physical activity or passive exercise as appropriate in a bowel-retraining regimen. These promote the urge to defecate by helping to move feces into the rectum.

(4) Help patients to maintain usual bowel habits during hospitalization. Provide privacy and comfort.

(5) Increase fluids and fiber and begin management with oral medications to help constipated patients with neutropenia or thrombocytopenia.

(6) Avoid performing rectal exams or using suppositories or enemas in patients with neutropenia; these could introduce bacteria into the rectum or lead to anal tears, fissures, or abscesses.

(7) Do not perform rectal exams or use suppositories or enemas in patients with thrombocytopenia; doing so may increase the risk of bleeding (Tuchmann, 2001).

(8) Clinical trials are under way examining the use of methylnaltrexone. This drug has shown efficacy in preventing opioid-induced constipation without diminishing pain palliation or precipitating opioid withdrawal (Yuan, 2004).

g) Patient and family education

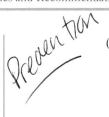

(1) Increase fluid intake: Encourage patients to drink at least eight glasses of fluid daily unless medically contraindicated. Warm liquids before a defecation attempt may be helpful to stimulate bowel movement. Consumption of coffee, tea, and grapefruit juice usually is discouraged because these beverages act as diuretics (Tuchmann, 2001).

(2) Increase fiber in diet: Fiber causes feces to pass through intestines more rapidly and decreases the occurrence of fecal impaction. High-fiber foods include bran, popcorn, corn, raisins, dates, vegetables, fruits, and whole grains. Warn patients that they may experience abdominal discomfort, flatulence, or erratic bowel habits in the first few weeks after increasing fiber. Fiber tolerance will develop, and such effects can be minimized by slowly titrating fiber consumption, starting with the addition of 3–4 g/day and increasing to 6–10 g/day. This approach is contraindicated in cases of structural bowel blockage because increasing bulky intraluminal contents may increase the obstruction (Tuchmann, 2001).

(3) Encourage patients to exercise regularly: Regular exercise stimulates GI motility.

(4) Teach diaphragmatic breathing and abdominal muscle exercises: These help to increase muscle tone, which is necessary for defecation (Tuchmann, 2001).

(5) Help patients to develop a regular bowel program.

(6) Instruct patients to report constipation and to be aware of the complications associated with constipation, such as fecal impaction. Stress that patients should call a physician if three days pass without a bowel movement (Camp-Sorrell, 2000).

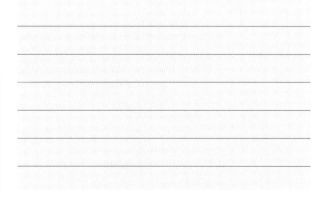

References

Avila, J. (2004). Pharmacologic treatment of constipation in cancer patients. *Cancer Control, 11,* 10–18.

Bisanz, A. (1997). Managing bowel elimination problems in patients with cancer. *Oncology Nursing Forum, 24,* 679–688.

Camp-Sorrell, D. (2000). Chemotherapy: Toxicity management. In C.H. Yarbro, M.H. Frogge, M. Goodman, & S.L. Groenwald (Eds.), *Cancer nursing: Principles and practice* (5th ed., pp. 444–486). Sudbury, MA: Jones and Bartlett.

Chu, E., & DeVita, V.T. (2004). *Physician's cancer chemotherapy drug manual 2004.* Sudbury, MA: Jones and Bartlett.

Clinical Pharmacology. (2004a). *Bortezomib online monograph.* Tampa, FL: Gold Standard. Retrieved September 29, 2004, from http://cpip.gsm.com

Clinical Pharmacology. (2004b). *Thalidomide online monograph.* Tampa, FL: Gold Standard. Retrieved September 29, 2004, from http://cpip.gsm.com

Clinical Pharmacology. (2004c). *Vinblastine online monograph.* Tampa, FL: Gold Standard. Retrieved September 29, 2004, from http://cpip.gsm.com

GlaxoSmithKline. (2003). Navelbine [Package insert]. Research Triangle Park, NC: Author.

Massey, R.L., Haylock, P.J., & Curtiss, C. (2004). Constipation. In C.H. Yarbro, M.H. Frogge, & M. Goodman (Eds.), *Cancer symptom management* (3rd ed., pp. 512–527). Sudbury, MA: Jones and Bartlett.

National Cancer Institute. (2004). *Gastrointestinal complications.* Retrieved September 29, 2004, from http://www.nci.nih.gov/cancertopics/ pdq/supportivecare/gastrointestinalcomplications/Patient/page3

Pace, J. (1999). Symptom management. In C. Miaskowski & P. Buchsel (Eds.), *Oncology nursing: Assessment and clinical care* (pp. 275–304). St. Louis, MO: Mosby.

Robinson, C., Fritch, M., Hullett, L., Petersen, M., Sikkema, S., Theuninck, L., et al. (2000). Development of a protocol to prevent opioid-induced constipation in patients with cancer: A research utilization project. *Clinical Journal of Oncology Nursing, 4,* 79.

Tuchmann, L. (2001). Constipation. In R. Gates & R. Fink (Eds.), *Oncology nursing secrets* (2nd ed., pp. 298–309). Philadelphia: Hanley & Belfus.

Wright, P., & Thomas, S. (1995). Constipation and diarrhea: The neglected symptoms. *Seminars in Oncology Nursing, 11,* 289–297.

Yuan, C. (2004). Clinical status of methylnaltrexone, a new agent to prevent and manage opioid-induced side effects. *Journal of Supportive Oncology, 2*(2), 111–117.

6. Perirectal cellulitis: Inflammation and edema of the perineal and rectal area
   a) Pathophysiology
      (1) Minimal tears of the anorectal mucosa allow infection. Most common infective organisms include gram-negative aerobic bacilli, enterococci, and bowel anaerobes (Alexander, Walsh, Freifeld, & Pizzo, 2002).
      (2) Infection starting as a local abscess can lead to systemic sepsis.
   b) Incidence: Overall incidence has decreased in recent years, presumably because of the early use of empiric antibiotics in febrile neutropenic patients.
   c) Risk factors
      (1) Neutropenia or thrombocytopenia that is chronic (the condition lasts for more than seven days) or profound (ANC < 100/mm^3) places patients at high risk of developing infection (Alexander et al., 2002; Wujcik, 2004).
      (2) Constipation: The passage of hard stool causes trauma to the rectal mucosa.
      (3) Diarrhea: Caustic fluid irritates and breaks down perirectal tissue.
      (4) Perirectal mucositis caused by chemotherapy and/or radiation therapy
      (5) Any rectal trauma, such as rectal stimulation or the use of rectal thermometers or suppositories
      (6) Hemorrhoids or anal fissures
   d) Assessment
      (1) Ask patients if they are experiencing perineal and/or rectal discomfort. Be alert to fear of defecation, which may signal discomfort that they are hesitant to mention.
      (2) Monitor for the presence of fever.
      (3) Perform a physical examination of the perineal area.
         (a) The entrance site for the infective agent may be a small tear that shows minimal irritation. Or you may see gross swelling and inflammation of the perirectal area.
         (b) Look for and document tissue sloughing and necrosis.
   e) Collaborative management (Alexander et al., 2002; Kline, 2002)
      (1) Ensure that antibiotic coverage includes a specific antianaerobic agent, such as clindamycin or metronidazole, in addition to broad-spectrum aerobic coverage.
      (2) Administer antipyretic medications to relieve fever.
      (3) Encourage patients to take sitz baths or use perineal irrigation to help to heal the area.
      (4) Administer stool softeners and encourage patients to eat a low-bulk diet.
      (5) Inspect the perirectal mucosa frequently for any signs of irritation or skin breakdown.
   f) Patient and family education
      (1) Teach patients and significant others to
         (a) Maintain meticulous perineal hygiene, especially in the presence of neutropenia.

(b) Apply appropriate barrier creams and medicated creams.
(c) Monitor carefully for any signs of infection or worsening of tissue integrity.
(2) Ensure that patients and significant others are able to
(a) Identify the risk factors for perirectal cellulitis.
(b) Implement measures that minimize the risk of developing perirectal cellulitis.
(c) Identify situations that require prompt professional intervention (Wujcik, 2004).
i) Pain, redness, or swelling in the affected area
ii) Body temperature ≥ 38.5°C (101.3°F)

References

Alexander, S.W., Walsh, T.J., Freifeld, A.G., & Pizzo, P.A. (2002). Infectious complications in pediatric cancer patients. In P.A. Pizzo & D.G. Poplack (Eds.), *Principles and practice of pediatric oncology* (4th ed., pp. 1239–1283). Philadelphia: Lippincott Williams & Wilkins.

Kline, N.E. (2002). Prevention and treatment of infections. In C.R. Baggott, K.P. Kelly, D. Fochtman, & G.V. Foley (Eds.), *Nursing care of children and adolescents with cancer* (3rd ed., pp. 266–278). Philadelphia: Saunders.

Wujcik, D. (2004). Infection. In C.H. Yarbro, M.H. Frogge, & M. Goodman (Eds.), *Cancer symptom management* (3rd ed., pp. 252–272). Sudbury, MA: Jones and Bartlett.

C. Alopecia
1. Pathophysiology: The pathobiology of the response of human hair follicles to chemotherapy remains largely unknown. Cells responsible for hair growth have high mitotic and metabolic rates. Certain cytotoxic agents disrupt the proliferative phase of hair growth. Approximately 90% of hair follicles on the scalp are in the anagen (growth) phase of the hair cycle (Fischer, Knobf, & Durivage, 1993). Recent studies discuss the role of p53 and its target genes that mediate responses of hair follicle cells; it is suggested that pharmacologic inhibition of p53 may serve as an effective treatment to prevent chemotherapy-induced hair loss (Botchkarev, 2003).
a) The sensitivity of hair to damage from cytotoxic agents, in order of decreasing sensitivity, is as follows: scalp hair; male beard; hair of the eyebrows, axilla, and pubis; and fine hair (Strohl, 1998).
b) Hair damage occurs either to the shaft or the root.
(1) Hair shaft damage results in partial atrophy or necrosis of the bulb, which causes constriction. Hair breaks off at the damaged area. The result of such damage is a head of hair that looks patchy and thin (Welch & Lewis, 1980).
(2) Root damage is associated with complete alopecia. Hair falls out spontaneously or during washing and/or combing. The more potent epilators (e.g., cyclophosphamide, daunorubicin, doxorubicin, etoposide, ifosfamide, paclitaxel) are associated with root damage (DeSpain, 1992).
2. Incidence
a) Many chemotherapy drugs are associated with some degree of alopecia.
b) The extent of alopecia depends on the mechanism of action of the drug, drug dose, serum half-life, infusion technique (e.g., bolus versus continuous infusion), and the use of combination chemotherapy (Fischer et al., 1993).
3. Risk factors (Strohl, 1998)
a) Type of cytotoxic drug(s) administered. The drugs that present the highest risk of alopecia are cyclophosphamide, daunorubicin, doxorubicin, etoposide, ifosfamide, and paclitaxel.
b) Certain noncytotoxic medications (e.g., propanolol hydrochloride, heparin sodium, lithium carbonate, prednisone, vitamin A, androgen preparations)
c) High-dose chemotherapy
d) Certain medical conditions (e.g., hypothyroidism, aging)
e) Nutritional status
f) Poor hair condition before cytotoxic treatment
g) Concomitant radiotherapy to head (local effect)
4. Clinical manifestations (Fischer et al., 1993)

a) Degrees of alopecia
  (1) Grade 0—No hair loss
  (2) Grade 1—Mild hair loss
  (3) Grade 2—Pronounced or total hair loss

b) Expected time frame (Fischer et al., 1993)
  (1) Hair loss begins approximately two weeks after administration of the drug.
  (2) Hair regrowth may take three to five months after cytotoxic therapy is complete.

5. Collaborative management: Alopecia can be so traumatic for patients that they might consider refusing therapy because of it. There is no known preventive or treatment strategy for alopecia caused by cytotoxic therapy.
  a) Scalp hypothermia, although used in the past with mixed results, is not currently recommended. There is longstanding concern that reducing circulation to the scalp through vasoconstriction may create a sanctuary site for cancer cells (DeSpain, 1992). Recent studies have explored the clinical benefit of using a digitized scalp cooling system in anthracycline-treated patients (Ridderheim, Bjurberg, & Gustavsson, 2003) and in patients receiving epirubicin and docetaxel (MacDuff, MacKenzie, Hutcheon, Melville, & Archibald, 2003). Randomized trials are needed to determine the efficacy and safety of scalp cooling in preventing chemotherapy-induced alopecia.
  b) Vitamin E is ineffective in preventing alopecia (Martin-Jimenez, Diaz-Rubio, Larriba, & Sangra, 1986; Perez et al., 1986).

6. Patient and family education: Advise patients and significant others about the following (Strohl, 1998).
  a) The cause of alopecia and the time frame of hair loss and regrowth
  b) Strategies to manage hair loss (e.g., instruction about gentle hair care and the need to avoid permanent waves and coloring agents, vigorous brushing, roller and hair-dryer use)
  c) The need to protect the scalp from cold and sun
  d) Local resources for support (e.g., wig salons, scarf and turban catalogs, support groups); refer interested patients to "Look Good . . . Feel Better," a program offered by the American Cancer Society (2004) to provide guidance and support regarding wigs and other head coverings, makeup, and skincare.

References

American Cancer Society. (2004). *Look good . . . feel better.* Retrieved December 6, 2004, from http://www.lookgoodfeelbetter.org

Botchkarev, V.A. (2003). Molecular mechanisms of chemotherapy-induced hair loss. *Journal of Investigational Dermatology Symposium Proceedings, 8*(1), 72–75.

DeSpain, J.D. (1992). Dermatologic toxicity of chemotherapy. *Seminars in Oncology, 19,* 501–507.

Fischer, D.S., Knobf, M.T., & Durivage, H.J. (Eds.). (1993). *The cancer chemotherapy handbook* (4th ed.). St. Louis, MO: Mosby.

MacDuff, C., MacKenzie, T., Hutcheon, A., Melville, L., & Archibald, H. (2003). The effectiveness of scalp cooling in preventing alopecia for patients receiving epirubicin and docetaxel. *European Journal of Cancer Care, 12,* 154–161.

Martin-Jimenez, M., Diaz-Rubio, E., Larriba, J.L., & Sangra, L. (1986). Failure of high-dose tocopherol to prevent alopecia induced by doxorubicin. *New England Journal of Medicine, 315,* 894–895.

Perez, J.E., Macchiavelli, M., Leone, B.A., Romero, A., Rabinovich, M.G., Goldar, D., et al. (1986). High-dose alpha-tocopherol as a preventive of doxorubicin-induced alopecia. *Cancer Treatment Reports, 70,* 1213–1214.

Ridderheim, M., Bjurberg, M., & Gustavsson, A. (2003). Scalp hypothermia to prevent chemotherapy-induced alopecia is effective and safe: A pilot study of new digitized scalp-cooling system in 74 patients. *Supportive Care in Cancer, 11,* 371–377.

Strohl, R.A. (1998). Alopecia. In F.A. Preston & R.S. Cunningham (Eds.), *Clinical guidelines for symptom management in oncology—A handbook for advanced practice nurses* (pp. 275–278). New York: Clinical Insights Press.

Welch, D., & Lewis, K. (1980). Alopecia and chemotherapy . . . the ice turban. *American Journal of Nursing, 80,* 903–905.

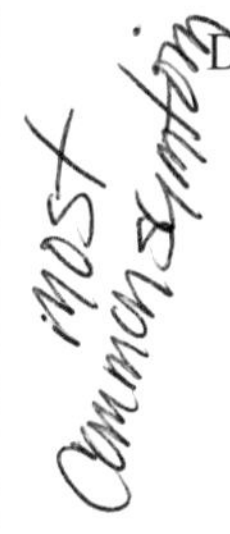

D. Fatigue: *Cancer-related fatigue* is defined by NCCN (2004) as "a persistent, subjective sense of tiredness related to cancer or cancer treatment that interferes with usual functioning" (p. FT-1). See Hinds et al. (1999) and Hockenberry-Eaton et al. (1998) for a discussion of how children, adolescents, and parents perceive fatigue.

1. Pathophysiology: The precise cause of fatigue is unknown, but theorists suggest several etiologies.

a) Biochemical: Changes in the production and balance of muscle proteins, glucose, electrolytes, and hormones (Nail, 1997)
b) Deconditioning: A catabolic process resulting from decreased daily energy expenditure and bed rest (Winningham, 2000)
c) Stress: Physiologic, psychological, or situational factors influence an individual's resistance and response to stress. It is the interaction of these factors that ultimately determines the manifestation of the stress response.
d) Disease, especially disease of the bone marrow, that results in anemia
e) Treatment-related factors: Fatigue is associated with surgery, chemotherapy, radiation therapy, and biotherapy (Nail, 1997; Winningham et al., 1994).
f) Nutritional factors: Anorexia, cachexia, poor nutrition intake, and weight loss contribute to fatigue (Nail, 1997).
g) Quality of sleep and rest (Nail, 1997)
h) Chronic or uncontrolled comorbid conditions or physical problems such as pain or nausea and vomiting (Nail, 1997)
i) Psychosocial factors: Depression, anxiety, lack of motivation and perceived social support, financial concerns, cultural beliefs, and altered coping mechanisms can contribute to fatigue (Curt et al., 2000; Jacobs & Piper, 1996; Nail, 1997; Winningham, 2001).
j) Attentional fatigue: This type of mental fatigue involves the loss or decline in the capacity to direct attention (Cimprich, 1995; Cimprich & Ronis, 2003).
k) Biologic characteristics (e.g., age, gender, genetics, allergies)
l) Environmental factors (e.g., noise, temperature, lighting)

2. Incidence: Fatigue is the most common and most distressing symptom associated with cancer and cancer therapies (Broeckel, Jacobsen, Horton, Balducci, & Lyman, 1998; Curt et al., 2000; Schwartz, 1998). Various studies indicate that patients with cancer can experience intense levels of fatigue that can interfere with daily living and quality of life (Curt et al., 2000; Ferrell, Grant, Dean, Fun, & Ly, 1996). For survivors of childhood cancer, fatigue remains the most common symptom one to five years after the completion of therapy (Crom, Hudson, Hinds, Gattuso, & Tyc, 2000).
3. Risk factors (Mock & Olsen, 2003; NCCN, 2004; Winningham, 2000)
a) Poor nutrition
b) Immobility
c) Insomnia
d) Stress
e) Emotional distress
(1) Depression
(2) Anxiety
f) Anemia
g) Comorbidities
h) Hypoxia
i) Infection and/or fever
j) Pain
k) Therapy, including surgery, chemotherapy, radiation, and biotherapy
4. Assessment
a) Recognize fatigue as a subjective experience that should be actively assessed using the patient self reports (Mock, 2003).
b) Ensure that patients are screened for fatigue at their initial clinical visit, at appropriate intervals, and as clinically indicated (Mock & Olsen, 2003).
c) Use a numeric rating scale to measure the intensity of fatigue (McDaniel & Rhodes, 2000; Nail, 2004) (see Figure 21).
d) Assess coexisting medical conditions, including anemia, hypertension, diabetes, thyroid or metabolic disorders, electrolyte imbalances, infection, and menopause.
e) Assess for use or nonuse of medications that contribute to symptoms, including vitamins, caffeine, alcohol, and recreational drugs.
f) Assess for benefits and risks if patient is using complementary and/or alternative therapy (e.g., diet modification, herbal therapy, mind-body interventions, bioelectromagnetic therapies) (Decker, 1999; Krebs, 1999; Murray & Decker, 1999; Myers, 1999).
g) Assess fatigue level.
(1) In adults (Mock, 2003)
(a) Solicit the patient's description of fatigue according to a linear analog scale (0–10, with 0 = not tired, full of energy, and peppy and 10 = total exhaustion).

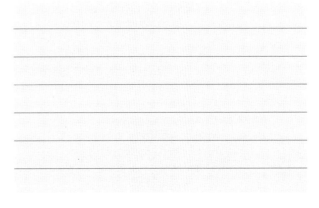

Figure 21. Oncology Nursing Society Fatigue Scale

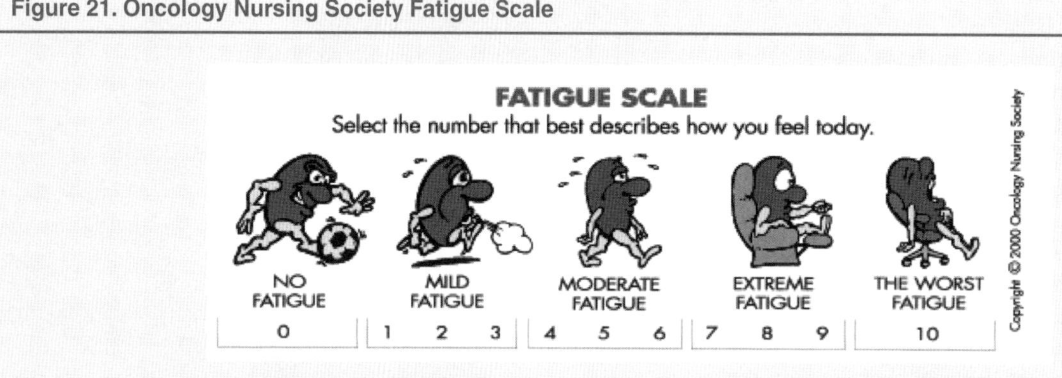

Note. Copyright 2000 by the Oncology Nursing Society.

(*b*) Determine the onset and duration of fatigue.

(*c*) Determine the pattern of fatigue (i.e., intermittent versus constant).

(*d*) Determine enhancing and alleviating factors.

(*e*) Determine primary factors associated with the fatigue experience. These primary factors include pain, emotional distress, sleep disturbance, anemia, nutritional status, activity level, and comorbidity (Mock, 2004; Mock & Olsen, 2003).

(*f*) A more comprehensive assessment is indicated if fatigue is rated as moderate to severe. A comprehensive assessment includes a systems review, medications and medication interactions, and the individual's clinical status (Mock & Olsen, 2003; NCCN, 2004).

(2) In children

(*a*) Assessment of fatigue has been shown to require a multidimensional approach in adults and has been found to be no different in children (Hockenberry-Eaton & Hinds, 2000a).

(*b*) Child Fatigue Instrument is a 14-item scale that measures the frequency of fatigue with a series of yes/no questions and the intensity of fatigue with a 1–5 Likert-type rating scale (Hockenberry-Eaton & Hinds, 2000a).

5. Collaborative management

a) Evaluate ability to perform ADLs and encourage patients to balance exercise, rest, and energy-enhancing activities (Nail, 1997; Winningham, 2001).

b) Correct the potential causes of fatigue (e.g., dehydration, anemia, electrolyte imbalances, oxygenation, hypothyroidism).

c) Provide anticipatory guidance about symptoms. Develop an individualized care plan (Jacobs & Piper, 1996).

(1) Encourage patients and significant others to reorganize activities and work schedules to decrease or eliminate low-priority activities.

(2) Evaluate medications that may contribute to fatigue, and develop strategies to offset the effects.

d) Obtain a nutritional consultation as needed.

e) Discuss and/or pursue a rehabilitation and/or physical therapy consultation, as needed.

f) Discuss and/or pursue a consultation with a psychiatric nurse, social worker, psycho-oncologist, or psychiatrist, as needed.

g) Collaborate with the healthcare team to reduce demands (e.g., interruptions, competing stimuli) on pediatric patients (Hockenberry-Eaton & Hinds, 2000b).

h) Collaborate with the parents of pediatric patients to identify the causes of fatigue (e.g., treatment environment, family schedule) and factors that could alleviate it (e.g., planning events when the child is at peak energy level; providing distractions that are pleasing to the child; offering food supplements, such as milkshakes or finger foods) (Hockenberry-Eaton & Hinds, 2000a).

6. Patient and family education

a) Provide information about the causes and contributing factors of fatigue (Jacobs & Piper, 1996; Mock et al., 2000).

b) Encourage patients and significant others to set goals based on realistic abilities and limitations.

c) Encourage patients to keep an activity-fatigue journal to identify patterns of energy and fatigue during the day.

d) Provide instruction about strategies for dealing with and alleviating fatigue based on baseline functional status (Nail, 1997; Winningham, 2001).

e) Strategies should include energy conservation, distraction, and stress management (Barsevick et al., 2004; Mock et al., 2000). Energy conservation includes

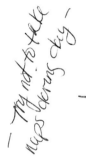

(1) Having patients and significant others prioritize activities and plan high-priority activities for times of increased energy.

(2) Having patients ask for help with personal responsibilities as needed.

f) Encourage patients to do aerobic exercises regularly if not medically contraindicated (e.g., lytic bone lesions, thrombocytopenia, cachexia) (Dimeo, 2001; Mock, 2003; Winningham, 2001).

g) Encourage patients to keep a regular sleep schedule and to take short, frequent rest periods.

h) Encourage patients to perform energy-enhancing activities (e.g., progressive muscle relaxation, visualization, listening to relaxation tapes, relaxing in a pleasant outdoor place) (Cimprich & Ronis, 2003; Mock, 2004; Mock & Olsen, 2003).

i) Encourage patients to maintain adequate dietary intake (e.g., appropriate caloric intake of carbohydrates, fat, and protein; adequate hydration) (Nail, 2002; Winningham, 2001).

j) Encourage patients and significant others to maintain a moderate-temperature home environment.

k) Instruct patients to report changes in energy level to their healthcare provider (Nail, 1997).

References

Barsevick, A.M., Dudley, W., Beck, S., Sweeney, C., Whitmer, K., & Nail, L. (2004). A randomized clinical trial of energy conservation for patients with cancer-related fatigue. *Cancer, 100,* 1302–1310.

Broeckel, J.A., Jacobsen, P.B., Horton, J., Balducci, L., & Lyman, G.H. (1998). Characteristics and correlates of fatigue after adjuvant chemotherapy for breast cancer. *Journal of Clinical Oncology, 16,* 1689–1696.

Cimprich, B. (1995). Symptom management: Loss of concentration. *Seminars in Oncology Nursing, 11,* 279–288.

Cimprich, B., & Ronis, R.L. (2003). An environmental intervention to restore attention in women with newly diagnosed breast cancer. *Cancer Nursing, 26,* 284–292.

Crom, D., Hudson, M., Hinds, P., Gattuso, J., & Tyc, V. (2000). *Perceived vulnerability among survivors of Hodgkin's disease.* Unpublished data. Memphis, TN: St. Jude Children's Research Hospital.

Curt, A.G., Breitbart, W., Cella, D., Groopman, J.E., Horning, S.J., Itri, L.M., et al. (2000). Impact of cancer-related fatigue on the lives of patients: New findings from the fatigue coalition. *Oncologist, 5,* 353–360.

Decker, G.M. (1999). Bioelectromagnetic therapies. In G.M. Decker (Ed.), *An introduction to complementary and alternative therapies* (pp. 29–41). Pittsburgh, PA: Oncology Nursing Society.

Dimeo, G.C. (2001). Effects of exercise on cancer-related fatigue. *Cancer, 92*(Suppl.), 1689–1693.

Ferrell, B.R., Grant, M., Dean, G.E., Funk, B., & Ly, J. (1996). Bone tired: The experience of fatigue and its impact on quality of life. *Oncology Nursing Forum, 23,* 1539–1547.

Hinds, P., Hockenberry-Eaton, M., Gilger, E., Kline, N., Burleson, C., Bottomley, S., et al. (1999). Comparing patient, parent, and staff perspectives on fatigue in pediatric oncology patients. *Cancer Nursing, 22,* 227–289.

Hockenberry-Eaton, M., & Hinds, P. (2000a). Fatigue in children and adolescents with cancer: Evolution of a program of study. *Seminars in Oncology Nursing, 16,* 261–271.

Hockenberry-Eaton, M., & Hinds, P. (2000b). Fatigue in children and adolescents with cancer. In M.L. Winningham & M. Barton-Burke (Eds.), *Fatigue in cancer: A multidimensional approach* (pp. 71–85). Sudbury, MA: Jones and Bartlett.

Hockenberry-Eaton, M., Hinds, P., Alcoser, P., O'Neill, J., Euell, K., Howard, V., et al. (1998). Fatigue in children and adolescents with cancer. *Journal of Pediatric Oncology Nursing, 15,* 172–182.

Jacobs, L.A., & Piper, B.F. (1996). The phenomenon of fatigue and the cancer patient. In R. McCorkle, M. Grant, M. Frank-Stromborg, & S. Baird (Eds.), *Cancer nursing: A comprehensive textbook* (2nd ed., pp. 1193–1208). Philadelphia: Saunders.

Krebs, L.U. (1999). Mind-body interventions. In G.M. Decker (Ed.), *An introduction to complementary and alternative medicine* (pp. 1–27). Pittsburgh, PA: Oncology Nursing Society.

McDaniel, R.W., & Rhodes, V.A. (2000). Fatigue. In C.H. Yarbro, M.H. Frogge, M. Goodman, & S.L. Groenwald (Eds.), *Cancer nursing: Principles and practice* (5th ed., pp. 737–753). Sudbury, MA: Jones and Bartlett.

Mock, V. (2003). Clinical excellence through evidence-based practice: Fatigue management as a model. *Oncology Nursing Forum, 29,* 537–544.

Mock, V. (2004). Evidence-based treatment of cancer-related fatigue. *Journal of the National Cancer Institute Monographs, 32,* 112–118.

Mock, V., & Olsen, M. (2003). Current management of fatigue and anemia in patients with cancer. *Seminars in Oncology Nursing, 19,* 36–41.

Mock, V., Atkinson, A., Barsevick, A., Cella, D., Cimprich, B., Cleeland, C., et al. (2000). NCCN practice guidelines for cancer-related fatigue. *Oncology, 14*(11A), 151–161.

Murray, M., & Decker, G.M. (1999). Diet, nutrition, and lifestyle changes. In G.M. Decker (Ed.), *An introduction to complementary and alternative therapies* (pp. 187–225). Pittsburgh, PA: Oncology Nursing Society.

Myers, J.S. (1999). Herbal medicine. In G.M. Decker (Ed.), *An introduction to complementary and alternative therapies* (pp. 159–185). Pittsburgh, PA: Oncology Nursing Society.

Nail, L.M. (2002). Fatigue in patients with cancer. *Oncology Nursing Forum, 29,* 537–544.

Nail, L.M. (1997). Fatigue. In C.H. Yarbro, M.H. Frogge, M. Goodman, & S.L. Gorenwald (Eds.), *Cancer nursing: Principles and practice* (4th ed., pp. 640–654). Sudbury, MA: Jones and Bartlett.

Nail, L.M. (2004). Fatigue. In C.H. Yarbro, M.H. Frogge, & M. Godman (Eds.), *Cancer symptom management* (3rd ed., pp. 47–60). Sudbury, MA: Jones and Bartlett.

National Comprehensive Cancer Network. (2004). *Practice guidelines in oncology: Cancer-related fatigue.* Retrieved October 13, 2004, from http://www.nccn.org

Schwartz, A.L. (1998). Patterns of exercise and fatigue in physically active cancer survivors. *Oncology Nursing Forum, 25,* 485–491.

Winningham, M.L. (2000). The foundations of energetics: Fatigue, fuel and functioning. In M.L. Winningham & M. Barton-Burke (Eds.), *Fatigue in cancer* (pp. 31–53). Sudbury, MA: Jones and Bartlett.

Winningham, M.L. (2001). Strategies for managing cancer-related fatigue syndrome. *Cancer, 92*(Suppl.), 988–997.

Winningham, M.L., Nail, L.M., Burke, M.B., Brophy, L., Cimprich, B., Jones, L.S., et al. (1994). Fatigue and the cancer experience: The state of the knowledge. *Oncology Nursing Forum, 21,* 23–36.

E. Cardiac toxicity (Table 24 lists cardiotoxic chemotherapeutic drugs by category.)
  1. Pathophysiology
    a) Decreased contractility of the heart leads to increased workload, hypertrophy, and progressive left ventricular systolic dysfunction (Krischer et al., 1997). These effects are related to direct insult of myofibrils by drugs such as the antitumor antibiotics doxorubicin, daunorubicin, epirubicin, and idarubicin, which also are known as DNA intercalators or anthracyclines.
    b) Oxidative stress in the presence of increased free radicals and decreased antioxidants results in myocyte injury and/or death (Santos, Moreno, Leino, Froberg, & Wallace, 2002; Singal & Iliskovic, 1998; Speyer & Wasserheit, 1998).
    c) With the use of some drugs in high doses (e.g., 5-FU), coronary artery spasm leads to ischemia and, possibly, infarction (Anand, 1994; Becker, Erckenbrecht, Haussinger, & Frieling, 1999; Gradishar & Vokes, 1990; Labianca, Beretta, Clerici, Fraschini, & Luporini, 1982; Pottage, Holt, Ludgate, & Langlands, 1978). Kleiman, Lehane, Geyer, Pratt, and Young (1987) reported on a type of angina similar to Prinzmetal angina that is associated with high-dose chemotherapy.
    d) Endothelial damage leading to myocardial necrosis has been reported with use of high-dose cyclophosphamide (Mills & Roberts, 1979; Wujcik & Downs, 1992).
    e) Cardiac events have occurred with the use of taxanes (e.g., paclitaxel). Some studies assert that an administration additive, Cremophor® EL emulsifier, may activate cardiac histamine receptors, producing coronary artery vasoconstriction (D'Incalci, Schuller, Colombo, Zucchetti, & Riva, 1998; Platel, Pouna, Bonoron-Adele, & Robert, 2000; Soe, Berkman, & Mardelli, 1996). Cardiac toxicity can be potentiated when taxanes are given with other cardiotoxic drugs such as doxorubicin. Paclitaxel (but not docetaxel) appears to interfere with the pharmacokinetic elimination of doxorubicin (D'Incalci et al.; Sparano, 1999).
    f) Occasional cases of hemorrhagic myocarditis have been reported in adults who received very high doses of cyclophosphamide, such as patients who are being prepared for BMT (Ewer & Benjamin, 1997). High-dose cyclophosphamide is considered potentially cardiotoxic for children. The effects may be additive with those of anthracyclines.
    g) One study of children associated respiratory-phase heart-rate variation with use of vincristine (Steinherz & Yahalom, 1997).
    h) Capillary leak syndrome, a condition associated with the use of IL-2, involves extravasation of fluids and albumin into body issues. The results are decreased peripheral vascular resistance, hypotension, and decreased intravascular volume (Gale, 2005; Newton, Jackowski, & Marrs, 2002).
    i) Renal retention of sodium, associated with IL 11, leads to fluid retention.

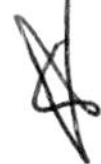

  2. Anthracycline-induced cardiotoxicity: Chemotherapy-induced cardiac toxicity in pediatric patients is almost always attributable to the group of antineoplastic drugs known as anthracyclines. These drugs are widely used and are particularly effective in treating many childhood cancers. However, the cardiac toxicity caused by anthracyclines limits their therapeutic potential. Researchers continue to look for ways to reduce or prevent anthracycline-related cardiac toxicity. In children and adults, cardiac toxicity has been associated with all anthracyclines in clinical use, including doxorubicin, daunorubicin, epirubicin, and idarubicin. The cumulative dose at which cardiac toxicity occurs varies from drug to drug. Doxorubicin is the most widely used anthracycline and the most extensively studied (Loerzel & Dow, 2003; Speyer & Wasserheit, 1998). Doxorubicin serves as a model for anthracycline-related cardiomyopathies (Ewer & Benjamin, 1997).
    a) Exposure to other agents may potentiate anthracycline-induced cardiac toxicity.
      (1) Amsacrine: Krischer et al. (1997) reported that administration of amsacrine

Table 24. Cardiotoxicity of Chemotherapeutic Drugs —

Classification	Drug	Incidence	Characteristic Effects	Comments
Antitumor antibiotic (anthracycline)	Doxorubicin	If total dose < 550 mg/m², incidence is 0.1%–1.2% (Kaszyk, 1986; Von Hoff et al., 1979). If total dose > 550 mg/m², incidence rises exponentially (Von Hoff et al., 1979). If total dose is 1,000 mg/m², incidence is nearly 50% (Carlson, 1992; Von Hoff et al., 1979). Incidence may manifest during therapy, for months to years afterward (Mead Johnson Oncology Products, 2001). Late effects for pediatric patients: In one study, some relevant cardiac impairments (12% of 129 patients) occurred, three of which required cardiac drug therapy (Langer et al., 2004).	ECG changes; nonspecific ST-T wave changes; premature ventricular and atrial contraction; low-voltage QRS changes; sinus tachycardia (Kaszyk, 1986) Decreased ejection fraction, sinus tachycardia, premature ventricular and atrial contractions, cardiomyopathy with symptom of CHF (Carlson, 1992)	Chronic effects seen with cumulative doses may result in CHF. Concomitant administration of other antineoplastics (e.g., cyclophosphamide) has been implicated as a risk factor, although exact synergism is unclear (Burns, 1992). Cardiotoxicity at lower doses may occur in mediastinally irradiated patients and/or patients with preexisting heart disease (Adams et al., 2003).
	Doxorubicin liposomal Pegylated liposomal doxorubicin	Effects on the myocardium have not been confirmed. In studies of patients with AIDS-related Kaposi's sarcoma, 4.3% experienced cardiac-related adverse effects possibly related to Doxil® (Ortho Biotech, 2004). Irreversible toxicity may occur as the total dose nears 550 mg/m²; patients receiving mediastinal radiotherapy or previous or concomitant cardiotoxic therapy may experience heart failure at 400 mg/m² (Ortho Biotech, 2004).	Nonspecific arrhythmia, tachycardia, cardiomyopathy, and/or CHF. Acute left ventricular failure can occur with high doses. CHF may be unresponsive to treatment. At cumulative doses at or above 450 mg/m², a sevenfold greater mean percent decrease in LVEF was observed with doxorubicin versus Doxil (–17.2% versus –2.3%; mean percent change from baseline in LVEF in doxorubicin-treated patients and Doxil-treated patients, respectively). Ten Doxil-treated patients developed protocol-defined cardiac events, compared with 48 doxorubicin-treated patients (O'Brien et al., 2004).	Because experience with large cumulative doses is limited, consider the cardiac risk posed by doxorubicin hydrochloride liposomal to be comparable to that of conventional doxorubicin formulation. Doxil (pegylated liposomal doxorubicin), although categorized as an anthracycline, is believed to be associated with less risk of cardiotoxicity than the other anthracyclines (Escobar et al., 2003; Rivera et al., 2003). Irreversible cardiac damage is dose-limiting. Cardiotoxicity of Doxil is indicated to be lower than with conventional doxorubicin. Long-term cardiac safety is unknown (Safra, 2003).
	Daunorubicin	If total dose < 600 mg/m², incidence is 0%–41% (Kaszyk, 1986). If total dose 1,000 mg/m², incidence is 12% (Kaszyk, 1986).	Nonspecific arrhythmia, tachycardia, cardiomyopathy, and/or CHF. Acute left ventricular failure can occur with high doses. CHF may be unresponsive to treatment. Acute toxicity unrelated to dose may occur within hours. Although rare, myocarditis-pericarditis syndrome may be fatal (Wilkes & Burke, 2004).	Chronic effects are similar to those of doxorubicin, but higher cumulative doses may be tolerated (Von Hoff et al., 1977). Liposomal form (see below) is less cardiotoxic.

(Continued on next page)

Table 24. Cardiotoxicity of Chemotherapeutic Drugs *(Continued)*

Classification	Drug	Incidence	Characteristic Effects	Comments
Antitumor antibiotic (anthracycline) *(cont.)*	Daunorubicin citrate liposomal	Chronic therapy > 300 mg/m^2 has increased the incidence of cardiomyopathy and CHF. In a phase III study, 13.8% of patients reported a triad of back pain, flushing, and chest tightness (Nextar Pharmaceuticals, 1999).	Cardiomyopathy associated with a decrease in LVEF, especially in patients with prior anthracycline experience or preexisting cardiac disease (Nextar Pharmaceuticals, 1999).	Ensure that the patient undergoes a cardiac exam before each course and at total cumulative doses of 320 mg/m^2 (160 mg/m^2 for higher risk patients) and at every 160 mg/m^2 thereafter. Triad usually occurs during the first five minutes of infusion, subsides with infusion interruption, and generally does not recur if the infusion is resumed at a slower rate (Nextar Pharmaceuticals, 1999).
	Dactinomycin	Incidence is rare (Kaszyk, 1986).	–	Assessment is complicated by concomitant combination chemotherapy (including anthracyclines) or prior mediastinal radiation. Monitor vital signs before, during, and four hours after infusion.
	Epirubicin hydrochloride	The probability of developing clinically evident CHF is estimated as approximately 0.9% at a cumulative dose of 550 mg/m^2, 1.6% at 700 mg/m^2, and 3.3% at 900 mg/m^2. The total cumulative dose has been established at 400 mg/m^2. The risk of developing CHF increases rapidly with increasing total cumulative doses in excess of 900 mg/m^2; cumulative dose only should be exceeded with extreme caution (Berchem et al., 1996; Pfizer, 2003a).	Myocardial toxicity, manifested in its most severe form by potentially fatal CHF, may occur either during therapy with epirubicin or months to years after termination of therapy (Pfizer, 2003a).	Active or dormant cardiovascular disease, prior or concomitant radiotherapy to the mediastinal /pericardial area, previous therapy with other anthracyclines or anthracenediones, or concomitant use of other cardiotoxic drugs may increase the risk of cardiac toxicity. In the adjuvant treatment of breast cancer, the maximum cumulative dose used in clinical trials was 720 mg/m^2. Cardiac toxicity with Ellence® may occur at lower cumulative doses whether or not cardiac risk factors are present (Pfizer, 2003a).
Alkylating agent	Estramustine (estradiol and nornitrogen mustard)	CHF occurred in 3 in 93 patients. MI occurred in 3 in 93 patients. The recommended daily dose is 14 mg per kg of body weight (i.e., one 140 mg capsule for each 10 kg or 22 lb of body weight) given in three or four divided doses. Most patients in studies in the United States have been treated at a dosage range of 10–16 mg/kg/day (Pfizer, 2003b).	General fluid retention; exacerbation of preexisting or incipient peripheral edema or CHF has been seen in some patients. Men receiving estrogens for prostatic cancer are at increased risk for thrombosis, including fatal and nonfatal myocardial infarction (Pfizer, 2003b).	Emcyt® capsules should be used with caution in patients with a history of cerebral vascular or coronary artery disease. Because hypertension may occur, blood pressure should be monitored periodically (Pfizer, 2003b).

(Continued on next page)

Table 24. Cardiotoxicity of Chemotherapeutic Drugs *(Continued)*

Classification	Drug	Incidence	Characteristic Effects	Comments
High-dose therapy	Cyclophosphamide	Toxicity is rare with cumulative or standard doses. Some reports of increased frequency with high-dose therapy, > 180–200 mg/kg/day x four days (Allen, 1992; Bristol-Myers Squibb Oncology/Immunology, 2000) Pediatric patients with thalassemia have been shown to have a potential for cardiac tamponade when cyclophosphamide is given with busulfan (FDA, 1998).	ECG: Diminished QRS complex Cardiomegaly; pulmonary congestion; cardiac tamponade in children often is preceded by complaints of abdominal pain and vomiting (FDA, 1998).	May result in acute lethal pericarditis, pericardial effusion, cardiac tamponade, and hemorrhagic myocardial necrosis (Mills & Roberts, 1979; Wujcik & Downs, 1992). Cardiotoxicity usually is related to high doses for short intervals prior to BMT (Allen, 1992). Cases of cardiomyopathy with subsequent death have been reported following experimental high-dose therapy with cytarabine in combination with cyclophosphamide when used for BMT preparation (FDA, 1998).
	5-fluorouracil	Incidence is 1.6% (Labianca et al., 1982). One death was reported from myocardia ischemia (Soe et al., 1996).	Angina, palpitations, sweating, and/or syncope (Akhtar et al., 1993) Severe but reversible cardiogenic shock (Akhtar et al., 1996)	May be treated prophylactically or therapeutically with long-acting nitrates or calcium channel blockers (Eskilsson et al., 1988)
	Capecitabine	Incidence is rare; incidence of cardiotoxicity associated with fluorinated pyrimidine therapy is 1% (Bertolini et al., 2001; Roche Pharmaceuticals, 2004; Van Cutsem et al., 2002).	Myocardial infarction, angina, dysrhythmias, cardiogenic shock, sudden death, and electrocardiograph changes	These adverse events may be more common in patients with a prior history of coronary artery disease. Interrupt drug if grade II or III adverse reactions occur; discontinue drug if grade IV (FDA, 2001; Roche Pharmaceuticals, 2004).
Taxane	Paclitaxel	Asymptomatic bradycardia occurred in almost 30% of patients with ovarian cancer; cardiac ischemia occurred in 5% (Rowinsky et al., 1991). Other disturbances: 5% (not associated with clinical symptoms). Significant cardiac events occurred in 3% of all cases (Bristol-Myers Squibb Oncology/Immunology, 2000). It has been speculated that Cremophor EL® activates histamine receptors. Rare reports of MI. CHF has been reported in cases of patients receiving other chemotherapy agents (Bristol-Myers Squibb, 2000; D'Incalci et al., 1998; Platel et al., 2000).	Asymptomatic bradycardia, hypotension, asymptomatic ventricular tachycardia, atypical chest pain	Toxicity has been documented as asymptomatic bradycardia (40–60 bpm), hypotension, asymptomatic ventricular tachycardia, and atypical chest pain. Obtain a baseline ECG, patient history, and cardiac assessment before treatment; however, routine cardiac monitoring during infusion is not recommended (Arbuck et al., 1992; Fischer et al., 1993; Rowinsky et al., 1991).
	Docetaxel	Few reports Hypotension is 2.8% (1.8% required treatment). Incidence related to high-dose treatment is unknown (Aventis Pharmaceuticals, 2003).	CHF occurred in patients also treated with doxorubicin (> 360 mg/m^2) (Sparano, 1999). Heart failure, sinus tachycardia, atrial flutter, dysrhythmia, unstable angina, pulmonary edema, and/or hypertension (Aventis Pharmaceuticals, 2003)	Well tolerated in elderly patients with non-small cell lung cancer (Hainsworth et al., 2000)

(Continued on next page)

Table 24. Cardiotoxicity of Chemotherapeutic Drugs *(Continued)*

Classification	Drug	Incidence	Characteristic Effects	Comments
Monoclonal antibody	Gemtuzumab ozogamicin	Effects are infrequent and acute infusion related at 9 mg/m² (all grade incidents): hypertension, 16% of participants; hypotension, 20%; and tachycardia, 11% (often in the first 24 hours of infusion) (Wyeth Pharmaceuticals, 2004).	Hypertension, tachycardia, hypotension	Monitor vital signs before, during, and four hours after infusion. See comments about dactinomycin.
	Trastuzumab	Incidence with Herceptin® as a single agent: 7% Incidence with paclitaxel: 11% When combined with anthracycline and cyclophosphamide: 28% The data suggest that advanced age may increase the probability of cardiac dysfunction (Genentech, Inc., 2003).	Signs and symptoms of cardiac dysfunction observed in patients treated with Herceptin include dyspnea, increased cough, paroxysmal nocturnal dyspnea, peripheral edema, S_3 gallop, or reduced ejection fraction (Genentech, Inc., 2003). Reducing the rate decreased infusion-related events for first infusion by 80%; 40% for subsequent infusions (Genentech, Inc., 2003).	CHF has been associated with disabling cardiac failure, death, and mural thrombosis leading to stroke. Discontinuation of therapy is strongly considered for those with significant CHF or asymptomatic ejection fraction decreases. Extreme caution should be exercised in treating patients with preexisting cardiac dysfunction. Patients receiving Herceptin should undergo frequent monitoring for deteriorating cardiac function (Genentech, Inc., 2003). Some severe reactions have been treated successfully with interruption of the Herceptin infusion and administration of supportive therapy including oxygen, IV fluids, beta agonists, and corticosteroids (Genentech, Inc., 2003).
	Rituximab	Cardiac toxicity when used as a single agent is unknown. Infusion-related deaths within 24 hours: 0.04%–0.07% (Genentech/IDEC Pharmaceuticals, 1999) Incidence of mild to moderate hypotension requiring treatment interruption: 10% Incidence of angioedema: 13%	Hypotension and angioedema Infusion-related complex includes these cardiac events: myocardial infarction, ventricular fibrillation, or cardiogenic shock (Genentech/IDEC Pharmaceuticals, 1999).	Nearly all fatalities have occurred on first infusion. Discontinue and medically treat patients who develop clinically significant cardiopulmonary reactions. After symptoms resolve, resume treatment by reducing the infusion rate by 50% (e.g., reduce an initial infusion rate of 100 mg/hour to 50 mg/hour).
Antimetabolite	Gemcitabine hydrochloride	CHF and MI have been reported rarely with the use of gemcitabine. Arrhythmias, predominantly supraventricular in nature, have been reported very rarely. Incidence of hypotension is 11% when given with cisplatin. Hypotension study of Gemzar® maximum tolerated dose above 1,000 mg/m² on a daily x 5 dose schedule showed that patients developed significant hypotension (Eli Lilly & Co., 2004).	Hypotension, myocardial infarction, arrhythmia, hypertension (Eli Lilly & Co., 2004)	Age, gender, and infusion time factors: Lower clearance in women and the elderly results in higher concentrations of gemcitabine for any given dose. Increased toxicity when administered more frequently than once weekly or with infusions longer than 60 minutes (Eli Lilly & Co., 2004)

(Continued on next page)

Table 24. Cardiotoxicity of Chemotherapeutic Drugs *(Continued)*

Classification	Drug	Incidence	Characteristic Effects	Comments
Antimetabolite *(cont.)*	Cladribine	Serious side effects are rare (Bryson & Sorkin, 1993). Incidence of edema and tachycardia is 6%. Incidence of chest pain has been reported (Ortho Biotech, 2002; Wilkes & Burke, 2004).	Tachycardia, edema, chest pain	Most events occured in patients with a history of cardiovascular disease or chest tumors (Bryson & Sorkin, 1993).
Plant alkaloid	Vinorelbine tartrate	There have been rare reports of MI with Navelbine®. Chest pain was reported in 5% of patients (GlaxoSmithKline, 2002).	Hypertension, hypotension, vasodilation, tachycardia, and pulmonary edema have been reported (GlaxoSmithKline, 2002).	Most reports of chest pain were in patients who had either a history of cardiovascular disease or tumor within the chest (GlaxoSmithKline, 2002).
Interleukin	Interleukin-2	Side effects following the use of Proleukin® IL-2 (aldesleukin) appear to be dose-related. Risk increases with doses > 100,000 U/kg (Wilkes & Burke, 2004). Average dose is 600,000 IU/kg (Chiron Corporation, 2004). Most adverse reactions are self-limiting and usually, but not invariably, reverse or improve within two to three days of discontinuation of therapy. Aldesleukin administration has been associated with CLS. The rate of drug-related deaths in the 255 patients with metastatic renal cell carcinoma who received single-agent aldesleukin was 4% (11/255); the rate of drug-related deaths in the 270 patients with metastatic melanoma who received single-agent aldesleukin was 2% (6/270).	Alteration in cardiac output resulting from CLS (loss of vascular tone and extravasation of plasma proteins and fluid into the extravascular space). CLS results in hypotension and reduced organ perfusion, which may be severe and can result in death. CLS may be associated with cardiac arrhythmias (supraventricular and ventricular), CHF, angina, pleural and pericardial effusion, myocarditis, chest pain, and (rarely) MI (Chiron Corporation, 2004; Wilkes & Burke, 2004). CLS begins immediately after aldesleukin treatment starts. In most patients, this results in a concomitant drop in mean arterial blood pressure within 2–12 hours after the start of treatment. With continued therapy, clinically significant hypotension (systolic blood pressure 90 mmHg or a 20 mmHg drop from baseline systolic pressure) and hypoperfusion will occur (Chiron Corporation, 2004).	Aldesleukin administration should be withheld in patients developing moderate to severe lethargy or somnolence; continued administration may result in coma. Should adverse events that require dose modification occur, dosage should be withheld rather than reduced. Patients should have normal cardiac, pulmonary, hepatic, and CNS function at the start of therapy. Medical management of CLS begins with careful monitoring of the patient's fluid and organ perfusion status; this is achieved by frequent determination of blood pressure and pulse and by monitoring organ function, which includes assessment of mental status and urine output. Hypovolemia is assessed by catheterization and central pressure monitoring. Dose modification for toxicity should be accomplished by withholding or interrupting a dose rather than reducing the dose to be given.

BMT—bone marrow transplant; CHF—congestive heart failure; CLS—capillary leak syndrome; CNS—central nervous system; ECG—electrocardiogram; LVEF—left ventricular ejection fraction; MI—myocardial infarction after anthracycline therapy resulted in a risk of cardiac toxicity that was 2.5 times higher than the risk associated with an anthracycline alone. [Note: Amsacrine is not available in the United States.]

(2) Mitoxantrone: This agent is known to be cardiotoxic; reports indicate that it potentiates cardiotoxicity when administered following anthracyclines or radiation to the mediastinal area (Cleri & Haywood, 2002; Kaszyk, 1986).

(3) Very high dose cyclophosphamide

(4) Dactinomycin

(5) Mitomycin C (rarely used in pediatric patients)

(6) Dacarbazine

(7) Vincristine

(8) Bleomycin

(9) Diethylstilbestrol diphosphate (DES): Cardiac toxicity has been reported 10 times more frequently with combined therapy than with doxorubicin alone (6.75% compared to 0.7%) (Leaf et al., 2003).

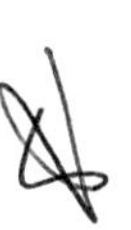

b) Types of anthracycline toxicity

(1) Early-onset anthracycline toxicity: Krischer et al. (1997) reported an incidence of early-onset anthracycline toxicity in 1.6% of 6,000 children with cancer who had been treated with anthracycline chemotherapy according to Pediatric Oncology Group protocols.

(a) Occurs during or within one year of completion of anthracycline therapy (Krischer et al., 1997)

(b) Is presumably related to myocyte damage or death, causing left ventricular dysfunction (Krischer et al., 1997)

(c) Varies in severity; some cases involve stable, asymptomatic abnormalities in left ventricular function. Other cases are progressive and involve ECG changes, associated signs of cardiomyopathy, changes in exercise-stress capacity, and overt CHF (Grenier & Lipshultz, 1998).

(d) Is dose-related; toxicity increases with higher cumulative doses and higher maximal doses (Grenier & Lipshultz, 1998).

(2) Late-onset anthracycline toxicity

(a) Occurs one year or more after completion of anthracycline therapy

(b) Is presumably caused by decreased left ventricular contractility and inappropriately thin left ventricular wall, elevated wall stress, and progressive ventricular dysfunction (Grenier & Lipshultz, 1998)

(c) Is dose-related; incidence increases with higher cumulative doses as well as higher maximal dose (Speyer & Wasserheit, 1998).

(d) Is more common than early-onset anthracycline toxicity

c) Anthracycline-toxicity diagnosis

(1) Cardiac toxicity associated with anthracycline therapy can be diagnosed by serial endocardial biopsy (Loerzel & Dow, 2003). The means for doing such a biopsy are not available in all institutions, however, and obtaining the tissue needed for the biopsy is an invasive procedure. Serial endocardial biopsy is seldom used in pediatrics.

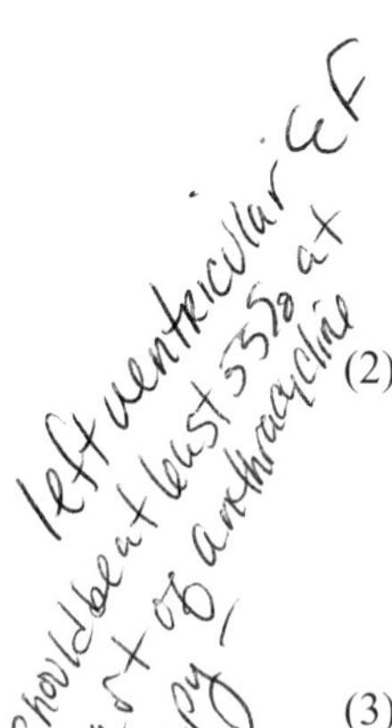
left ventricular EF
should be at least 55% at
start of anthracycline
therapy

(2) Multiple-gated acquisition (MUGA) scans are widely used as a means of detecting early-onset anthracycline cardiac toxicity. They are reliable indicators of cardiac damage (Speyer & Wasserheit, 1998).

(3) Two-dimensional echocardiography also is widely used to diagnose anthracycline toxicity. It has the advantage of being noninvasive and can measure left ventricular ejection fraction, fractional shortening, and left ventricular wall thickness (Speyer & Wasserheit, 1998).

(4) Blood levels of cardiac troponin can detect early myocardiocyte injury (Speyer & Wasserheit, 1998) caused by anthracycline toxicity.

(5) Electrocardiogram (ECG) can detect abnormalities in cardiac electrophysiology caused by anthracycline toxicity.

3. Acuity
   a) Acute (Loerzel & Dow, 2003)
      (1) Occurs within 24 hours of drug administration
      (2) Is self-limiting
      (3) Is not dose-related (Camp-Sorrell, 2000)
      (4) May cause electrical changes in the heart that an ECG may reflect
         (a) Electrical changes caused by chemotherapy: The most frequent electrical change is decreased voltage (Steinherz & Yahalom, 1997). Chemotherapy has led to cardiac decompensation and collapse (Kaszyk, 1986); however, transient changes usually do not call for discontinuation of therapy (Allen, 1992). Following are two exceptions.
            i) Acute changes associated with 5-FU warrant immediate discontinuation of the drug (Akhtar, Salim, & Bano, 1993).
            ii) Serious arrhythmias resulting from a drug warrant immediate discontinuation of the drug (Barton-Burke, Wilkes, & Ingwersen, 2001).
         (b) Electrical changes caused by biotherapy: Electrical changes associated with biotherapeutic agents generally necessitate discontinuation of the biotherapeutic drug.
      (5) In pediatric patients, elevated blood cardiac troponin T (a specific marker for myocardiocyte damage) has been observed after the patient received the initial dose of anthracycline (Grenier & Lipshultz, 1998).
   b) Subacute (Story, 2005)
      (1) Symptoms appear four to five weeks following therapy.
      (2) Causes fibrinous pericarditis and myocardial dysfunction, which may be diagnosed with a radionuclide cardiac MUGA scan (Kaszyk, 1986)
      (3) Usually reversible
      (4) Chemotherapy may or may not be stopped, depending on the patient.
      (5) Biotherapy usually is discontinued if symptoms of subacute cardiac toxicity appear.
   c) Chronic (Story, 2005)
      (1) Nonreversible cardiomyopathy may occur weeks or months after administration of an anthracycline (Camp-Sorrell, 2000).
      (2) Seen with cumulative doses of cardiotoxic drugs (e.g., anthracyclines) that cause myocardial weakening because of direct damage to myocytes (Speyer & Freedberg, 2000; Yahalom & Portlock, 2005)
      (3) Enhanced if radiation therapy has been given to the left chest or thorax and/or mediastinum (Carlson, 1992; Loerzel & Dow, 2003)
      (4) Cardiotoxic chemotherapy is stopped if chronic toxicity occurs (Yahalom & Portlock, 2005).
      (5) See Table 24 for information about chronic cardiac effects.
4. Incidence
   a) Acute and subacute toxicity occur infrequently (Allen, 1992; Story, 2005); approximately 10% of acute toxicity consists of transient electrical changes in the heart (Camp-Sorrell, 2000).
   b) Chronic toxicity is related to cumulative dose (Allen, 1992; Loerzel & Dow, 2003).
   c) Studies show that some drugs (e.g., epirubicin, idarubicin, mitoxantrone) produce less cardiac toxicity than do other anthracyclines (Hurteloup & Ganzina, 1986; Loerzel & Dow, 2003; Shenkenberg & Von Hoff, 1986).
   d) Of patients with ovarian cancer who were treated with paclitaxel, 30% developed asymptomatic bradycardia. More profound cardiac events (i.e., ventricular tachycardia and left-bundle branch block) have been observed in 5% of patients (Rowinsky et al., 1991). A death resulting from myocardial ischemia has been documented (Soe et al., 1996).

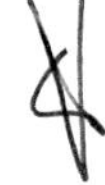

5. Risk factors (note that these risk factors do not always apply for patients undergoing biotherapy)

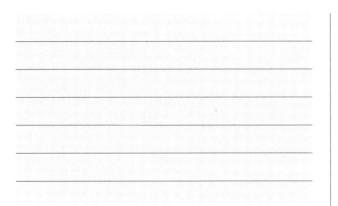

a) Cardiotoxic drugs (see Tables 24 and 25)
b) High-dose therapy
c) Administration schedule: Higher doses over a shorter period increase toxicity (Allen, 1992). Dividing doses into smaller boluses has been shown to decrease toxicity (Von Hoff et al., 1979).
d) Infusion rate: Longer infusion times have been shown to reduce the risk of toxicity (Doroshow, 1991). A 75% decrease in CHF was seen when doxorubicin, at total cumulative doses less than or equal to 450 mg/m^2, was administered as a continuous infusion rather than a bolus infusion (Hortobagyi et al., 1989; Loerzel & Dow, 2003).
e) Thoracic irradiation to the lungs or mediastinum (Adams, Hardenbergh, Constine, & Lipshulz, 2003; Blatt, Copeland, & Bleyer, 1997; Bottomley, 2004; Carlson, 1992): Cardiac toxicity may occur at lower radiation doses when patients receive anthracyclines and mediastinal radiation (Chronowski et al., 2003).
f) Age
  (1) In cases of preexisting malnutrition, children are at higher risk than adults because of biologic and metabolic differences, the high tissue sensitivity of children, and the intensity of pediatric chemotherapy regimens (Carlson, 1992; Kaszyk, 1986).
  (2) Conflicting evidence regarding the elderly
    (a) Some researchers maintain that the elderly are at higher risk than other adults because of the inability of an elderly person's body to self-repair and the greater likelihood of preexisting cardiac disease (Carlson, 1992; Kaszyk, 1986; Speyer & Freedberg, 2000; Von Hoff et al., 1977).
    (b) Other studies indicate that the elderly can tolerate aggressive treatment and that, in regard to treatment for solid tumors, geriatric patients tolerate chemotherapy as well as young people do (Damon, 1992). Elderly people with non-small cell lung cancer tolerate docetaxel well (Hainsworth et al., 2000). However, advanced age may increase the chances of cardiac dysfunction with selected drugs (e.g., trastuzumab).
g) Preexisting cardiac disease (Kaszyk, 1986), cardiac abnormalities, or tumors in the chest (Blatt et al., 1997; Bottomley, 2004)
h) Smoking, because of its association with cardiac changes (Kaszyk, 1986)
i) Malnutrition, which may increase cardiotoxicity (Ewer & Benjamin, 1997)

6. Assessment before biotherapy (Loerzel & Dow, 2003)
  a) Before treatment with IL-2: Ensure that patients have undergone a baseline cardiac evaluation of left ventricular function to determine eligibility for treatment with IL-2.
  b) Before treatment with certain monoclonal antibodies (e.g., trastuzumab) and chemotherapy agents: Ensure that patients have undergone a MUGA or ECG to establish baseline cardiac function.
7. Assessment throughout therapy, especially for high-risk patients (Loerzel & Dow, 2003)
  a) Check the results of baseline cardiac studies (e.g., ejection fraction) before administering the drug.
  b) Observe for clinical manifestations of CHF (e.g., tachycardia, shortness of breath, nonproductive cough, neck-vein distention, ankle edema, gallop rhythm, rales, hepatomegaly, cardiomegaly).
  c) Calculate and assess the cumulative dose of the applicable drug (e.g., doxorubicin) and document it in the patient's records.
  d) Assess heart rate, rhythm, and regularity, including murmurs, split sounds, and extra sounds (a gallop or third heart sound may indicate insufficiency).
  e) Assess electrolytes (e.g., potassium, calcium); abnormal electrolytes can interfere with cardiac function.
8. Collaborative management
  a) Administer, if part of the protocol in your institution, the cardiac-protective iron-chelating agent dexrazoxane during or prior to the administration of doxorubicin to prevent cardiotoxicity in some patients (e.g., patients with metastatic breast cancer who

Table 25. Nursing Management of General Side Effects of Biotherapy

Side Effects	Associated Agents	Pattern of Occurrence or Frequency	Pathophysiology or Rationale (if known)	Monitoring Parameters	Interventions	Comments
Cardiovascular						
Hypertension	Bevacizumab	Uncommon	–	Monitor blood pressure as needed based on clinical status.	Provide medical management with angiotensin-converting enzyme inhibitors, beta blockers, diuretics, or calcium channel blockers.	Worsening hypertension may require discontinuation of therapy.
Hypotension	Interferons	Dose dependent, uncommon	Decreased systemic vascular resistance	Monitor blood pressure as needed based on clinical status.	Teach patients to report signs and symptoms of dizziness or lightheadedness; change positions gradually; and avoid hot showers and excessive heat.	IL-2: Use IV fluid boluses carefully. The idiosyncratic first-dose reaction with GM-CSF may be accompanied by transient flushing, tachycardia, and hypoxia. Slow initial infusions of monoclonal antibodies may help to prevent hypotensive reactions.
	IL-1	Dose dependent				
	IL-2	Common dose-dependent effect: Increased frequency with high-dose or bolus administration				
	GM-CSF	First-dose effect				
	G-CSF	Rare				
	TNF	Dose dependent				
	Monoclonal antibodies	May occur as allergic response; rapid infusion may precipitate side effect.				
Arrhythmia	IL-2 Interferons IL 11	Common transient ventricular and supraventricular arrhythmias Atrial fibrillation Dose, schedule, and route dependent	Most likely secondary to sustained hyperdynamic state induced by capillary leak syndrome	Continuous telemetry is needed in cases of severe hypotension or in the presence of arrhythmia. Assess rhythm, vital signs, and heart sounds on a regular basis. Assess patients for chest pain or palpitations. Assess cardiac isoenzymes as indicated.	Treat arrhythmias with appropriate medications as ordered. Explain all interventions to patients and significant others.	Dose may need to be held or discontinued.

(Continued on next page)

Table 25. Nursing Management of General Side Effects of Biotherapy *(Continued)*

Side Effects	Associated Agents	Pattern of Occurrence or Frequency	Pathophysiology or Rationale (if known)	Monitoring Parameters	Interventions	Comments
Capillary leak syndrome	IL-2 TNF Fusion proteins	Dose dependent; common	An intravascular fluid shift may occur secondary to endothelial membrane inflammation from the cytokine cascade release. Decreased capillary hydrostatic pressure causes a drop in arterial pressure. Concomitantly, the decrease in perfusion and oxygen supply to tissues results in the release of vasodilators.	Monitor intake and output, weight (daily), abdominal girth, electrolytes, and oxygen saturation.	Interstitial fluid mobilizes 24–48 hours after discontinuation of IL-2. Ensure that complaints of chest pain are medically evaluated to determine etiology. Position patients to maximize ventilation and perfusion. Provide comfort measures. Provide oxygen therapy. Use vasopressors to maintain blood pressure.	Dose may need to be held or discontinued.
Cardiomyopathy	Trastuzumab	Highest in patients receiving trastuzumab plus anthracyclines and patients with advanced age	–	Monitor patients for dyspnea, increased cough, paroxysmal nocturnal dyspnea, peripheral edema, S3 gallop, and reduced ejection fraction.	Perform thorough baseline cardiac assessment (ECG, echocardiogram, MUGA scan).	Use extreme caution in patients with preexisting cardiac dysfunction.
Hypersensitivity reactions	Monoclonal antibodies	Most often occurs with first infusion; manifests with hypotension, angioedema, bronchospasm, or hypoxia; if severe, can manifest in pulmonary infiltrates, acute respiratory distress syndrome, or myocardial infarction	The mouse or chimeric component induces the hypersensitivity response.	Follow specific package insert for appropriate initial and subsequent rates of infusion.	Interrupt infusion; administer supportive care as medically indicated (e.g., IV fluids, vasopressors, oxygen, bronchodilators, antihistamines).	Most severe reactions occur with the first infusion.

(Continued on next page)

Table 25. Nursing Management of General Side Effects of Biotherapy *(Continued)*

Side Effects	Associated Agents	Pattern of Occurrence or Frequency	Pathophysiology or Rationale (if known)	Monitoring Parameters	Interventions	Comments
Cutaneous						
Acneform rash	Cetuximab	> 80% of patients; occurs in the first two weeks of treatment	–	–	Instruct patients to limit sun exposure, wear sunscreen, perform meticulous skin care, and avoid topical steroids. Treat with topical and oral antibiotics. Delay dose as needed.	Sunlight can exacerbate any skin reactions.
	Erlotinib	75% of patients	–	–	Delay dose as needed. Treat with antihistamines and antibiotics.	Incidence of rash may correlate to survival benefit.
Dry desquamation	IL-2	Common	Proposed: Eosinophilia	Assess skin color, pigmentation, texture, turgor, vascularity, skin integrity, presence of lesions, eruptions, petechiae, purpura, edema, and pruritus. Assess injection site to ascertain dermatologic effect or infectious etiology.	Instruct patients to use mild soaps and rinse thoroughly; avoid lotions with alcohol, perfumes, and chemicals; use emollients and creams generously; and avoid steroid creams.	Antihistamines may be contraindicated in certain regimens.
	Interferon	Infrequent	–			
	Monoclonal antibodies	Infrequent	May be an allergic response	–	Antihistamines may provide relief.	Antihistamines may be contraindicated in certain regimens.
Pruritus	IL-2	Common; can be severe	–	–	Antihistamines may provide relief. Adjust room humidity to 30%–40%. Ensure that the patients avoid frequent hot showers and baths; use mild soaps and rinse thoroughly; and keep nails short. Cleanse ulcerations frequently and expose them to air. Apply cool towels.	Antihistamines may be contraindicated in certain regimens.
	Interferons	–	–	–		
	Levamisole	–	–	–		
	Monoclonal antibodies	–	May be an allergic response	–		

(Continued on next page)

Table 25. Nursing Management of General Side Effects of Biotherapy *(Continued)*

Side Effects	Associated Agents	Pattern of Occurrence or Frequency	Pathophysiology or Rationale (if known)	Monitoring Parameters	Interventions	Comments
Transient flushing, flare reaction	IL-2 CSFs TNF IL-12 Vaccines	Common; dose and agent dependent	Release of cytokines clustering in immediate vicinity of injection Inflammatory response secondary to activation of cytokine cascade	Assess for signs and symptoms of dermatologic effects: skin color, pigmentation, texture, turgor, vascularity, skin integrity, presence of lesions, eruptions, petechiae, purpura, edema, and pruritus.	Rotate injection sites. Split high-volume doses into two syringes for two separate injections. Ask physician whether to apply ice or heat to site pre- and postinjection. Premedicate patient with diphenhydramine if pruritus develops.	–
Alopecia	Interferons	Infrequent	Unknown	–	Before treatment, alert patients to the potential for alopecia.	–
Flu-like symptoms						
Fever	IL-2	Delayed onset; almost universal	Activation of IL-1, interferon-gamma, and TNF release	Monitor temperature pattern. If fever is unresponsive to acetaminophen, assess for infectious etiology.	Premedicate with acetaminophen or NSAIDs; 24-hour administration may be needed. Maintain adequate fluid intake. Promote measures to decrease fever including sponge baths, removal of extra clothing and blankets, and use of cooling blanket as needed.	Route, dose, and frequency of agent will determine temperature pattern and intensity. Fever associated with interferon administration diminishes in intensity with continued treatments. A sharp elevation in temperature after an afebrile period without changes in drug administration, or fever unresponsive to acetaminophen, may indicate infection.
	Interferons	Rapid-onset tachyphylaxis; almost universal	Activation of IL-1 release			
	Monoclonal antibodies	Rapid for 1–2 hours after treatment begins	Activation of IL-1, -6, and TNF			
	CSFs	Dependent on agent, low-grade fever; more common with multilineage CSFs	Activation of IL-1 release			

(Continued on next page)

Table 25. Nursing Management of General Side Effects of Biotherapy *(Continued)*

Side Effects	Associated Agents	Pattern of Occurrence or Frequency	Pathophysiology or Rationale (if known)	Monitoring Parameters	Interventions	Comments
Chills or rigors (shaking chills)	IL-2 Interferons TNF Monoclonal antibodies	Occur prior to fever spike; common Tachyphylaxis may occur with daily treatment.	Compensation mechanism to adjust to increased temperature	Monitor temperature and comfort.	Administer opiates to relieve rigors (IV meperidine, IV morphine, sublingual hydromorphone). Antipyretic premedications may be used with some treatment regimens. Minimize chills/rigors by using heating pads, hot water bottles, and extra blankets.	Opiate administration may potentiate decreased blood pressure. Predictable pattern occurs with rise in temperature.
Myalgia or arthralgia	Interferons	Common	–	Assess patient for presence of myalgia or arthralgia.	Administer NSAIDs and/or oral analgesics. Provide comfort measures. Provide local moist heat.	–
	ILs	Common	–			
	CSFs	Common	Bone pain secondary to rapid growth of neutrophils in bone marrow before release to periphery			
	Monoclonal antibodies	Causes more arthralgia than it does myalgia	–			
Headache	Interferons	Common	Unknown	–	Provide analgesics. Maintain a quiet, dark room.	–
	ILs	Common	Multicausal			
	TNF	Common	–			
	Monoclonal antibodies	Unusual	–			
Malaise	Interferons	Common	Unknown; possibly related to release of TNF	Assess objective and subjective indicators of patient's activity status.	Employ energy-conservation strategies.	–
	ILs	Common				
	TNF	Common				
	Monoclonal antibodies	Common				

(Continued on next page)

Table 25. Nursing Management of General Side Effects of Biotherapy *(Continued)*

Side Effects	Associated Agents	Pattern of Occurrence or Frequency	Pathophysiology or Rationale (if known)	Monitoring Parameters	Interventions	Comments
Fatigue	Interferons ILs TNF	Interferons, ILs, and TNF: Cumulative and dose-related effect, may be a dose-limiting toxicity; common	Etiology is poorly understood; fatigue may be the result of central nervous system or frontal lobe toxicity.	Perform subjective and objective assessment of patient's ability to participate in activities of daily living (performance status). Monitor for presence and degree of immobility, sensory deprivation, and depression. Monitor for physical signs or symptoms of concurrent health problem(s) (e.g., anemia).	Help the patient to employ energy-conservation strategies, including priority setting. Help the patient to maintain an appropriate level of physical activity. Provide optimal fluid intake and nutrition. Control pain. Correct anemia if it is present.	Medications used to alleviate concurrent symptoms (e.g., antiemetics, narcotics) may compound fatigue.
	GM-CSF	Rare				
Gastrointestinal						
Gastrointestinal (GI) perforations/ wound healing complications	Bevacizumab	–	Antiangiogenesis	Wait a minimum of 28 days after major surgery before initiating bevacizumab therapy.	–	Wait an appropriate interval between bevacizumab termination and subsequent elective surgery, taking into account the drug's half-life (20 days).
Nausea and/ or vomiting	IL-2 IL 11 TNF Interferons G-CSF Erythropoietin Monoclonal antibodies GM-CSF Levamisole	IL-2 and interferons: Dose and schedule dependent. TNF: Tachyphylaxis may occur. Monoclonal antibodies: Dose dependent, rare; usually subsides within 24 hours of the discontinuation of therapy	IL-2: Unknown; toxicity may be related to capillary leak syndrome or the leakage of fluid and albumin into the GI tract. Interferons: Related to flu-like syndrome (the higher the dose, the more common the GI symptoms). Monoclonal antibodies: Nausea and/or vomiting may be related to cytokine release and/ or flu-like syndromes.	Assess patients for nausea. Monitor frequency and amount of nausea or vomiting.	Provide routine antiemetic coverage and frequent mouth care. Serve food at room temperature. Modify diet as needed to clear liquid or frequent light meals. Minimize triggering stimuli in the environment. Offer relaxation or distraction therapy. Obtain nutritional consult.	Steroids may be contraindicated because of their immunosuppressive effects. Phenothiazines are effective. Metoclopramide may potentiate diarrhea. For denileukin diftitox: Nausea and vomiting are dose-limiting toxicities.

(Continued on next page)

Table 25. Nursing Management of General Side Effects of Biotherapy *(Continued)*

Side Effects	Associated Agents	Pattern of Occurrence or Frequency	Pathophysiology or Rationale (if known)	Monitoring Parameters	Interventions	Comments
Anorexia	IL-2 Interferons TNF GM-CSF IL 11 Monoclonal antibodies Levamisole	Dose and schedule dependent	May be related to cytokine release syndrome. Cytokine-induced anorexia involves both peripheral and central nervous system mechanisms. TNF: Receptors in the brain induce anorexia in response to various stimuli.	Monitor weight loss or gain, calorie count (maintain intake), and lab indices of visceral protein (e.g., albumin) for evidence of fat and muscle wasting. Determine calorie and protein needs in collaboration with a dietitian.	Encourage patients to eat small, high-protein, high-calorie meals frequently; increase daily protein intake; and avoid filling or gas-forming foods. Teach patients to eat slowly. Obtain dietary evaluation in regard to protein depletion and weight loss.	Food may seem to have less taste or to taste salty, bitter, or metallic. Some patients develop intolerance to sweet tastes. For interferons: Anorexia may be dose limiting. Fatigue or depression may contribute to anorexic symptoms. Anorexia induced by gemtuzumab ozogamicin may be caused by metabolite from the calicheamicin derivative.
Diarrhea (more than three stools per day)	IL-2 IL 11 Interferons TNF G-CSF GM-CSF Erythropoietin Retinoids Monoclonal antibodies Levamisole	Dose and schedule dependent	All cited agents except erythropoietin and monoclonal antibodies: Unknown; may be related to intracellular levels of cyclic adenosine monophosphate Erythropoietin: May be related to underlying disease Monoclonal antibodies: May be related to cytokine release syndrome	Assess number of stools per day, for presence of fecal impaction, bowel sounds, and hydration and electrolyte status. Monitor intake and output and the frequency, duration, character, and amount of diarrhea. Administer replacement fluids as ordered.	Administer antidiarrheal medications as ordered. Provide perineal care to prevent skin breakdown.	Interferons used in conjunction with antimetabolites may increase diarrhea. Trastuzumab used in combination with chemotherapy increases severity of diarrhea. Diarrhea caused by biotherapy is more chronic but less severe than diarrhea caused by chemotherapy.
Stomatitis	IL-2 Interferons TNF G-CSF GM-CSF IL 11 Retinoids Monoclonal antibodies Levamisole	Dose and schedule dependent	Unknown	Assess oral cavity frequently.	Provide frequent oral hygiene, topical analgesics, and a high-protein diet. Increase fluid intake. Avoid trauma to mucous membranes.	Interferons may activate herpes simplex virus.

(Continued on next page)

Table 25. Nursing Management of General Side Effects of Biotherapy *(Continued)*

Side Effects	Associated Agents	Pattern of Occurrence or Frequency	Pathophysiology or Rationale (if known)	Monitoring Parameters	Interventions	Comments
Hematologic						
Neutropenia, thrombo-cytopenia, anemia	Interferons IL-2 TNF	Dose and schedule dependent	Neutropenia: Redistribution of white cell differential rather than myelosuppression	Monitor complete blood count, differential, and platelet count. Assess patient for signs and symptoms of infection, bleeding, and anemia.	Initiate precautions against bleeding and neutropenia. Administer blood or blood products as ordered.	Condition reverses rapidly upon cessation of therapy.
Neurologic						
Confusion or hallucinations	IL-2 (high-dose)	Related to dose and time	Activation of cytokine cascade; may directly affect central nervous system activity and function (neurotoxic, neuroendocrine, or neurotransmitter effects or hormone alterations)	Assess mental status, cranial nerves, neuro-motor function, and reflexes. Assess normal coping strategies. Obtain baseline assessment (should include contributing factors [e.g., age, performance status, psychological history, underlying disease processes]). Perform ongoing routine neurologic assessments.	Provide education regarding potential neurologic side effects and memory prompts for orientation in regard to time, date, and location. Take patient safety measures. Encourage expression of fears and concerns. Promote regular sleep routines. Caution patients against drinking alcohol. Evaluate providing treatment of the following types. • Behavioral • Pharmacologic • Antidepressant • Opioid antagonist • Psychostimulant	Differential diagnosis may include ICU psychosis. The elderly and patients with a psychiatric history are at increased risk. For these patients, treatment (particularly with IL-2, interferons) may be contraindicated. IL-2: Concurrent administration of psychotropic drugs (e.g., narcotics, analgesics, antiemetics, antihistamines) may exacerbate neurologic toxicities. Neurologic toxicities are common reasons for dose reduction or termination. When a drug is discontinued, the severity of the toxicity may increase before improvement occurs. Patients may not regain baseline neurologic status for two to four weeks after treatment ends.
	Interferons	Related to duration, dose, and route				
	TNF	Rare				
	Retinoids	–				

(Continued on next page)

Table 25. Nursing Management of General Side Effects of Biotherapy *(Continued)*

Side Effects	Associated Agents	Pattern of Occurrence or Frequency	Pathophysiology or Rationale (if known)	Monitoring Parameters	Interventions	Comments
Depression	IL-2 Interferons Levamisole	Cumulative effect; reversible	Activation of cytokine cascade; may directly affect central nervous system activity and function (neurotoxic, neuroendocrine, or neurotransmitter effects or hormone alterations)	Assess mental status, cranial nerves, neuromotor function, and reflexes. Assess normal coping strategies. Obtain baseline assessment (should include contributing factors; e.g., age, performance status, psychological history, underlying disease process). Perform ongoing and routine neurologic assessments.	Provide education regarding potential neurologic side effects and memory prompts for orientation in regard to time, date, and location. Take patient safety measures. Encourage expression of fears and concerns. Promote regular sleep routines. Caution patients against drinking alcohol. Evaluate providing treatment of the following types. • Behavioral • Pharmacologic • Antidepressant • Opioid antagonist • Psychostimulant	Differential diagnosis may include ICU psychosis. At increased risk: the elderly, patients with a psychiatric history. For these patients, treatment (particularly with IL-2, interferons) may be contraindicated. IL-2: Concurrent administration of psychotropic drugs (e.g., narcotics, analgesics, antiemetics, antihistamines) may exacerbate neurologic toxicities. Neurologic toxicities are common reasons for dose reduction or termination. When a drug is discontinued, the severity of the toxicity may increase before improvement occurs. Patients may not regain baseline neurologic status for two to four weeks after treatment ends.
Anxiety	IL-2 Erythropoietin Interferons GM-CSF Retinoids Levamisole	–				
Lethargy or somnolence	IL-2 Interferons Retinoids	Common; dose and schedule dependent				
Headache	IL-2 Interferons G-CSF GM-CSF Erythropoietin Retinoids Monoclonal antibodies IL 11 Levamisole	Dose and schedule dependent				
Decreased concentration	IL-2 Interferons	Common; dose and schedule dependent				
Insomnia	Retinoids Erythropoietin IL 11 Levamisole G-CSF Daclizumab	Dose and schedule dependent				
Irritability, mood changes	IL-2 Retinoids	–				

(Continued on next page)

Table 25. Nursing Management of General Side Effects of Biotherapy *(Continued)*

Side Effects	Associated Agents	Pattern of Occurrence or Frequency	Pathophysiology or Rationale (if known)	Monitoring Parameters	Interventions	Comments
Peripheral neuropathy	Interferons (low-dose) Levamisole Monoclonal antibodies Daclizumab Erythropoietin Retinoids IL 11	Dose and schedule dependent	Activation of cytokine cascade; may directly affect central nervous system activity and function (neurotoxic, neuroendocrine, or neurotransmitter effects or hormone alterations)	Assess mental status, cranial nerves, neuromotor function, and reflexes. Assess normal coping strategies. Obtain baseline assessment (should include contributing factors; e.g., age, performance status, psychological history, underlying disease process). Perform ongoing and routine neurologic assessments.	Position patients so they are comfortable. Provide oxygen per nasal cannula or face mask, per order. Provide comfort measures, effective analgesia, and anticipatory teaching regarding ICU transfer (intubation may be necessary). Limit patients' activity. Elevate head of bed. Administer diuretics and bronchodilators as ordered. Take aspiration precautions as indicated. Promote mucus clearance.	Differential diagnosis may include ICU psychosis. At increased risk: the elderly, patients with a psychiatric history. For these patients, treatment (particularly with IL-2, interferons) may be contraindicated. IL-2: Concurrent administration of psychotropic drugs (e.g., narcotics, analgesics, antiemetics, antihistamines) may exacerbate neurologic toxicities. Neurologic toxicities are common reasons for dose reduction or termination. When a drug is discontinued, the severity of the toxicity may increase before improvement occurs. Patients may not regain baseline neurologic status for two to four weeks after treatment ends.
Dizziness	Interferons Levamisole Monoclonal antibodies Daclizumab Erythropoietin Retinoids IL 11	Dose and schedule dependent				
Paresthesia	Retinoids Erythropoietin Levamisole Monoclonal antibodies GM-CSF	Dose and schedule dependent				
Hallucinations	IL-2 Retinoids	Dose and schedule dependent				
Seizures or coma	Interferons (high-dose cumulative) Erythropoietin (rare) TNF (rare)	Dose and schedule dependent				
Pulmonary						
Respiratory symptoms • Dyspnea • Pulmonary edema • Acute respiratory distress syndrome • Pleural effusion	IL-2	Dose dependent; common Addition to lymphokine-activated killer cells increases likelihood	Secondary to fluid accumulation in the lungs; related to capillary leak syndrome	Monitor lung sounds at least every four hours; rate, rhythm, and depth of respiration; for behavior changes; intake and output; and oxygen saturation. Assess use of accessory muscles and presence of retractions; symmetry of chest; cough (color, amount of sputum); chest or back pain; skin color; and level of consciousness.	Increase oral intake of fluids. Hydrate patients by using IV fluids or colloids. Administer diuretics if blood pressure is stable. Alter diet as appropriate. Encourage patients to void frequently.	Use assessment techniques and intervention outcomes to prevent severe respiratory distress and need for ventilatory support. IL-2 dose may be held or discontinued.

(Continued on next page)

Table 25. Nursing Management of General Side Effects of Biotherapy *(Continued)*

Side Effects	Associated Agents	Pattern of Occurrence or Frequency	Pathophysiology or Rationale (if known)	Monitoring Parameters	Interventions	Comments
Renal						
Elevated creatinine, blood urea, nitrogen, and uric acid	IL-2 Interferons	Dose-related	Concurrent disease pathology Alterations in hemodynamics Metabolic effects Compression or obstruction Neurogenic bladder Direct renal toxicity Dehydration	Monitor daily lab results (especially creatinine, blood urea nitrogen, chemistries), intake and output, specific gravity and pH of urine, and vital signs. Assess for proteinuria, hematuria, and flank pain.	–	For patients receiving high-dose IL-2: Maintain hydration at a minimal level because of the exacerbation caused by capillary leak syndrome. Use diuretics as indicated to "pull" excess accumulated fluid.
TLS	Rituximab	Occurs in the first 12–24 hours after the first rituximab infusion	Rapid reduction in tumor volume followed by acute renal failure	Patient education; monitor electrolyte levels.	Administer hydration. Correct electrolyte abnormalities. Monitor renal function and fluid balance.	Allopurinol remains the standard of care for TLS, but rasburicase (urate oxidase) currently is being studied as a more powerful agent in lowering uric acid levels to prevent complications of TLS.
Oliguria	IL-2	Dose-related anuria may develop. Secondary to hypotension and fluid volume depletion	Current disease pathology Alterations in hemodynamics Metabolic effects Compression or obstruction Neurogenic bladder Direct renal toxicity Dehydration	Monitor intake and output every four hours or per clinical status.	Administer low-dose dopamine (2–5 mcg/kg/minute) to assist in maintaining renal perfusion. Until output resumes, holding IL-2 dose may be necessary.	Dopamine is titrated based on vital signs and urine output. Low urine output is consistent with high-dose treatment regardless of interventions.
Proteinuria	Bevacizumab	–	–	Monitor urine with protein dipstick before each dose.	Dipstick results of 2+ or greater require 24-hour urine collection. Stop bevacizumab if results remain elevated at > 2+ protein.	Increase in proteinuria can lead to nephrotic syndrome.

CSF—colony-stimulating factor; ECG—electrocardiogram; G-CSF—granulocyte–colony-stimulating factor; GM-CSF—granulocyte macrophage–colony-stimulating factor; ICU—intensive care unit; IL—interleukin; MUGA—multiple gated acquisition; NSAID—nonsteroidal anti-inflammatory drug; TLS—tumor lysis syndrome; TNF—tumor necrosis factor

Note. Based on information from Battiato & Wheeler, 2000; Belldegrun et al., 1987; Bender, 1994; Bristol-Myers Squibb Oncology, 2005; Conrad & Dexter, 1990; Dawson, 1991; Del Toro et al., 2005; Demetri, 1992; Dewey, 1987; Dudjak & Fleck, 1991; Ettinghausen et al., 1987; Farrell, 1992; Fields & Koeller, 1993; Genentech, Inc., 2005; Haeuber, 1995; Hogan et al., 1990; Kozeny et al., 1988; Lee et al., 1989; Licinio et al., 1998; Quesada et al., 1986; Ream et al., 1990; Richardson, 2004; Rieger, 1999; Robinson & Posner, 1992; Rosenberg, 1991; Rust et al., 1990; Sandstrom, 1996; Sergi, 1991; Shelton & Sargent, 1990; Siegel & Puri, 1991; St. Pierre et al., 1992; Valentine et al., 1998.

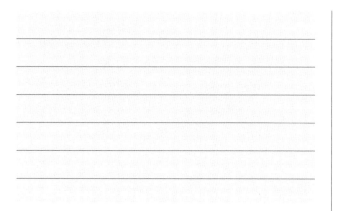

have received > 300 mg/m² doxorubicin) (Speyer et al., 1992). Iron-chelating agents inhibit the generation of free radicals. Speyer and Wasserheit (1998) reported that dexrazoxane significantly decreased cardiac toxicity in children when the drug was administered in pediatric trials. Additional trials involving pediatric patients are ongoing. Dexrazoxane is FDA-approved to reduce cardiac toxicity in adults (Pfizer, 2003c).

b) Administer medications as prescribed to treat CHF, and support cardiac output (e.g., use diuretics, inotropic cardiac medications, vasodilators, and/or oxygen).

c) Metoprolol tartrate, a beta blocker, has been used effectively to treat pediatric patients who have severe CHF following doxorubicin therapy (Shaddy et al., 1995).

d) Develop an activity or exercise plan.

e) Institute dietary modifications (e.g., a low-salt diet), as necessary for CHF.

f) Instruct patients to avoid tobacco and alcohol use because these agents stimulate cardiac muscle.

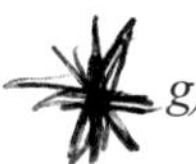

g) Expect to discontinue or reduce the dose of the cardiotoxic agent if the patient's ejection fraction is less than 55% (Kantrowitz & Bristow, 1984; Loerzel & Dow, 2003).

h) Monitor results of ECGs; for patients receiving chemotherapy, an ECG is recommended at three months, six months, and one year post–anthracycline therapy.

i) Monitor results of MUGA scans; for patients receiving chemotherapy, a scan is recommended every five years.

9. Patient and family education (Loerzel & Dow, 2003; Story, 2005)

a) Teach patients that cardiotoxicity is a possible side effect of the drug(s) (e.g., anthracyclines [doxorubicin, daunorubicin and liposomal daunorubicin, mitoxantrone]; high-dose 5-FU; high-dose cyclophosphamide; and interleukins, interferons, and some monoclonal antibodies); see Tables 24 and 25.

b) Instruct patients about the signs and symptoms of CHF and when to report to a nurse or physician; explain that close monitoring for possible late effects may be required even after treatment has ended.

c) Instruct patients that chronic cardiac toxicity usually is dose-related and possibly irreversible.

d) Inform patients and caregivers about strategies they can use to manage symptoms at home.

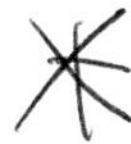

e) Ensure that patients are familiar with the ongoing protocol for follow-up care (Blatt et al., 1997).

(1) Each year, a standard physical and history

(2) Every two to five years, MUGA scans and/or ECG. The number of risk factors should determine the interval between such tests.

(3) Every three years, 24-hour Holter monitoring

(4) Before pregnancy, general anesthesia, or the start of a vigorous exercise program, a cardiology consult.

f) Encourage maintenance of a healthful lifestyle that eliminates tobacco and alcohol and includes exercising regularly and maintaining an appropriate weight and nutritious diet (Bottomley, 2004).

g) Stress the importance of lifelong follow-up care with a healthcare provider familiar with the patient's cancer history, treatment, and risk of late effects (Bottomley, 2004).

References

Adams, M.J., Hardenbergh, P.H., Constine, L.S., & Lipshultz, S.E. (2003). Radiation-associated cardiovascular disease. *Critical Reviews in Oncology/Hematology, 45,* 55–75.

Akhtar, S.S., Salim, K.P., & Bano, Z.A. (1993). Symptomatic cardiotoxicity with high-dose 5-fluorouracil infusion: A prospective study. *Oncology, 50,* 441–444.

Akhtar, S.S., Wani, B.A., Bano, Z.A., Salim, K.P., & Handoo, F.A. (1996). 5-fluorouracil-induced severe but reversible cardiogenic shock: A case report. *Tumori, 82,* 505–507.

Allen, A. (1992). The cardiotoxicity of chemotherapeutic drugs. In M.C. Perry (Ed.), *The chemotherapy source book* (2nd ed., pp. 582–597). Baltimore: Williams & Wilkins.

Anand, A.J. (1994). Fluorouracil cardiotoxicity. *Annals of Pharmacotherapy, 28,* 374–378.

Arbuck, S.G., Adams, J., & Strauss, H. (1992). *A reassessment of cardiac toxicity associated with Taxol.* Abstract presented at the Second National Cancer Institute Workshop on Taxol and Taxus, Alexandria, VA.

Aventis Pharmaceuticals. (2003). Taxotere [Package insert]. Collegeville, PA: Author.

Barton-Burke, M., Wilkes, G.M., & Ingwersen, K.C. (2001). *Cancer chemotherapy: A nursing process approach* (3rd ed.). Sudbury, MA: Jones and Bartlett.

Battiato, L.A., & Wheeler, V.S. (2000). Biotherapy. In C.H. Yarbro, M. Goodman, M.H. Frogge, & S.L. Groenwald (Eds.), *Cancer nursing: Principles and practice* (5th ed., pp. 543–579). Sudbury, MA: Jones and Bartlett.

Becker, K., Erckenbrecht, J.F., Haussinger, D., & Frieling, T. (1999). Cardiotoxicity of antiproliferative compound fluorouracil. *Drugs, 57,* 475–484.

Belldegrun, A., Webb, D.E., & Austin, H.A. (1987). Effects of interleukin-2 on renal function in patients receiving immunotherapy for advanced cancer. *Annals of Internal Medicine, 106,* 817–822.

Bender, C. (1994). Cognitive dysfunction associated with biological response modifier therapy. *Oncology Nursing Forum, 21,* 515–523.

Berchem, G.J., Ries, F., Hanfelt, J., Duhem, C., Keipes, M., Delagardelle, C., et al. (1996). Epirubicin cardiotoxicity: A study comparing low with high-dose-intensity weekly schedules. *Supportive Care in Cancer, 4,* 308–312.

Bertolini, A., Flumano, M., Fusco, O., Muffatti, A., Scarinici, A., Pontiggia, G., et al. (2001). Acute cardiotoxicity during capecitabine treatment: A case report. *Tumori, 87,* 200–206.

Blatt, J., Copeland, D.R., & Bleyer, A. (1997). Late effects of childhood cancer and its treatment. In P.A. Pizzo, M.D. Poplack, & D.G. Poplack (Eds.), *Principles and practice of pediatric oncology* (3rd ed., pp. 1303–1329). Philadelphia: Lippincott-Raven.

Bottomley, S.J. (2004). Late effects of childhood cancer: Cardiovascular system. In N.E. Kline (Ed.), *Essentials of pediatric oncology nursing: A core curriculum* (pp. 273–274). Glenview, IL: Association of Pediatric Oncology Nurses.

Bristol-Myers Squibb Oncology. (2005). Erbitux [Package insert]. Princeton, NJ: Author.

Bristol-Myers Squibb Oncology/Immunology. (2000). *A.S.K. BMSOI: Ask Bristol-Myers Squibb Oncology/Immunology medical information fax catalog*. Princeton, NJ: Author.

Bryson, H.M., & Sorkin, E.M. (1993). Cladribine: A review of its pharmacodynamic and pharmacokinetic properties and therapeutic potential in hematological malignancies. *Drugs, 46,* 872–894.

Burns, L. (1992). The cardiotoxicity of chemotherapeutic drugs. In M.C. Perry (Ed.), *The chemotherapy source book* (2nd ed., pp. 582–597). Baltimore: Williams & Wilkins.

Camp-Sorrell, D. (2000). Chemotherapy: Toxicity management. In C.H. Yarbro, M.H. Frogge, M. Goodman, & S.L. Groenwald (Eds.), *Cancer nursing: Principles and practice* (5th ed., pp. 444–486). Sudbury, MA: Jones and Bartlett.

Carlson, R.W. (1992). Reducing the cardiotoxicity of the anthracyclines. *Oncology, 6*(6), 95–108.

Chiron Corporation. (2004). Proleukin [Package insert]. Retrieved April 27, 2004, from http://www.proleukin.com

Chronowski, G.M., Wilder, R.B., Tucker, S.L., Ha, C.S., Younes, A., Fayad, L., et al. (2003). Analysis of in-field control and late toxicity for adults with early-stage Hodgkin's disease treated with chemotherapy followed by radiotherapy. *International Journal of Radiation Oncology, Biology, Physics, 55,* 36–43.

Cleri, L.B., & Haywood, R. (2002). *Oncology pocket guide to chemotherapy* (5th ed.). Philadelphia: Elsevier.

Conrad, K.J., & Dexter, L.J. (1990). Cutaneous alterations. In J.M. Yasko & L.A. Dudjak (Eds.), *Biological response modifier therapy: Symptom management* (pp. 129–134). New York: Park Row.

D'Incalci, M., Schuller, J., Colombo, T., Zucchetti, M., & Riva, A. (1998). Taxoids in combination with anthracyclines and other agents: Pharmacokinetic considerations. *Seminars in Oncology, 25*(Suppl. 13), 16–20.

Damon, L.E. (1992). Anemia of chronic disease in the aged: Diagnosis and treatment. *Geriatrics, 47,* 47–54, 57.

Dawson, M. (1991). *Lymphokines and interleukins.* Boca Raton, FL: CRC Press.

Del Toro, G., Morris, E., & Cairo, M.S. (2005). Tumor lysis syndrome: Pathophysiology, definition, and alternative treatment approaches. *Clinical Advances in Hematology and Oncology, 3*(1), 54–61.

Demetri, G. (1992). Hematopoietic growth factors: Current knowledge and future prospects. *Current Problems in Cancer, 16*(4), 177–259.

Dewey, D. (1987). Role of the nurse in the use of biological response modifiers. *AAOHN Journal, 35*(4), 163–167.

Doroshow, J.H. (1991). Doxorubicin-induced cardiac toxicity. *New England Journal of Medicine, 324,* 343–345.

Dudjak, L., & Fleck, A. (1991). BRMs: New drug therapy comes of age. *RN, 54*(10), 42–48.

Eli Lilly & Co. (2004). Gemzar [Package insert]. Indianapolis, IN: Author.

Escobar, P.F., Markman, M., Zanotti, K., Webster, K., & Belinson, J. (2003). Phase 2 trial of pegylated liposomal doxorubicin in advanced endometrial cancer. *Journal of Cancer Research and Clinical Oncology, 129,* 651–654.

Eskilsson, J., Albertsson, M., & Mercke, C. (1988). Adverse cardiac effects during induction chemotherapy treatment with cisplatin and 5-fluorouracil. *Radiotherapy and Oncology, 13*(1), 41–46.

Ettinghausen, S., Moore, J., White, D., Plalanras, L., Young, N., & Rosenberg, S. (1987). Hematologic effects of immunotherapy with lymphokine-activated killer cells and recombinant interleukin-2 in cancer patients. *Blood, 69,* 1654–1660.

Ewer, M.S., & Benjamin, R.S. (1997). Cardiotoxicity of chemotherapeutic drugs. In M.C. Perry (Ed.), *The chemotherapy source book* (2nd ed., pp. 649–659). Baltimore: Williams & Wilkins.

Farrell, M.M. (1992). The challenge of adult respiratory distress syndrome during interleukin-2 immunotherapy. *Oncology Nursing Forum, 19,* 475–480.

Fields, S.M., & Koeller, M.S. (1993). Biologic agents. In G. Weiss (Ed.), *Clinical oncology* (pp. 119–123). Norwalk, CT: Appleton & Lange.

Fischer, D.S., Knobf, M.T., & Durivage, H.J. (Eds.). (1993). *The cancer chemotherapy handbook* (4th ed.). St. Louis, MO: Mosby.

Genentech, Inc. (2003). Herceptin (trastuzumab) [Package insert]. South San Francisco, CA: Author.

Genentech, Inc. (2005). *Oncology products: Herceptin, Rituxan, Avastin, Tarceva.* Retrieved January 31, 2005, from http://www.gene.com/gene/products

Genentech/IDEC Pharmaceuticals. (1999). Rituxan [Package insert]. South San Francisco, CA: Author.

GlaxoSmithKline. (2002). Navelbine [Package insert]. Retrieved April 30, 2004, from http://www.gsk.com

Gradishar, W.J., & Vokes, E.S. (1990). 5-fluorouracil cardiotoxicity: A critical review. *Annals of Oncology, 1,* 409–414.

Grenier, M.A., & Lipshultz, S.E. (1998). Epidemiology of anthracycline cardiotoxicity in children and adults. *Seminars in Oncology, 25*(Suppl. 10), 72–85.

Haeuber, D. (1995). The flu-like syndrome. In P.T. Rieger (Ed.), *Biotherapy: A comprehensive overview* (pp. 243–258). Sudbury, MA: Jones and Bartlett.

Hainsworth, J.D., Burris, H.A., III, Litchy, S., Morrissey, L.H., Barton, J.H., Bradhof, J.E., et al. (2000). Weekly docetaxel in the treatment of elderly patients with advanced nonsmall cell lung carcinoma: A Minnie Pearl Cancer Research Network phase II trial. *Cancer, 89,* 328–333.

Hogan, C.M., Colao, D.M., & Horban-Shuster, M. (1990). Nausea and vomiting. In J.M. Yasko & L.A. Dudjak (Eds.), *Biological response modifier therapy: Symptom management* (pp. 75–90). New York: Park Row.

Hortobagyi, G.N., Frye, D., Buzdar, A.U., Ewer, M.S., Fraschini, G., Hug, V., et al. (1989). Decreased cardiac toxicity of doxorubicin administered by continuous intravenous infusion in combination chemotherapy for metastatic breast carcinoma. *Cancer, 63,* 37–45.

Hurteloup, P., & Ganzina, F. (1986). Clinical studies with new anthracyclines: Epirubicin, idarubicin, esorubicin [Abstract]. *Drugs Under Experimental Clinical Research, 12*(1–3), 233–246.

Kantrowitz, N.E., & Bristow, M.R. (1984). Cardiotoxicity of antitumor agents. *Progress in Cardiovascular Disease, 27,* 195–200.

Kaszyk, L.K. (1986). Cardiac toxicity associated with cancer therapy. *Oncology Nursing Forum, 13*(4), 81–88.

Kleiman, N.S., Lehane, D.E., Geyer, C.E., Jr., Pratt, C.M., & Young, J.G. (1987). Prinzmetal's angina during 5-fluorouracil chemotherapy. *American Journal of Medicine, 82,* 566–568.

Kozeny, G.A., Nicolas, J.D., Creekmore, S., Sticklin, L., Hano, J.E., & Fisher, R.I. (1988). Effects of interleukin-2 immunotherapy on renal function. *Journal of Clinical Oncology, 7,* 1170–1176.

Krischer, J.P., Epstein, S., Cuthbertson, D.D., Goorin, A.M., Epstein, M.L., & Lipshultz, S.E. (1997). Clinical cardiotoxicity following anthracycline treatment for childhood cancer: The pediatric oncology group experience. *Journal of Clinical Oncology, 15,* 1544–1552.

Labianca, R., Beretta, G., Clerici, M., Fraschini, P., & Luporini, G. (1982). Cardiac toxicity of 5-fluorouracil: A study of 1083 patients. *Tumori, 68,* 505–510.

Langer, T., Stohr, W., Bielack, S., Paulussen, M., Treuner, J., & Beck, J.D. (2004). Late effects surveillance system for sarcoma patients. *Pediatric Blood Cancer, 42,* 373–379.

Leaf, A.N., Propert, K., Corcoran, C., Catalano, P.J., Trump, D.L., Harris, J.E., et al. (2003). Phase III study of combined chemohormonal therapy in metastatic prostate cancer (ECOG 3882): An Eastern Cooperative Oncology Group study. *Medical Oncology, 20*(2), 137–146.

Lee, R., Lotze, M., Skibber, J., Tucker, E., Bonow, R., Ognibene, F., et al. (1989). Cardiorespiratory effects of immunotherapy with interleukins. *Journal of Clinical Oncology, 7*(1), 7–20.

Licinio, J., Kling, M., & Hauser, P. (1998). Cytokines and brain function: Relevance to interferon—An induced mood and cognitive changes. *Seminars in Oncology, 25*(Suppl. 1), 30–38.

Loerzel, V.W., & Dow, K.H. (2003). Cardiac toxicity related to cancer treatment. *Clinical Journal of Oncology Nursing, 7,* 557–562.

Mead Johnson Oncology Products. (2001). Rubex [Package insert]. Princeton, NJ: Author.

Mills, B.A., & Roberts, R.W. (1979). Cyclophosphamide-induced cardiomyopathy: A report of two cases and review of the English literature. *Cancer, 43,* 2223–2226.

Nextar Pharmaceuticals, Inc. (1999). DaunaXome [Package insert]. Retrieved August 28, 2004, from http://www.gilead.com

O'Brien, M.E.R., Wigler, N., Inbar, M., Rosso, R., Grischke, E., Santoro, A., et al. (2004). Reduced cardiotoxicity and comparable efficacy in a phase 3 trial of pegylated liposomal doxorubicin HCl (CAELYX/DOXIL) versus conventional doxorubicin for first-line treatment of metastatic breast cancer. *Annals of Oncology, 15,* 440–449.

Ortho Biotech. (2002). Leustatin [Package insert]. Raritan, NJ: Author.

Ortho Biotech. (2004). Doxil [Package insert]. Raritan, NJ: Author.

Pfizer. (2003a). Ellence [Package insert]. New York: Author. Retrieved January 10, 2005, from http://www.pfizer.com/do/medicines/mn_uspi.html

Pfizer. (2003b). Emcyt [Package insert]. Retrieved January 10, 2005, from http://www.pfizer.com/do/medicines/mn_uspi.html

Pfizer. (2003c). Zinecard [Package insert]. Retrieved January 10, 2005, from http://www.pfizer.com/do/medicines/mn_uspi.html

Platel, D., Pouna, P., Bonoron-Adele, S., & Robert, J. (2000, March 1). Preclinical evaluation of the cardiotoxicity of taxane-anthracycline combinations using the model of isolated perfused rat heart [Abstract]. *Toxicology and Applied Pharmacology, 163,* 135–140.

Pottage, A., Holt, S., Ludgate, S., & Langlands, A.O. (1978). Fluorouracil cardiotoxicity. *BMJ, 1,* 547.

Quesada, J.R., Talpaz, M., Rios, A., Kurzrock, R., & Gutterman, J.U. (1986). Clinical toxicity of interferons in cancer patients: A review. *Journal of Clinical Oncology, 4,* 234–243.

Ream, M.A., Colao, D.M., & Downs, M.A. (1990). Urinary system alterations. In J.M. Yasko & L.A. Dudjak (Eds.), *Biological response modifier therapy: Symptom management* (pp. 149–162). New York: Park Row.

Richardson, M.T. (2004). Electrolyte imbalances. In C.H. Yarbro, M.H. Frogge, & M. Goodman (Eds.), *Cancer symptom management* (3rd ed., pp. 440–460). Sudbury, MA: Jones and Bartlett.

Rieger, P.T. (Ed.). (1999). *Clinical handbook for biotherapy.* Sudbury, MA: Jones and Bartlett.

Rivera, E., Valero, V., Arun, B., Royce, M., Adinin, R., Hoelzer, K., et al. (2003). Phase II study of pegylated liposomal doxorubicin in combination with gemcitabine in patients with metastatic breast cancer. *Journal of Clinical Oncology, 21,* 3249–3254.

Robinson, K.D., & Posner, J.D. (1992). Patterns of self-care needs and interventions related to biologic response modifier therapy: Fatigue as a model. *Seminars in Oncology Nursing, 8*(Suppl. 4), 17–22.

Roche Pharmaceuticals. (2004). Xeloda [Package insert]. Nutley, NJ: Author. Retrieved April 5, 2004, from http://www.xeloda.com

Rosenberg, S.A. (1991). Immunotherapy and gene therapy of cancer. *Cancer Research, 51*(Suppl. 19), 5074S–5079S.

Rowinsky, E.K., McGuire, W.P., Guarnieri, T., Fisherman, J.S., Christian, M.C., & Donehower, R.C. (1991). Cardiac disturbances during the administration of Taxol. *Journal of Clinical Oncology, 9,* 1704–1712.

Rust, D., Miller, S., & Horbal-Shuster, M. (1990). Stomatitis. In J.M. Yasko & L.A. Dudjak (Eds.), *Biological response modifier therapy: Symptom management* (pp. 107–120). New York: Park Row.

Safra, T. (2003). Cardiac safety of liposomal anthracyclines. *Oncologist, 8,* 17–24.

Sandstrom, S.K. (1996). Nursing management of patients receiving biological therapy. *Seminars in Oncology Nursing, 12,* 152–162.

Santos, D.L., Moreno, A.J., Leino, R.L., Froberg, M.K., & Wallace, K.B. (2002). Carvedilol protects against doxorubicin-induced mitochondrial cardiomyopathy. *Toxicology Applied Pharmacology, 185,* 218–227.

Sergi, J. (1991). *The physiology of the flu-like syndrome and the cardiopulmonary and renal symptoms associated with BRM therapy* [Monograph]. Emeryville, CA: Cetus.

Shaddy, R.E., Olsen, S.L., Bristow, M.R., Taylor, D.O., Bullock, E.A., Tani, L.Y., et al. (1995). Efficacy and safety of metoprolol in the treatment of doxorubicin-induced cardiomyopathy in pediatric patients. *American Heart Journal, 129,* 197–199.

Shelton, B., & Sargent, C. (1990). Neurologic toxicity management with BRMs. *Oncology Nursing Forum, 17,* 964–965.

Shenkenberg, T.D., & Von Hoff, D.D. (1986). Mitoxantrone: A new anticancer drug with significant clinical activity. *Annals of Internal Medicine, 105,* 67–81.

Siegel, J.P., & Puri, R.K. (1991). Interleukin-2 toxicity. *Journal of Clinical Oncology, 9,* 694–704.

Singal, P.K., & Iliskovic, N. (1998). Doxorubicin-induced cardiomyopathy. *New England Journal of Medicine, 339,* 900–904.

Soe, M.S., Berkman, A., & Mardelli, J. (1996). Case report: Paclitaxel induced myocardial ischemia. *Maryland Medical Journal, 45,* 41–43.

Sparano, J.A. (1999, June). Doxorubicin/taxane combinations: Cardiac toxicity and pharmacokinetics. *Seminars in Oncology, 26*(Suppl. 9), 14–19.

Speyer, J., & Freedberg, R.S. (2000). Cardiac complications. In M.D. Abeloff, J.D. Armitage, A.S. Lichter, & J.E. Niederhuber (Eds.), *Clinical oncology* (2nd ed., pp. 1047–1060). New York: Churchill Livingstone.

Speyer, J., & Wasserheit, C. (1998). Strategies for reduction of anthracycline cardiac toxicity. *Seminars in Oncology, 25,* 525–537.

Speyer, J.L., Green, M.D., Zeleninch-Jacquotte, A., Wernz, J.C., Rey, M., Sanger, J., et al. (1992). ICRF-187 permits longer treatment with doxorubicin in women with breast cancer. *Journal of Clinical Oncology, 10,* 117–127.

St. Pierre, B.A., Kasper, C.E., & Lindsey, A.M. (1992). Fatigue mechanisms in patients with cancer: Effects of tumor necrosis factor and exercise on skeletal muscle. *Oncology Nursing Forum, 19,* 419–425.

Steinherz, L.J., & Yahalom, J. (1997). Adverse effects of treatment. In V.T. DeVita, S. Hellman, & S.A. Rosenberg (Eds.), *Cancer: Principles and practice of oncology* (5th ed., pp. 2739–2747). Philadelphia: Lippincott-Raven.

Story, K.T. (2005). Alterations in circulation. In J.K. Itano & K.N. Taoka (Eds.), *Core curriculum for oncology nursing* (4th ed., pp. 364–379). St. Louis, MO: Elsevier.

U.S. Food and Drug Administration. (1998). Busulfan [Product information]. Retrieved April 30, 2004, http://www.fda.gov/cder/cancer/index.htm

U.S. Food and Drug Administration. (2001). Xeloda [Product information]. Retrieved April 30, 2004, http://www.fda.gov/cder/cancer/index.htm

Valentine, A., Meyers, C.A., Kling, M.A., Richelson, E., & Hauser, P. (1998). Mood and cognitive side effects of interferon-a therapy. *Seminars in Oncology, 25*(Suppl. 1), 39–47.

Van Cutsem, E., Hoff, P.M., Blum, J.L., Abt, M., & Osterwalder, B. (2002). Incidence of cardiotoxicity with the oral fluoropyrimidine capecitabine is typical of that reported with 5-fluorouracil. *Annals of Oncology, 13,* 484–485.

Von Hoff, D.D., Layard, M.W., Basa, P., Davis, H.L., Von Hoff, A.L., Rozencweig, M., et al. (1979). Risk factors for doxorubicin-induced congestive heart failure. *Annals of Internal Medicine, 91,* 710–717.

Von Hoff, D.D., Rozencweig, M., Layard, M., Slavik, M., & Muggia, F.M. (1977). Daunomycin-induced cardiotoxicity in children and adults: A review of 110 cases. *American Journal of Medicine, 62,* 200–208.

Wilkes, G.M., & Burke, M.B. (2004). *2004 oncology nursing drug handbook.* Sudbury, MA: Jones and Bartlett.

Wujcik, D., & Downs, S. (1992). Bone marrow transplantation. *Critical Care Nursing Clinics of North America, 4*(1), 149–166.

Wyeth Pharmaceuticals. (2004). Mylotarg [Package insert]. Philadelphia: Author.

Yahalom, J., & Portlock, C.S. (2005). Cardiac toxicity. In V.T. DeVita, S. Hellman, & S.A. Rosenberg (Eds.), *Cancer: Principles and practice of oncology* (7th ed., pp. 2545–2555). Philadelphia: Lippincott Williams & Wilkins.

F. Pulmonary toxicity: Pulmonary toxicity and damage usually are irreversible and progressive as a result of chemotherapy administration. Diagnosing pulmonary signs and symptoms in patients with cancer can be challenging because toxicity can mimic a broad spectrum of pathogenic causes including infectious agents and neoplastic lung disorders (Tietjen & Stover, 2002). Consequently, it is imperative to detect evidence of pulmonary toxicity as early as possible and have a clear understanding of potential for toxicity (Camp-Sorrell, 2000).

1. Pathophysiology
    a) Toxic effects of chemotherapy
        (1) Direct damage: Some chemotherapy causes direct damage to the alveoli and capillary endothelium (Kriesman & Wolkove, 1992; Wickham, 1986).
        (2) Immunologic mechanism may cause damage. Either the lung or the drug may act as an antigen, causing an allergic-like response that results in an inflammatory-type reaction (Koh & Castro, 1996).
        (3) Metabolic damage: Cyclophosphamide metabolism in the lung leads to the formation of alkylating metabolites and acrolein (a reactive aldehyde), which may cause toxicity (Barton-Burke, Wilkes, & Ingwersen, 2001).
        (4) Mechanism of the clinical antitumor action is not fully characterized (i.e., gefitinib inhibits intracellular phosphorylation of numerous tyrosine kinases associated with transmembrane cell surface receptors, including the epidermal growth factor receptor [EGFR-TK]; studies are lacking to confirm any correlation) (AstraZeneca Pharmaceuticals, 2004).
    b) Toxic effect of biotherapy: Progressive development of noncardiogenic interstitial pulmonary edema is related to capillary leak syndrome induced by IL-2 (Schwartzentruber, 2000).
2. Most common types of pulmonary toxicity
    a) Pulmonary edema (noncardiogenic): Acute onset is related to capillary leak syndrome. Docetaxel is associated with fluid retention

that is treatable with diuretics (Pronk, Stoter, & Verweij, 1995).

b) Hypersensitivity pneumonitis

c) Pulmonary interstitial fibrosis and pneumonitis

(1) Caused by inflammatory-type reaction (Kachel & Martin, 1994; Koh & Castro, 1996)

(2) Occurrence of delayed or abnormal tissue regeneration

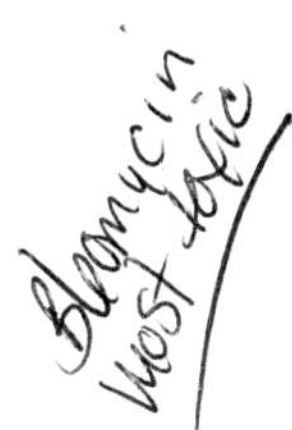

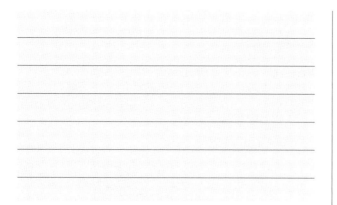

(3) Destruction of the alveolar-capillary endothelium, leading to changes in interstitial fibroblast (Kachel & Martin, 1994; Koh & Castro, 1996); honeycomb-like changes can occur from chronic exposure to chemotherapy agents resulting in extensive alteration of pulmonary parenchyma. Changes in the connective tissue, obliteration of alveoli, and dilatation of air spaces result in "honeycombing" pathophysiology (Koh & Castro).

3. Incidence: Incidence varies according to agent. The incidence associated with specific agents may be difficult to determine because of combination therapies. Pulmonary toxicity increases with thoracic radiation therapy and if the patient is a smoker (Comis, 1992; Senan, Paul, Thompson, & Kay, 1992) (see Table 26).

a) The chemotherapy drugs most commonly associated with pulmonary toxicity

(1) Pulmonary toxicity is commonly associated with bleomycin, busulfan, carmustine, cyclophosphamide, cytosine arabinoside, gemcitabine, methotrexate, and mitomycin (Tiejen & Stover, 2002). Newer agents also are associated with toxicity (e.g., gefitinib) (AstraZeneca Pharmaceuticals, 2004).

(2) Other agents associated with pulmonary dyspnea include azathioprine, chlorambucil, chlorozotocin, erlotinib, etoposide, gemcitabine, lomustine, melphalan, mercaptopurine, procarbazine, semustine, teniposide, trans-retinoic acid, vinblastine, vindesine, and teniposide (Camp, Gullatte, Gilmore, & Hutcherson, 2001; Tiejen & Stover, 2002).

(3) The primary pulmonary toxicity associated with paclitaxel is acute pneumonitis, which appears to be a rare hypersensitivity reaction to Cremophor EL emulsifier (Camp et al., 2001; Goldberg & Vannice, 1995; Ramanathan & Belani, 1996; Read, Mortimer, & Picus, 2002).

(4) Use of hydroxyurea has resulted in rare reports of interstitial pulmonary infiltrates and acute alveolitis (Hennemann, Bross, Reichle, & Andreessen, 1993; Kavuru, Gadsden, Lichtin, & Gephardt, 1994).

(5) Patients who develop cyclophosphamide-associated pulmonary toxicity have a poor prognosis—a 50% mortality rate. However, the incidence of related pneumonitis or fibrosis appears to be low (Twohig & Matthay, 1990).

(6) Medications such as imatinib mesylate cause cardiac problems related to severe fluid retention. Pleural effusion, pericardial effusion, pulmonary edema, and ascites were reported in 2%–6% of patients. These events appear to be dose related, were more common in the blast crisis and accelerated phase studies (where the dose was 600 mg/day), and were more common in the elderly. These events usually were managed by interrupting imatinib mesylate treatment and using diuretics or other appropriate supportive care measures. However, a few of these events may be serious or life-threatening, and one patient with blast crisis died with pleural effusion, CHF, and renal failure (Deininger, O'Brien, Ford, & Drukcer, 2003; Novartis Pharmaceuticals, 2004).

b) Biotherapy agents most commonly associated with pulmonary toxicity (Schwartzentruber, 2000; Siegel & Puri, 1991)

(1) A high incidence of pulmonary edema is associated with IL-2 associated with capillary leak syndrome. It commonly occurs with the administration of IL-2 and resolves quickly after therapy ends and diuresis begins. Pulmonary edema is a dose-limiting toxicity of high-dose IL-2 therapy; severity depends on

Table 26. Pulmonary Toxicity of Chemotherapeutic Drugs

Classification	Drug	Incidence	Characteristic Effects and Comments
Alkylating agents	Busulfan	Incidence is rare but serious. Busulfan is associated with pulmonary damage and pneumonitis. It occurs in between 2.5% and 11.5% of patients, usually those on long-term treatment, although it can occur more acutely. A progressive and often untreatable pneumonitis is an important complication of therapy. Bronchopulmonary dysplasia with pulmonary fibrosis occurs with chronic therapy (GlaxoSmithKline, 2004).	Insidious onset cough, dyspnea, and low-grade fever; bronchodysplasia progressing to interstitial pulmonary fibrosis ("busulfan lung") (Wilkes & Burke, 2004) Bronchopulmonary dysplasia with pulmonary fibrosis is a rare but serious complication following chronic busulfan therapy. The average onset of symptoms is four years after therapy; delayed onsets have occured (range = 4 months–10 years) (GlaxoSmithKline, 2004). Chest x-rays show diffuse linear densities, sometimes with reticular nodular or nodular infiltrates or consolidation. Pleural effusions have occured (GlaxoSmithKline, 2004; Smalley & Wall, 1966).
	Chlorambucil	Incidence is low. Respiratory dysfunction is reported at high doses (GlaxoSmithKline, 2003c).	Pulmonary fibrosis; bronchopulmonary dysplasia in patients receiving long-term therapy (GlaxoSmithKline, 2003c)
	Cyclophosphamide	The incidence of cyclophosphamide pulmonary toxicity is rare. Diffuse alveolar damage is the most common manifestation of cyclophosphamide-induced lung disease (Rossi et al., 2000). There is no relationship between development of lung injury and dose or duration of administration (Erasmus, 2000).	Edema, fibrosis, alveolar hemorrhage, and fibrin deposition (Twohig & Matthay, 1990); onset can be six months or longer. Interstitial pneumonitis has been reported as part of the postmarketing experience. Interstitial pulmonary fibrosis has been reported in patients receiving high doses of cyclophosphamide over a prolonged period (Mead Johnson Oncology, 2000). Anaphylactic reactions and death also have been reported in association with this event. Possible cross-sensitivity with other alkylating agents has been reported (Mead Johnson Oncology, 2000). Treatment is discontinuation of the agent, and steroids have good to variable response (Mead Johnson Oncology, 2000).
	Melphalan	Reports of bronchopulmonary dysplasia (GlaxoSmithKline, 2003a) Acute hypersensitivity reactions including anaphylaxis were reported in 2.4% of 425 patients receiving the injected drug for myeloma (GlaxoSmithKline, 2003a).	Pulmonary fibrosis, interstitial pneumonia, bronchospasm, and dyspnea also may be a sign of rare hypersensitivity, not pulmonary toxicity. These patients appeared to respond to antihistamine and corticosteroid therapy. If a hypersensitivity reaction occurs, IV or oral melphalan should not be readministered because hypersensitivity reactions also have been reported with oral melphalan (GlaxoSmithKline, 2003a).
	Oxaliplatin	Associated with pulmonary fibrosis (< 1% of study patients), which may be fatal Incidence of events increase with combined therapy. An acute syndrome of pharyngolaryngeal dysesthesia seen in 1%–2% (grade 3 or 4) of patients previously untreated for advanced colorectal cancer. Previously treated patients experienced subjective sensations of dysphagia or dyspnea, without laryngospasm or bronchospasm (no stridor or wheezing) (Sanofi-Synthelabo, Inc., 2004).	Anaphylactic-like reactions are treatable with epinephrine, corticosteroids, and antihistamines. The combined incidence of cough, dyspnea, and hypoxia was 43% (any grade) and 7% (grades 3 and 4) in the oxaliplatin plus 5-FU/LV arm compared to 32% (any grade) and 5% (grades 3 and 4) in the irinotecan plus 5-FU/LV arm of unknown duration for patients with previously untreated colorectal cancer. In case of unexplained respiratory symptoms such as nonproductive cough, dyspnea, crackles, or radiologic pulmonary infiltrates, oxaliplatin should be discontinued until further pulmonary investigation excludes interstitial lung disease or pulmonary fibrosis (Sanofi-Synthelabo, Inc., 2004).
	Temozolomide	Upper respiratory tract infection: 8% Pharyngitis: 8% Sinusitis: 6% Coughing: 5% (Schering Corporation, 2004)	Allergic reactions, including rare cases of anaphylaxis; used with nitrosoureas and procarbazine (Schering Corporation, 2004)

(Continued on next page)

Table 26. Pulmonary Toxicity of Chemotherapeutic Drugs *(Continued)*

Classification	Drug	Incidence	Characteristic Effects and Comments
Anticancer cytokines	Aldesleukin (IL-2)	Life-threatening grade IV: • Dyspnea: 1% • Respiratory disorders: 3% (acute respiratory distress syndrome [ARDS], respiratory failure, intubation); 1% (apnea) Adverse events occurring in ≥ 10% of patients (N = 525) (Chiron Corporation, 2002) • Dyspnea: 43% • Lung disorder: 24% (physical findings associated with pulmonary congestion, rales, rhonchi) • Respiratory disorder: 11% (ARDS, chest x-ray infiltrates, unspecified pulmonary changes) • Increased cough: 11% • Rhinitis: 10%	Pulmonary congestion, dyspnea, pulmonary edema, respiratory failure, tachypnea, pleural effusion, wheezing, apnea, pneumothorax, hemoptysis (Chiron Corporation, 2002)
	Interferon alfa-2b	Rare (Schering Corporation, 2002)	Fever, cough, dyspnea, pulmonary infiltrates, pneumonitis, pneumonia
	Oprelvekin (IL 11)	Dyspnea: 48% Rhinitis: 42% Increased cough: 29% Pharyngitis: 25% Pleural effusions: 10% (Wyeth Pharmaceuticals, 2004b)	Peripheral edema, dyspnea; preexisting fluid collections, including pericardial effusions or ascites, should be monitored. Fluid retention is reversible within several days following discontinuation of the oprelvekin. Fluid balance should be monitored, and appropriate medical management is advised. Closely monitor fluid and electrolyte status in patients receiving chronic diuretic therapy (Wyeth Pharmaceuticals, 2004b). Patients should be advised to immediately seek medical attention if any of the following signs or symptoms develop: swelling of the face, tongue, or throat; difficulty breathing, swallowing, or talking; shortness of breath; wheezing (Wyeth Pharmaceuticals, 2004b).
Antimetabolites	Capecitabine	Dyspnea: 14% (Roche Pharmaceuticals, 2003) Not considered a major toxicity but has demonstrated these side effects: 0.1% cough; 0.1% epistaxis and hemoptysis and respiratory distress; 0.2% asthma	Manage toxicities with symptomatic treatment, dose interruptions, and dose adjustment. Once dose has been adjusted, it should not be increased at a later time (Roche Pharmaceuticals, 2003).
	Cytarabine	"Cytarabine syndrome" in doses > 5 g/m² (6–12 hours after dose) (Castleberry et al., 1981; Spratto & Woods, 2004) Cytarabine liposomal: No pulmonary data (Chiron Corporation, 2000).	A syndrome of sudden respiratory distress, rapidly progressing to pulmonary edema, capillary leak syndrome, respiratory failure, and adult respiratory disease (Haupt et al., 1981)
	Fludarabine phosphate	Cough: 10%*; 44%** Pneumonia: 16%*; 22%** Dyspnea: 9%*; 22%** Sinusitis: 5%*; 0%** Pharyngitis: 0%*; 9%** Upper respiratory infection: 2%*; 16%** Allergic pneumonitis: 0%*; 6%** *N = 101; **N = 32 (Berlex Laboratories, 2003)	Pulmonary hypersensitivity reactions such as dyspnea, cough, and interstitial pulmonary infiltrate have been observed. In a clinical investigation using fludarabine phosphate injection in combination with pentostatin for the treatment of refractory chronic lymphocytic leukemia in adults, there was an unacceptably high incidence of fatal pulmonary toxicity. Therefore, this combination is not recommended (Berlex Laboratories, 2003).

(Continued on next page)

Table 26. Pulmonary Toxicity of Chemotherapeutic Drugs *(Continued)*

Classification	Drug	Incidence	Characteristic Effects and Comments
Antimetabolites *(cont.)*	Gemcitabine hydrochloride	Dyspnea: 23% (severe dyspnea in 3%) (Eli Lilly & Co., 2004) Parenchymal lung toxicity, including interstitial pneumonitis, pulmonary fibrosis, pulmonary edema, and adult respiratory distress syndrome, has been reported rarely (Eli Lilly & Co., 2004).	Dyspnea, cough, bronchospasm, and parenchymal lung toxicity (rare) may occur. If such effects develop, gemcitabine should be discontinued. Early use of supportive care measures may help to ameliorate these conditions (Eli Lilly & Co., 2004). Prolonged infusion time beyond 60 minutes and doses more than once weekly increase toxicities (Castleberry et al., 1981; Spratto & Woods, 2004). Respiratory failure and death occurred very rarely in some patients despite discontinuation of therapy (Pavlakis et al., 1997). Some patients experienced the onset of pulmonary symptoms up to two weeks after the last dose (Eli Lilly & Co., 2004).
	Methotrexate	Pulmonary edema: 1%–2% (Immunex, 1999) The incidence of pulmonary toxicity in patients receiving methotrexate is 5%–10% (Rossi et al., 2000). The toxicity is not dose related, although patients who receive treatment more frequently may be more susceptible to lung injury (Aronchick & Gefter, 1991).	Fever, dyspnea, cough (especially dry nonproductive), nonspecific pneumonitis, or a chronic interstitial obstructive pulmonary disease (deaths have been reported); pulmonary infiltrates (Immunex, 1999)
Antitumor antibiotics	Bleomycin sulfate	10% of treated patients (Bristol-Myers Squibb Oncology/Immunology, 1999). Nonspecific pneumonitis in approximately 1% progresses to pulmonary fibrosis and death. More common in patients older than 70 years of age receiving more than 400 units total dose. Toxicity is unpredictable and has been seen occasionally in young patients receiving low doses (Bristol-Myers Squibb Oncology/Immunology, 1999). Possible lower toxicity if not given IV bolus (Bristol-Myers Squibb Oncology/Immunology, 1999; Chisholm et al., 1992)	The characteristics of bleomycin-induced pneumonitis include dyspnea and fine rales. Bleomycin-induced pneumonitis produces patchy x-ray opacities usually of the lower lung fields that look the same as infectious bronchopneumonia or even lung metastases in some patients. Early toxicity may be self-resolving. Monitor for early warning signs of toxicity to avoid irreversible pulmonary damage. Chest x-rays should be taken every one to two weeks. If pulmonary changes are noted, treatment should be discontinued. Conflicting studies regarding exposure to increasing concentrations of oxygen-increasing toxicity warrants prudently maintaining oxygen levels at room air (25%) (Bristol-Myers Squibb Oncology/Immunology, 1999). Carbon monoxide diffusion capacity may be abnormal before other symptoms appear (Sleijfer et al., 1995).
	Doxorubicin hydrochloride liposome	Serious and sometimes life-threatening or fatal allergic/anaphylactoid-like infusion reactions have been reported (Ortho Biotech Corporation, 2003).	Acute infusion-related pulmonary reactions include shortness of breath and tightness of the throat (other reactions include, but are not limited to, flushing, facial swelling, headache, chills, back pain, tightness in the chest, and/or hypotension). In most patients, these reactions resolve over the course of several hours to a day once the infusion is terminated. In some patients, the reaction has resolved with slowing of the infusion rate. Doxil® should be administered at an initial rate of 1 mg/minute to minimize the risk of infusion reactions (Ortho Biotech Corporation, 2003).

(Continued on next page)

Table 26. Pulmonary Toxicity of Chemotherapeutic Drugs *(Continued)*

Classification	Drug	Incidence	Characteristic Effects and Comments
Antitumor antibiotics *(cont.)*	Mitomycin	Pulmonary toxicity has been reported with both single-agent therapy and combination chemotherapy, 3%–36%, 6–12 months after therapy. Prior treatment with mitomycin, cumulative doses > 30 mg/m^2, and other anticancer drugs may increase risk of toxicity (Bristol-Myers Squibb Oncology, 2000).	Dyspnea, nonproductive cough, diffuse alveolar damage, capillary leak, and pulmonary edema; severe bronchospasm has been reported following administration of vinca alkaloids in patients who previously or simultaneously received mitomycin. Acute respiratory distress occurred within minutes to hours after the vinca alkaloid injection. The total doses for each drug varied considerably (Bristol-Myers Squibb Oncology, 2000). Signs and symptoms of pneumonitis associated with mitomycin may be reversed if appropriate therapy is instituted early. Drug may be discontinued if dyspnea occurs even with normal chest radiograph (Luedke et al., 1985). Caution should be exercised using oxygen, because oxygen itself is toxic to the lungs. Pay careful attention to fluid balance and avoid overhydration (Bristol-Myers Squibb Oncology, 2000).
	Mitoxantrone	Reports of pulmonary toxicity (Immunex, 2000)	Interstitial pneumonitis
Miscellaneous antineoplastic agents	Arsenic trioxide	Incidence of respiratory events (all grades, N = 40): • Cough: 65% • Dyspnea: 53% • Epistaxis: 25% • Hypoxia: 23% • Pleural effusion: 20% • Wheezing: 13% Grade 3 and 4: • Dyspnea: 10% • Hypoxia: 10% • Pleural effusion: 3% (Cell Therapeutics, 2004)	These adverse effects have not been observed to be permanent or irreversible, nor do they usually require interruption of therapy (Cell Therapeutics, 2004).
	Gefitinib	Cases of interstitial lung disease have been observed in patients at an overall incidence of about 1%. Approximately one-third of the cases have been fatal. Reports indicated that interstitial lung disease has occurred in patients who have received prior radiation therapy (31%), prior chemotherapy (57%), and no previous therapy (12%) (AstraZeneca Pharmaceuticals, 2004).	Interstitial pneumonia, pneumonitis, and alveolitis. Patients often present with the acute onset of dyspnea, sometimes associated with cough or low-grade fever, often becoming severe within a short time and requiring hospitalization. If acute onset or worsening of pulmonary symptoms (dyspnea, cough, fever) occurs, therapy should be interrupted and promptly investigated. If interstitial lung disease is confirmed, discontinue Iressa®. Increased mortality has been observed in patients with concurrent idiopathic pulmonary fibrosis whose condition worsens while receiving gefitinib (AstraZeneca Pharmaceuticals, 2004).
	Imatinib mesylate	Severe superficial edema and severe fluid retention (pleural effusion, pulmonary edema, and ascites) were reported in 1%–6% of patients taking imatinib for gastrointestinal stromal tumors. 14%–15% reported dyspnea. Interstitial pneumonitis and pulmonary fibrosis are rare (Novartis Pharmaceuticals, 2004).	54%–74% of patients (two studies) had fluid retention, making pulmonary events difficult to identify. Other fluid retention events include pleural effusion, ascites, pulmonary edema, pericardial effusion, anasarca, edema aggravated, and fluid retention not otherwise specified. The overall safety profile of pediatric patients (39 children studied) was similar to that found in studies with adult patients treated with imatinib; however, no peripheral edema has been reported (Novartis Pharmaceuticals, 2004).

(Continued on next page)

Table 26. Pulmonary Toxicity of Chemotherapeutic Drugs *(Continued)*

Classification	Drug	Incidence	Characteristic Effects and Comments
Miscellaneous antineoplastic agents *(cont.)*	Irinotecan hydrochloride	Severe pulmonary events are rare, 4% grades 3 and 4; dyspnea (Pharmacia & Upjohn, 2002).	Dyspnea, increased coughing, rhinitis, and pneumonia Actual toxicity caused by the drug alone is unknown because more than half of patients had malignant or preexisting lung disease, and many were on combination therapy (Pharmacia & Upjohn, 2002). Irinotecan should not be used in combination with the "Mayo Clinic" regimen of 5-FU/leucovorin (administration for four to five consecutive days every four weeks) because of reports of increased toxicity, including toxic deaths (Pharmacia & Upjohn, 2002).
	Topotecan hydrochloride	The incidence of grades 3 and/or 4 dyspnea was 4% in patients with ovarian cancer and 12% in patients with small cell lung cancer. All grades, dyspnea: 22% (GlaxoSmithKline, 2003b)	Dyspnea, coughing, and pneumonia are the main pulmonary side effects (GlaxoSmithKline, 2003b).
Monoclonal antibodies	Alemtuzumab	Infusion-rate–related dyspnea: 17% Acute infusion-related events were most common during the first week of therapy. Incidence (N = 149) • Dyspnea: 26% • Cough: 25% • Bronchitis/pneumonitis: 21% • Pneumonia: 16% • Pharyngitis: 12% • Bronchospasm: 9% • Rhinitis: 7% (Berlex Laboratories, 2002)	Alemtuzumab has been associated with infusion-related events, including hypotension, rigors, fever, shortness of breath, bronchospasm, chills, and/or rash. To ameliorate or avoid infusion-related events, patients should be premedicated with an oral antihistamine and acetaminophen prior to dosing and monitored closely for infusion-related adverse events. Side effects include asthma, bronchitis, chronic obstructive pulmonary disease, hemoptysis, hypoxia, pleural effusion, pleurisy, pneumothorax, pulmonary edema, pulmonary fibrosis, pulmonary infiltration, respiratory depression, respiratory insufficiency, sinusitis, stridor, and throat tightness (Berlex Laboratories, 2002).
	Gemtuzumab ozogamicin	Hypoxia: 5% Pharyngitis: 12% Pneumonia: 13% Increased cough: 17% Epistaxis: 28% Dyspnea: 32% (often during the first 24 hours) Severe pulmonary events leading to death have been reported infrequently (Wyeth Pharmaceuticals, 2004a).	Signs, symptoms, and clinical findings include dyspnea, pulmonary infiltrates, pleural effusions, noncardiogenic pulmonary edema, pulmonary insufficiency and hypoxia, and ARDS. These events occur as sequelae of infusion reactions. Monitor for increased cough, dyspnea, pharyngitis, and pneumonia, and check vital signs before, during, and four hours after infusion. Patients with white cell counts > 30,000 µl may be at increased risk; also, patients with symptomatic intrinsic lung disease may have more severe pulmonary reactions. Do not administer as an IV push or bolus (Wyeth Pharmaceuticals, 2004a).

(Continued on next page)

Table 26. Pulmonary Toxicity of Chemotherapeutic Drugs *(Continued)*

Classification	Drug	Incidence	Characteristic Effects and Comments
Monoclonal antibodies *(cont.)*	Rituximab	38% (N = 135) experienced pulmonary events in clinical trials. Infusion-related deaths involving pulmonary function: 0.04%–0.07%. Bronchospasm: 8% (Genentech, Inc., 2003b)	Most common respiratory system adverse events experienced were increased cough, rhinitis, bronchospasm, dyspnea, and sinusitis. Infusion-related symptom complex includes pulmonary effects: hypoxia, bronchospasm, dyspnea, pulmonary infiltrates, and ARDS (Genentech, Inc., 2003b). There have been reports of bronchiolitis obliterans presenting up to six months postinfusion and a limited number of reports of pneumonitis (including interstitial pneumonitis) presenting up to three months postinfusion, some of which resulted in fatal outcomes. Treatment should be interrupted for severe reactions and resumed at 50% reduced infusion rate when symptoms resolve. The safety of resuming or continuing administration of rituximab in patients with pneumonitis or bronchiolitis obliterans is unknown (Genentech, Inc., 2003b).
	Trastuzumab	As a single agent: Increased cough: 26% Dyspnea: 22% Pharyngitis: 12% In the postmarketing setting, severe hypersensitivity reactions (including anaphylaxis), infusion reactions, and pulmonary adverse events have been reported (Severe pulmonary events leading to death have been reported rarely.) (Genentech, Inc., 2003a).	Increased cough, dyspnea, rhinitis, pharyngitis, pulmonary infiltrates, pleural effusions, noncardiac edema, pulmonary insufficiency, hypoxia, and ARDS (Genentech, Inc., 2003a) Other severe events reported rarely in the postmarketing setting include pneumonitis and pulmonary fibrosis (Genentech, Inc., 2003a). Patients with symptomatic intrinsic lung disease or with extensive tumor involvement of the lungs, resulting in dyspnea at rest, may be at greater risk for severe reactions. Adverse effects increase with combined drug therapy (Genentech, Inc., 2003a).
Nitrosoureas	Carmustine	Although rare, cases of fatal pulmonary toxicity have been reported. Most of these patients were receiving prolonged therapy with total doses of carmustine greater than 1,400 mg/m^2. However, there have been reports of pulmonary fibrosis in patients receiving lower total doses (Bristol-Myers Squibb Oncology, 1998a). In a long-term study of carmustine, all those initially treated at younger than five years of age died of delayed pulmonary fibrosis (Bristol-Myers Squibb Oncology, 1998a).	Pulmonary infiltrates and/or fibrosis have been reported to occur from 9 days to 43 months after treatment and appear to be dose-related. Fibrosis may be slowly progressive (Bristol-Myers Squibb Oncology, 1998a). When used in *high doses* (300–600 mg/m^2) prior to bone marrow transplantation, pulmonary toxicity may occur and may be dose limiting. The pulmonary toxicity of high-dose carmustine may manifest as severe interstitial pneumonitis, which occurs most frequently in patients who have had recent radiation to the mediastinum. Perform baseline and regular pulmonary function tests, especially in patients with risk factors or who have received > 800 mg/m^2. There is a linear relationship between total dose and pulmonary toxicity at doses > 1,000 mg/m^2, with 50% of patients developing pulmonary toxicity at total cumulative doses of 1,500 mg/m^2. Risk factors include preexisting lung disease, smoking, cyclophosphamide therapy, and recent (within months) thoracic radiation. Patients with baseline forced vital capacity and/or pulmonary diffusion capacity for carbon monoxide that are less than 70% of the predicted value are at high risk (Bristol-Myers Squibb Oncology, 1998a).

(Continued on next page)

Table 26. Pulmonary Toxicity of Chemotherapeutic Drugs *(Continued)*

Classification	Drug	Incidence	Characteristic Effects and Comments
Nitrosoureas *(cont.)*	Lomustine	Rare, usually in doses > 1,100 mg/m^2 (one reported case at a dose of 600 mg) (Bristol-Myers Squibb Oncology, 1998b) There appeared to be some late reduction of pulmonary function of all long-term survivors. This form of lung fibrosis may be slowly progressive and has resulted in death in some cases (Bristol-Myers Squibb Oncology, 1998b).	Pulmonary toxicity characterized by pulmonary infiltrates and/or fibrosis has been reported rarely with lomustine. Onset of toxicity has occurred after an interval of six months or longer from the start of therapy with cumulative doses of lomustine usually > 1,100 mg/m^2 (Bristol-Myers Squibb Oncology, 1998b). Delayed onset pulmonary fibrosis occurring up to 17 years after treatment has been reported in patients who received nitrosoureas in childhood and early adolescence (1–16 years) combined with cranial radiotherapy for intracranial tumors (Bristol-Myers Squibb Oncology, 1998b).
Plant alkaloids	Docetaxel	Unknown if drug is actual cause of toxicity (Aventis Pharmaceuticals, 2003; Merad et al., 1997)	Pulmonary infiltrates, pleural effusion, pulmonary edema Reversible with diuretics (Aventis Pharmaceuticals, 2003)
	Etoposide	Reported cases of pulmonary events have been infrequently reported: interstitial pneumonitis/pulmonary fibrosis; anaphylactic-like reactions characterized by chills, fever, tachycardia, bronchospasm, dyspnea, and/or hypotension have been reported to occur in 0.7%–2% of patients receiving IV etoposide and in less than 1% of patients treated with the oral capsules (Bristol Laboratories, 1998).	Anaphylactic-like reactions have occurred during the initial infusion of etoposide. Facial/tongue swelling, coughing, diaphoresis, cyanosis, tightness in throat, laryngospasm, back pain, and/or loss of consciousness have sometimes occurred in association with the above reactions. In addition, an apparent hypersensitivity-associated apnea has been reported rarely. Higher rates of anaphylactic-like reactions have been reported in children who received infusions at concentrations higher than those recommended. The role that concentration of infusion (or rate of infusion) plays in the development of anaphylactic-like reactions is uncertain. Treatment is symptomatic. The infusion should be terminated immediately, followed by the administration of pressor agents, corticosteroids, antihistamines, or volume expanders at the discretion of the physician (Bristol Laboratories, 1998).
	Paclitaxel	Rare for single agent: 2% dyspnea Rare reports of interstitial pneumonia, lung fibrosis, and pulmonary embolism (Bristol-Myers Squibb Oncology, 2003) 8.5%–9% combined therapy Events occur usually in high doses or in combined therapy (Bristol-Myers Squibb Oncology, 2003; Dunsford et al., 1999).	Hypersensitivity pneumonitis (Dunsford et al., 1999) Rare reports of radiation pneumonitis have been received in patients receiving concurrent radiotherapy (Bristol-Myers Squibb Oncology, 2003).
	Vinorelbine tartrate	Shortness of breath was reported in 3% of patients; it was severe in 2% receiving vinorelbine. Rare but severe: Reported cases of interstitial pulmonary changes and ARDS, most of which were fatal, occurred in patients treated with single-agent vinorelbine (GlaxoSmithKline, 2002).	Acute shortness of breath and severe bronchospasm, most commonly when vinorelbine was used in combination with mitomycin. These adverse events may require treatment with supplemental oxygen, bronchodilators, and/or corticosteroids, particularly when there is preexisting pulmonary dysfunction. The mean time to onset of these symptoms after vinorelbine administration was one week (range = 3–8 days). Patients with alterations in their baseline pulmonary symptoms or with new onset of dyspnea, cough, hypoxia, or other symptoms should be evaluated promptly (GlaxoSmithKline, 2002).

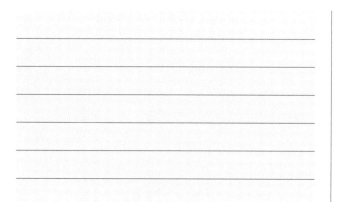

the route, dose, and administration schedule (Conant, Fox, & Miller, 1989; Schwartzentruber, 2000).

(2) Pulmonary function testing is a prerequisite for the following patients being evaluated for biotherapy (particularly for treatment with IL-2) (Chiron Corporation, 2002; Letizia & Conway, 1996).

(a) Heavy smokers

(b) Patients with extensive pulmonary disease

(c) Patients with symptoms suggesting decreased pulmonary reserve

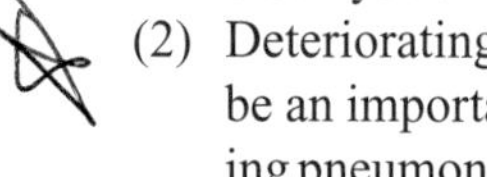

4. Risk and predisposing factors (Comis, 1992; Matthews, 2005; Senan, Paul, Thompson, & Kay, 1992)

a) Smoking

b) Impaired drug excretion

(1) Renal dysfunction may cause delayed drug excretion and increased pulmonary toxicity, especially with bleomycin.

(2) Deteriorating creatinine clearance can be an important parameter in predicting pneumonitis (Van Barneveld et al., 1984).

c) High oxygen concentrations, such as those used during administration of general anesthesia, can enhance the pulmonary toxicity of bleomycin (Ginsberg & Comis, 1984).

d) Multidrug regimens may increase the incidence and severity of pulmonary toxicity, but this is not clearly defined. Typically, these chemotherapy regimens include bleomycin, mitomycin, cyclophosphamide, methotrexate, or carmustine. It has not been determined whether any single drug is the causative agent or if the interaction of these antineoplastics results in enhanced toxicity (DeVita, Hellman, & Rosenberg, 2000).

e) Concurrent chemotherapy and radiation therapy, especially employing agents such as bleomycin, carmustine, cyclophosphamide, or doxorubicin, has been associated with interstitial pulmonary pneumonitis (Hydzik, 1990; Wickham, 1986).

f) Cumulative dose: Cytotoxic agents that are directly toxic to the lungs generally exhibit increasing toxicity with increasing dose. This is believed to be a result of drug accumulation in the lung itself. Two patterns of dose-related pulmonary toxicity usually are clinically observed.

(1) A definite increase in risk for development of pulmonary toxicity occurs once a threshold effect has been reached (e.g., total lifetime dose of bleomycin exceeds 450–500 units). Pulmonary toxicity secondary to busulfan, in the absence of other predisposing factors, only has been noted with total doses > 500 mg (DeVita et al., 2000).

(2) With linear effect, there is a constantly increasing risk for the development of pulmonary toxicity as more drug is administered (e.g., carmustine) (DeVita et al., 2000).

g) Long-term treatment (e.g., busulfan treatment) (Barton-Burke et al., 2001)

h) Age: A normal physiologic phenomenon that has been observed with aging is a decrease in the effectiveness of the antioxidant defense system. Therefore, as the patients age, they would be expected to be more susceptible to pulmonary toxicity from certain cytotoxic drugs. To date, however, age has been shown to be a risk factor only for the development of bleomycin-induced pulmonary disease (DeVita et al., 2000). The risk of pulmonary toxicity increases significantly after age 70 (Hydzik, 1990; Wickham, 1986).

i) Underlying lung disease: Chronic obstructive pulmonary disease (COPD), asthma, bronchitis, and a history of smoking contribute to chemotherapy-induced pulmonary toxicity (Wickham, 1986).

j) Radiation: Radiation therapy results in the production of oxidant species that lead to pulmonary damage (DeVita et al., 2000).

5. Clinical manifestations: Detection may be difficult when clinical manifestations are subtle.

a) Onset of hypersensitivity pneumonitis usually occurs 7–10 days after drug administration.

b) Pulmonary fibrosis can be an acute or chronic reaction.

c) Delayed toxicity may occur 8 months to 10 years after therapy initiation (Tenenbaum, 1994).

d) Presenting clinical signs and symptoms: Dyspnea; dry, nonproductive cough; crackles; rhonchi; tachypnea; fatigue; and restlessness (hypoxia). Arterial blood gases may reveal hypoxia with hypocapnia and respiratory alkalosis. The most sensitive pulmonary function test is the carbon monoxide diffusion capacity measurement that becomes abnormal before the onset of clinical symptoms (Bahhady & Unterborn, 2003).

e) Radiographic tests may be within normal limits but also may show a pattern of diffuse interstitial markings and honeycombing.

f) In biotherapy patients (Berthiaume et al., 1995; Letizia & Conway, 1996; Muehlbauer & White, 1998; Sandstrom, 1996; Schwartzentruber, 2000)

(1) Pleural effusions can be detected radiographically in 42%–52% of patients receiving IL-2. In general, no intervention is required; effusions resolve after IL-2 is discontinued.

(2) Changes suggesting pulmonary edema are observed in approximately 20% of radiographs of patients receiving high-dose IL-2 (Berthiaume et al., 1995).

(3) Tachypnea

(4) Dyspnea

(5) Crackles

(6) Decreased transcutaneous oxygen saturations

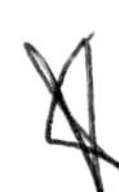

6. Assessment: The following assessment steps may not apply if the patient is an inpatient receiving IV IL-2 or vasopressors or is an outpatient receiving SQ IL-2 (Letizia & Conway, 1996; Muehlbauer & White, 1998; Sandstrom, 1996; Schwartzentruber, 2000).

a) Percuss and auscultate the lungs. Assess location and degree of adventitious breath sounds (e.g., rales, rhonchi, wheezes, rubs).

b) Assess depth, rhythm, and effort of respiratory breathing.

c) Note chest symmetry and retraction of intercostal muscles.

d) Note accessory muscle use.

e) Determine the presence of a cough and the amount, color, and productive nature of sputum.

f) Note skin and mucous membrane color (dusky, ashen, or cyanotic).

g) Monitor the results of pulse oximetry and arterial blood-gas tests.

h) Observe the abdomen for distention. If the abdomen presses on the diaphragm, breathing is more difficult.

i) Assess for chest and/or back pain and evaluate possible causes. Possible causes include pleural effusion, pulmonary embolism, and pneumothorax, all of which require medical attention.

j) Assess and document level of consciousness (LOC).

k) Obtain chest radiographs. Frequency depends on patient and therapy.

l) Monitor pulmonary function tests.

7. Collaborative management: Because lung damage is often irreversible, early detection and prevention of pulmonary toxicity are imperative (Comis, 1992).

a) If pulmonary toxicity is suspected, hold chemotherapy and notify a physician.

b) Do not use fluid boluses if patient is in respiratory distress (e.g., showing signs of dyspnea, or increasing crackles).

c) Initiate fluid restriction if pulmonary edema is problematic; administer IV colloidal therapy as ordered.

d) Keep strict intake and output records for all patients receiving IV IL-2.

e) Administer corticosteroids and antibiotics as ordered. Corticosteroids usually are contraindicated for patients receiving biotherapy.

f) Elevate the head of the bed if signs of respiratory compromise appear.

g) Provide supportive therapy (e.g., vasopressors, diuretics, artificial ventilation) for acute episodes.

h) Provide oxygen therapy when ordered; however, when using bleomycin, be aware of reports of oxygen-induced lung damage (Bristol-Myers Squibb Oncology/Immunology, 1999).

i) Monitor patients' weight.

j) Monitor the adequacy of diuresis after the patient has finished IL-2 therapy. Heart rate and blood pressure should be within acceptable limits.

k) Follow-up recommendations

(1) Monitor pulmonary function tests as indicated.

(2) Obtain chest radiographs; a radiograph may be recommended every one to two weeks to monitor for bleomycin toxicity (Bristol-Myers Squibb Oncology/Immunology, 1999).

8. Patient and family education (Camp-Sorrell, 2000; Hood & Harwood, 2004; Padburg & Padburg, 2000)

a) Provide education regarding symptoms associated with pulmonary toxicity (e.g., cough, dyspnea, chest pain, shallow breathing, chest-wall discomfort). Make sure all patients, including outpatients receiving subcutaneous IL-2, know to seek medical assistance immediately if symptoms begin.

b) Ensure that a biotherapy patient knows the effects of cytokines before biotherapy begins.
c) Make sure that patients receiving biotherapy know that IL-2 may be delayed or held until pulmonary symptoms resolve.
d) Explore with patients their wishes regarding intubation and resuscitation status; establish advance directives.
e) Teach patients that raising the head of the bed may facilitate breathing.
f) Instruct patients to conserve energy by performing daily activities when their energy level is highest.
g) Teach patients and significant others methods to decrease symptoms of dyspnea by exercising to tolerance, practicing pursed-lip breathing, refraining from smoking, and using a small fan.
h) Teach patients to take an opioid (in most cases, morphine) as prescribed by a physician; opioids may relieve the discomfort caused by air hunger.
i) If at risk for pulmonary edema, teach patients to restrict fluid.
j) Review the safety issues (e.g., flammability) related to oxygen administration.
k) Upon discharge, ensure that patients know to notify the physician if dyspnea, cough, or fever develops.

References

Aronchick, J.M., & Gefter, W.B. (1991). Drug-induced pulmonary disease: An update. *Journal of Thoracic Imaging, 6*(1), 19–29.

AstraZeneca Pharmaceuticals. (2004). Iressa [Package insert]. Wilmington, DE: Author.

Aventis Pharmaceuticals. (2003). Taxotere [Package insert]. Collegeville, PA: Author.

Bahhady, I.J., & Unterborn, J. (2003). What pulmonary function tests can and cannot tell you: Results help assess disease severity in ILD and COPD. *Journal of Respiratory Diseases, 24*(4), 170–176.

Barton-Burke, M., Wilkes, G.M., & Ingwersen, K.C. (2001). *Cancer chemotherapy: A nursing process approach* (3rd ed.). Sudbury, MA: Jones and Bartlett.

Berlex Laboratories. (2002). Campath [Package insert]. Richmond, CA: Author.

Berlex Laboratories. (2003). Fludara [Package insert]. Richmond, CA: Author.

Berthiaume, Y., Boiteau, P., Fick, G., Kloiber, R., Sinclair, G.D., Fong, C., et al. (1995). Pulmonary edema during IL-2 therapy: Combined effect of increased permeability and hydrostatic pressure. *American Journal of Respiratory Critical Care Medicine, 152,* 329–335.

Bristol Laboratories. (1998). VePesid [Package insert]. Princeton, NJ: Author.

Bristol-Myers Squibb Oncology. (1998a). BiCNU [Package insert]. Princeton, NJ: Author.

Bristol-Myers Squibb Oncology. (1998b). CeeNU [Package insert]. Princeton, NJ: Author.

Bristol-Myers Squibb Oncology. (2000). Mutamycin [Package insert]. Princeton, NJ: Author.

Bristol-Myers Squibb Oncology. (2003). Taxol [Package insert]. Princeton, NJ: Author.

Bristol-Myers Squibb Oncology/Immunology. (1999). Blenoxane [Package insert]. Princeton, NJ: Author.

Camp, M.J., Gullatte, M.M., Gilmore, J.W., & Hutcherson, D.A. (2001). Antineoplastic agents. In M.M. Gullatte (Ed.), *Clinical guide to antineoplastic therapy: A chemotherapy handbook* (pp. 71–279). Pittsburgh, PA: Oncology Nursing Society.

Camp-Sorrell, D. (2000). Chemotherapy: Toxicity management. In C.H. Yarbro, M.H. Frogge, M. Goodman, & S.L. Groenwald (Eds.), *Cancer nursing: Principles and practice* (5th ed., pp. 444–486). Sudbury, MA: Jones and Bartlett.

Castleberry, R.P., Grist, W.M., Holbrook, T., Malluh, A., & Gaddy, D. (1981). The cytosine arabinoside (Ara-C) syndrome. *Medical Pediatric Oncology, 9,* 257–264.

Cell Therapeutics. (2004). Trisenox [Package insert]. Seattle, WA: Author.

Chiron Corporation. (2002). Proleukin [Package insert]. Emeryville, CA: Author.

Chisholm, R.A., Dixon, A.K., Williams, M.V., & Oliver, R.T. (1992). Bleomycin lung: The effect of different chemotherapeutic regimens. *Cancer Chemotherapy and Pharmacology, 30,* 158–160.

Comis, R.L. (1992). Bleomycin pulmonary toxicity: Current status and future directions. *Seminars in Oncology, 19,* 64–70.

Conant, E.F., Fox, K.R., & Miller, W.T. (1989). Pulmonary edema as a complication of interleukin-2 therapy. *American Journal of Roentgenology, 15,* 749–752.

Deininger, M., O'Brien, S.G., Ford, J.M., & Druker, B.J. (2003). Practical management of patients with chronic myeloid leukemia receiving imatinib. *Journal of Clinical Oncology, 21,* 1637–1647.

DeVita, V.T., Hellman, S., & Rosenberg, S.A. (Eds.). (2000). *Cancer: Principles and practice of oncology* (6th ed.). Philadelphia: Lippincott-Raven.

Dunsford, M.L., Mead, G.M., Bateman, A.C., Cook, T., & Tung, K. (1999). Severe pulmonary toxicity in patients treated with a combination of docetaxel and gemcitabine for metastatic transitional cell carcinoma. *Annals of Oncology, 10,* 943–947.

Eli Lilly & Co. (2004). Gemzar [Package insert]. Indianapolis, IN: Author.

Erasmus, J.J. (2000). Pulmonary drug toxicity: Pathogenesis and radiologic manifestations. *Society of Thoracic Radiology Annual Meeting 2000* [Course syllabus]. Retrieved June 5, 2004, from http://www.thoracicrad.org/str99/TI2000/sundaypm.htm

Genentech, Inc. (2003a). Herceptin (trastuzumab) [Package insert]. South San Francisco, CA: Author.

Genentech, Inc. (2003b). Rituxan [Package insert]. South San Francisco, CA: Author.

Ginsberg, S.J., & Comis, R.L. (1984). The pulmonary toxicity of antineoplastic agents. In M.C. Perry & J.W. Yarbro (Eds.), *Toxicity of chemotherapy* (pp. 227–268). New York: Grune & Stratton.

GlaxoSmithKline. (2002). Navelbine [Package insert]. Research Triangle Park, NC: Author. Retrieved April 30, 2004, from http://www.gsk.com

GlaxoSmithKline. (2003a). Alkeran [Package insert]. Research Triangle Park, NC: Author. Retrieved April 30, 2004, from http://www.gsk.com

GlaxoSmithKline. (2003b). Hycamtin [Package insert]. Research Triangle Park, NC: Author. Retrieved April 30, 2004, from http://www.gsk.com

GlaxoSmithKline. (2003c). Leukeran [Package insert]. Research Triangle Park, NC: Author. Retrieved April 30, 2004, from http://www.gsk.com

GlaxoSmithKline. (2004). Myleran [Package insert]. Research Triangle Park, NC: Author. Retrieved April 30, 2004, from http://www.gsk.com

Haupt, H.M., Hutchins, G.M., & Moore, G.W. (1981). Ara-C lung: Noncardiogenic pulmonary edema complicating cytosine arabinoside therapy of leukemia. *American Journal of Medicine, 70,* 256–261.

Hennemann, B., Bross, K.J., Reichle, A., & Andreesen, R. (1993). Acute alveolitis induced by hydroxyurea in a patient with chronic myeloproliferative syndrome. *Annals of Hematology, 67,* 133–134.

Hood, L.E., & Harwood, K.V. (2004). Dyspnea. In C.H. Yarbro, M.H. Frogge, & M. Goodman (Eds.), *Cancer symptom management* (3rd ed., pp. 29–46). Sudbury, MA: Jones and Bartlett.

Hydzik, C.A. (1990). Late effects of chemotherapy: Implications for patient management and rehabilitation. *Nursing Clinics of North America, 24,* 423–446.

Immunex. (1999). Methotrexate LPF sodium [Package insert]. Seattle, WA: Author.

Immunex. (2000). Novantrone [Package insert]. Seattle, WA: Author.

Kachel, D.L., & Martin, W.J., II. (1994). Cyclophosphamide-induced lung toxicity: Mechanism of endothelial cell injury. *Journal of Pharmacology and Experimental Therapeutics, 268*(1), 42–46.

Kavuru, M.S., Gadsden, T., Lichtin, A., & Gephardt, G. (1994). Hydroxyurea-induced acute interstitial lung disease. *Southern Medical Journal, 87,* 67–69.

Koh, D.W., & Castro, M. (1996). Pulmonary toxicity of chemotherapy drugs. In M.C. Perry (Ed.), *The chemotherapy source book* (3rd ed., pp. 665–695). Baltimore: Williams & Wilkins.

Kriesman, H., & Wolkove, N. (1992). Pulmonary toxicity of antineoplastic therapy. In M.C. Perry (Ed.), *The chemotherapy source book* (2nd ed., pp. 598–619). Baltimore: Williams & Wilkins.

Letizia, M., & Conway, A.M. (1996). Interleukin-2 therapy for renal cell cancer: Indications, effects, and nursing implications. *Critical Care Nurse, 16*(5), 20–35.

Luedke, D., McLaughlin, T.T., Daughaday, C., Luedke, S., Harrison, B., Reed, G., et al. (1985). Mitomycin C and vindesine associated pulmonary toxicity with variable clinical expression. *Cancer, 55,* 542–545.

Matthews, L.V. (2005). Alterations in ventilation. In J.K. Itano & K.N. Taoka (Eds.), *Core curriculum for oncology nursing* (4th ed., pp. 347–363). St. Louis, MO: Elsevier.

Mead Johnson Oncology. (2000). Cytoxan [Package insert]. Princeton, NJ: Author.

Merad, M., Le Cesne, A., Baldeyrou, P., Mesurolle, B., & Le Chevalier, T. (1997). Docetaxel and interstitial pulmonary injury. *Annals of Oncology, 8,* 191–194.

Muehlbauer, P.M., & White, R.L. (1998). Are you prepared for interleukin-2? *RN, 61*(2), 34–39.

Novartis Pharmaceuticals. (2004). Gleevec [Package insert]. East Hanover, NJ: Author.

Ortho Biotech Corporation. (2003). Doxil [Package insert]. Raritan, NJ: Author.

Padburg, L.F., & Padburg, R.M. (2000). Patient and family education. In C.H. Yarbro, M.H. Frogge, M. Goodman, & S.L. Groenwald (Eds.), *Cancer nursing: Principles and Practice* (5th ed., pp. 1609–1631). Sudbury, MA: Jones and Bartlett.

Pavlakis, N., Bell, D.R., Millward, M.J., & Levi, J.A. (1997). Fatal pulmonary toxicity redulting from treatment with gemcitabine. *Cancer, 80,* 286–291.

Pharmacia & Upjohn. (2002). Camptosar [Package insert]. Kalamazoo, MI: Author.

Pronk, L.C., Stoter, G., & Verweij, J. (1995). Docetaxel (Taxotere®): Single agent activity, development of combination treatment and reducing side effects. *Cancer Treatment Reviews, 21,* 463–478.

Ramanathan, R.K., Belani, C.P., & Reddy, V.V. (1996). Transient pulmonary infiltrates: A hypersensitivity reaction to paclitaxel. *Annals of Internal Medicine, 124,* 278.

Read, W.L., Mortimer, J.E., & Picus, J. (2002). Severe interstitial pneumonitis associated with docetaxel administration. *Cancer, 94,* 847–853.

Roche Pharmaceuticals. (2003). Xeloda [Package insert]. Nutley, NJ: Author. Retrieved April 5, 2004, from http://www.xeloda.com

Rossi, S.E., Erasmus, J.J., McAdams, H.P., Sporn, T.A., & Goodman, P.C. (2000). Pulmonary drug toxicity: Radiologic and pathologic manifestations. *Radiographics, 20,* 1245–1259.

Sandstrom, S.K. (1996). Nursing management of patients receiving biological therapy. *Seminars in Oncology Nursing, 12,* 152–162.

Sanofi-Synthelabo, Inc. (2004). Eloxatin [Package insert]. Bedford, OH: Author.

Schering Corporation. (2002). Intron-A [Package insert]. Kenilworth, NJ: Author.

Schering Corporation. (2004). Temodar [Package insert]. Kenilworth, NJ: Author.

Schwartzentruber, D.J. (2000). Interleukin-2: Clinical applications: Principles of administration and management of side effects. In S.A. Rosenberg (Ed.), *Principles and practice of the biologic therapy of cancer* (3rd ed., pp. 32–50). Philadelphia: Lippincott Williams & Wilkins.

Senan, S., Paul, J., Thompson, N., & Kay, S.B. (1992). Cigarette smoking is a risk factor for bleomycin-induced pulmonary toxicity. *European Journal of Cancer, 28A,* 2084.

Siegel, J.P., & Puri, R.K. (1991). Interleukin-2 toxicity. *Journal of Clinical Oncology, 9,* 694–704.

Sleijfer, S., van der Mark, T.W., Schraffordt Koops, S., & Mulder, N.H. (1995). Decrease in pulmonary function during bleomycin-containing combination chemotherapy for testicular cancer: Not only a bleomycin effect. *British Journal of Cancer, 71,* 120–123.

Smalley, R.V., & Wall, R.L. (1966). Two cases of busulfan toxicity. *Annals of Internal Medicine, 64,* 154–164.

Spratto, G.R., & Woods, A.L. (2004). *PDR nurse's drug handbook.* Clifton Park, NY: Delmar Learning.

Tenenbaum, L. (1994). *Cancer chemotherapy and biotherapy: A reference guide.* Philadelphia: Saunders.

Tietjen, P.E., & Stover, D.E. (2002). Lung injury associated with cancer treatment. *Pulmonary and Critical Care Update, 17*(Lesson 10). Retrieved March 24, 2005, from http://www.chestnet.org/education/online/pccu/vol17/lessons9_10/lesson10.php

Twohig, K.J., & Matthay, R.A. (1990). Pulmonary effects of cytotoxic agents other than bleomycin. *Clinics in Chest Medicine, 11*(1), 31–54.

Van Barneveld, P.W., van der Mark, T.W., Sleijfer, D.T., Mulder, N.H., Koops, H.S., Sluiter, H.J., et al. (1984). Predictive factors for bleomycin-induced pneumonitis. *American Review of Respiratory Disease, 130,* 1078–1081.

Wickham, R. (1986). Pulmonary toxicity secondary to cancer treatment. *Oncology Nursing Forum, 13*(5), 69–76.

Wilkes, G.M., & Burke, M.B. (2004). *2004 oncology nursing drug handbook.* Sudbury, MA: Jones and Bartlett.

Wyeth Pharmaceuticals. (2004a). Gemtuzumab ozogamicin [Package insert]. Philadelphia: Author.

Wyeth Pharmaceuticals. (2004b). Neumega [Package insert]. Philadelphia: Author.

G. Hemorrhagic cystitis: An irritation of the bladder that ranges from microscopic hematuria to acute exsanguinating hematuria (Strohl, 2000)

1. Pathophysiology: Irritation, inflammation, and ulceration occur as a result of the binding of drug metabolites or by-products to the bladder mucosa primarily related to cyclophosphamide and ifosfamide therapy (Strohl, 2000).
   a) Acrolein is a drug metabolite of cyclophosphamide.
   b) Acrolein and chloroacetaldehyde are metabolites of ifosfamide.
2. Incidence (American Society of Clinical Oncology [ASCO], 2002)
   a) Toxicity occurs in rare instances with bortezomib and with repeated cycles of gemcitabine and irinotecan.
   b) Toxicity primarily is associated with cyclophosphamide and ifosfamide.
      (1) In adults
         (a) Standard- or low-dose cyclophosphamide (< 1,000 mg): Associated with a 6%–10% incidence of toxicity usually manifested as microscopic hematuria that may or may not be symptomatic (Choudhury & Ahmed, 1997; Patterson & Reams, 2001)
         (b) High-dose cyclophosphamide (at least 120 mg/kg): Associated with up to a 40% incidence of toxicity ranging from microscopic to frank hematuria with clotting (ASCO, 2002; Patterson & Reams, 2001)
         (c) Ifosfamide: Associated with 18%–40% incidence of frank hematuria. Incidence of combined microscopic and frank hematuria is up to 50%. Mortality with severe hemorrhage is 2%–4% (ASCO, 2002).
      (2) In children: Symptoms occur as early as a few weeks following chemotherapy or as late as several years after treatment (McCarville, Hoffer, Gingrich, & Jenkins, 2000).
         (a) Mild dysuria to severe hemorrhage occurs in 5%–10% of children receiving low-dose cyclophosphamide (Balis, Holcenberg, & Blaney, 2001).
         (b) Mild dysuria to severe hemorrhage occurs in 20%–40% of children receiving ifosfamide (Balis et al., 2001).
3. Risk factors
   a) Cyclophosphamide (Stillwell & Benson, 1988)
      (1) IV administration presents a greater risk than does cyclophosphamide administered orally.
      (2) High-dose administration presents a greater risk than does low-dose administration.
      (3) Toxicity can occur with a single dose of IV cyclophosphamide or with up to 57 mg/kg administered cumulatively over two years.
   b) Cumulative doses of ifosfamide 45 g/m^2 or greater, especially for children younger than age three, are associated with increased incidence and severity of renal toxicity (Loebstein et al., 1999).
   c) Prior radiation therapy to the pelvis or bladder increases risk (ASCO, 2002; McCarville et al., 2000; Stillwell & Benson, 1988).
4. Clinical manifestations (Patterson & Reams, 2001; Stillwell & Benson, 1988; Strohl, 2000)
   a) Dysuria
   b) Frequency
   c) Burning during urination
   d) Nocturia or oliguria
   e) Microscopic or frank hematuria
5. Assessment: Obtain a baseline urinalysis before therapy, and regularly monitor subsequent urinalysis results and subjective reports.
6. Collaborative management—preventive strategies
   a) Preventive measures for hemorrhagic cystitis focus on assessment and monitoring, forced hydration and diuresis, and frequent voiding (Strohl, 2000; West, 1997).
      (1) Assess baseline blood urea nitrogen (BUN) and creatinine and the results of routine urinalysis and urine cultures as needed to rule out renal pathology and infection.

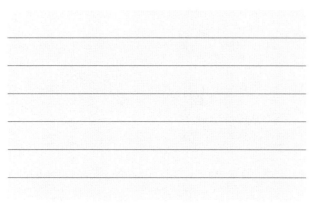

(2) Maintain and monitor intake and output; instruct patient and caregiver in this process.

(3) Instruct patients to increase oral fluid intake (adults: two to three liters/day); provide parenteral hydration if the patient is unable to drink and retain oral fluids. Encourage hydration to begin 12–24 hours prior to scheduled chemotherapy. Urinary output should be > 100 cc/hour/m^2 (West, 1997). Prevention includes forced diuresis and administration of chemoprotectants (e.g., mesna).

(4) Administer final daily dose of oral cyclophosphamide prior to 4 pm to allow the drug to pass through the bladder prior to bedtime.

(5) Encourage frequent voiding, day and night.

(6) Instruct the patient on visual observation of urine.

(7) Administer forced saline hydration and forced diuresis with ifosfamide and high-dose cyclophosphamide.

b) Administer the bladder protectant mesna with high-dose cyclophosphamide and any dose of ifosfamide. Mesna binds to drug metabolite, inactivating and detoxifying it, then allowing it to be flushed from the bladder (ASCO, 2002).

(1) For adults receiving standard-dose ifosfamide via short infusion, the total daily mesna dose should be equal to 60% of the total daily ifosfamide dose and administered 15 minutes before (0 hours) and at four and eight hours after each infusion dose of ifosfamide. Therefore, each bolus mesna dose is approximately 20% of the total daily dose of ifosfamide to equal 60% when three bolus mesna doses are complete (ASCO, 2002). Oral mesna is given in a dosage equal to 40% of the ifosfamide dose two and six hours after each dose of ifosfamide (Bristol-Myers Squibb Oncology, 2002).

(2) For adults receiving standard-dose ifosfamide via continuous infusion, mesna can be administered with ifosfamide, as a continuous infusion at 60%–100% of the ifosfamide dose, following a loading dose of 20% of the total daily ifosfamide dose.

(3) Another recommendation for adults receiving standard-dose ifosfamide by continuous infusion is to include one bolus loading dose of 20% of the total daily ifosfamide dose followed by a continuous infusion of mesna up to 40% of the total daily ifosfamide dose and continuing the mesna infusion for 12–24 hours following completion of the ifosfamide. Note: No relevant clinical data are available to support a mesna dose of > 60% of the ifosfamide dose, and doses above 60% have been associated with increased GI toxicity (ASCO, 2002; Fischer, Knobf, Durivage, & Beaulieu, 2003).

(4) For adults with high-dose ifosfamide (> 2.5g/m^2/d), no guidelines have yet been established regarding the concomitant mesna dosing. Some studies indicate more frequent and prolonged mesna dosing is needed for maximum uroprotection with high-dose ifosfamide (ASCO, 2002).

(5) For adults receiving high-dose cyclophosphamide therapy, mesna dosing as protection should be at 40% of the total cyclophosphamide dose. Doses of up to 60%–120% of the cyclophosphamide dose have been administered, but the efficacy of higher mesna dosing has not yet been established. Administer mesna 15 minutes before and at four and eight hours after the cyclophosphamide dose (ASCO, 2002; Shepherd et al., 1991).

(6) For children, an IV mesna dose is typically 60% of the ifosfamide or cyclophosphamide dose; some studies recommend a 1:1 ratio. The most common pediatric administration schedule consists of IV mesna 15 minutes prior to chemotherapy and at four and eight hours after chemotherapy (Katz et al., 1995; Links & Lewis, 1999).

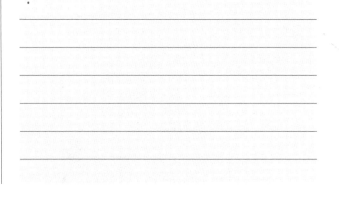

(7) The initial loading bolus dose of mesna should be administered IV, but

subsequent doses can be administered intravenously or orally. SQ dosing also has been utilized. Oral dosing may be higher, and the dose can be mixed with juices or beverages to mask the taste (ASCO, 2002).

(8) Adverse effects of mesna include nausea, vomiting, diarrhea, abdominal pain, altered taste, rash, urticaria, headache, and hypotension (Bristol-Myers Squibb Oncology, 2002).

7. Management of hemorrhagic cystitis
   a) Discontinue ifosfamide or cyclophosphamide administration if evidence of gross hematuria or cystitis is noted.
   b) Insert a urinary catheter.
      (1) In adult patients, place a three-way Foley catheter to provide continuous irrigation with saline or acetylcysteine (Patterson & Reams, 2001).
      (2) In patients who have clots obstructing their ability to void, place a large-bore urethral catheter to provide irrigation with a saline solution (West, 1997).
   c) Administer an antifibrinolytic agent, such as aminocaproic acid, to promote clotting. Other agents aiding in the formation of a protein precipitate over bleeding surfaces include saline, potassium aluminum sulfate, silver nitrate, and formalin (Choudhury & Ahmed, 1997; West, 1997).
   d) Obtain a urology consultation. Cystoscopy with electrocautery or cryosurgery may be used to control bleeding. Cystectomy may be necessary for last-resort cases.
   e) Follow-up is needed because prolonged mucosal irritation, inflammation, and bleeding can lead to persistent cystitis, irreversible bladder fibrosis, and an increased risk for bladder cancer (ASCO, 2002). Follow-up recommendations include (Stillwell & Benson, 1988)
      (1) Periodic and at least annual urinalysis, urine cytology, and cystoscopy
      (2) Periodic excretory urograms for patients with gross hematuria, new microhematuria, abnormal cytologic findings regarding the urine, or persistent irritative voiding.
8. Patient and family education
   a) Tell patients about the possibility of hemorrhagic cystitis with ifosfamide and cyclophosphamide regimens.
   b) Ensure that patients know the signs and symptoms to report.
   c) Encourage patients to void at least every two hours and to take oral cyclophosphamide early in the day, with the last dose before 4 pm.
   d) Instruct patients to increase fluid intake daily.

References

American Society of Clinical Oncology. (2002). *2002 update of recommendations for the use of chemotherapy and radiotherapy protectants: Clinical practice guidelines of the American Society of Clinical Oncology.* Retrieved January 13, 2005, from http://www.asco.org/ac/1,1003,_12-002306,00.asp

Balis, F.M., Holcenberg, J.S., & Blaney, S.M. (2001). General principles of chemotherapy. In P.A. Pizzo & D.G. Poplack (Eds.), *Principles and practice of pediatric oncology* (4th ed., pp. 237–308). Philadelphia: Lippincott Williams & Wilkins.

Bristol-Myers Squibb Oncology. (2002). Mesnex [Package insert]. Princeton, NJ: Author. Retrieved January 13, 2005, from http://www.bms.com/products/data

Choudhury, D., & Ahmed, Z. (1997). Drug-induced nephrotoxicity. *Medical Clinics of North America, 81,* 705–717.

Fischer, D.S., Knobf, M.T., Durivage, H.J., & Beaulieu, N.J. (Eds.). (2003). *The cancer chemotherapy handbook* (6th ed.). St Louis, MO: Mosby.

Katz, A., Epelman, S., Anelli, A., Gorender, E.F., Cruz, S.M., Oliveira, R.M., et al. (1995). A prospective randomized evaluation of three schedules of mesna administration in patients receiving an ifosfamide-containing chemotherapy regimen: Sustained efficiency and simplified administration. *Journal of Cancer Research in Clinical Oncology, 121,* 128–131.

Links, M., & Lewis, C. (1999). Chemoprotectants: A review of their clinical pharmacology and therapeutic efficacy. *Drugs, 57,* 293–306.

Loebstein, R., Atanackovic, G., Bishai, R., Wolpin, J., Khattak, S., Hashemi, G., et al. (1999). Risk factors for long-term outcome of ifosfamide-induced nephrotoxicity in children. *Journal of Clinical Pharmacology, 39,* 454–461.

McCarville, M.B., Hoffer, F.A., Gingrich, J.R., & Jenkins, J.J. (2000). Imaging findings of hemorrhagic cystitis in pediatric oncology patients. *Pediatric Radiology, 30,* 131–138.

Patterson, W.P., & Reams, G.P. (2001). Renal and electrolyte abnormalities due to chemotherapy. In M.C. Perry (Ed.), *The chemotherapy source book* (3rd ed., pp. 494–503). Philadelphia: Lippincott Williams & Wilkins.

Shepherd, J.D., Pringle, L.E., Barnett, M.J., Klingemann, H.G., Reece, D.E., & Phillips, G.L. (1991). Mesna versus hyperhydration for the prevention of cyclophosphamide-induced hemorrhagic cystitis in bone marrow transplantation. *Journal of Clinical Oncology, 9,* 2016–2020.

Stillwell, T.J., & Benson, R.C. (1988). Cyclophosphamide-induced hemorrhagic cystitis: A review of 100 patients. *Cancer, 61,* 451–457.

Strohl, R. (2000). Hemorrhagic cystitis. In D. Camp-Sorrell & R.A. Hawkins (Eds.), *Clinical manual for the oncology advanced practice nurse* (pp. 547–549). Pittsburgh, PA: Oncology Nursing Society.

West, N.J. (1997). Prevention and treatment of hemorrhagic cystitis. *Pharmacotherapy, 17,* 696–706.

H. Hepatotoxicity
   1. Pathophysiology (McDonald & Tirumali, 1984)

   a) Hepatotoxicity is a direct toxic effect to the liver as a result of drugs being metabolized. It is usually transient and asymptomatic.
   b) Pediatric considerations
      (1) The organ systems of preterm and term infants and children are immature, causing many drugs, including antineoplastics, to have a different disposition from that seen in adults.
      (2) The clearance rates of adolescents may be lower than the high rates typical of toddlers and higher than typical adult rates. Toxicity alters drug clearance (Grochow & Baker, 1998).
      (3) Liver injury may manifest as fatty changes, hepatocellular necrosis, cholestasis, peliosis hepatitis, veno-occlusive disease (McDonald, Hinds, Fisher, & Schooch, 1993), nodular regenerative hyperplasia, hepatic neoplasms, hepatic fibrosis, and parenchymal cell damages.
2. Incidence (see Table 27)
3. Risk factors (Weiss, 2005)
   a) Prior liver infection or damage (cirrhosis, hepatitis)
   b) Hepatotoxic chemotherapeutic drugs (risk increases with higher dosing)
   c) High dose intensity and/or frequent cycles of dactinomycin
   d) Prior tumor involvement of the liver
   e) Past medical history of transplant (liver, kidney, bone marrow, peripheral blood stem cell)
   f) Prior radiation therapy to the liver or right side of abdomen
   g) History of alcohol abuse, especially with cirrhosis
   h) Use of illicit drugs
   i) Concurrent administration of noncytotoxic hepatotoxic drugs
   j) Intrahepatic chemotherapy administration
   k) Advancing age

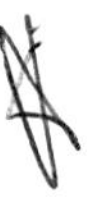

4. Clinical manifestations (Horrell, 2000)
   a) Varying degrees of jaundice
   b) Hyperpigmentation of the skin
   c) Ascites
   d) Fatigue, malaise, and other flu-like symptoms
   e) Anorexia
   f) Nausea and/or vomiting
   g) Dyspepsia
   h) Diarrhea, weight loss, dehydration, cachectic appearance
   i) Right upper quadrant pain
   j) Hepatosplenomegaly
   k) Dark-orange urine, clay-colored stools
   l) Pruritus
   m) Elevated transaminases (aspartate aminotransferase, alanine aminotransaminase), prolonged prothrombin times
   n) Bruising and/or bleeding
   o) Portal hypertension
   p) Encephalopathy
   q) Arthralgia/myalgia

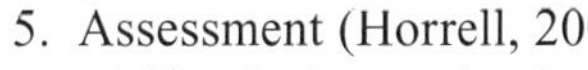

5. Assessment (Horrell, 2000)
   a) Physical examination to find and document the preceding clinical manifestations
   b) Obtain baseline liver function tests (LFTs) prior to initiation of therapy
   c) History of hepatotoxic drug and/or alcohol use
6. Collaborative management: Few guidelines exist for the dosing of drugs based on elevated liver function studies.
   a) Avoid using hepatotoxic drugs other than chemotherapy agents if LFT results are abnormal.
   b) It may be necessary to adjust the dose of chemotherapy in the presence of impaired hepatic function (Wilkes, Ingwersen, & Barton-Burke, 2003).
   c) Monitor the full blood chemistry, CBC, and clotting factor results.
   d) Assist the patient in following a low-fat, high-glucose diet containing vitamin B and C additives.
   e) Assess the patient's level of consciousness and for signs of bleeding.
   f) Monitor subsequent LFT results.
7. Patient and family education (Horrell, 2000)
   a) If appropriate, inform patients and significant others that hepatotoxicity is a possible side effect of the chemotherapy agent.
   b) Instruct patients to avoid alcoholic beverages if hepatotoxicity is noted.

Table 27. Hepatotoxicity of Chemotherapeutic and Biotherapeutic Drugs

Medication Name	Incidence	Comments
6-mercaptopurine	–	If daily dose is > 2 mg/kg, hepatocellular or cholestatic liver effects may occur (Perry, 1992). Hepatotoxicity usually is mild and reversible. Elevated transaminases and cholestatic jaundice may occur.
Asparaginase	42%–87% (Capizzi et al., 1970) Asparaginase increases the indicators of hepatic function (transaminases, alkaline phosphatase, and hyperbilirubinemia). These changes rarely reach critical significance (Muller & Boos, 1998). 50% experience abnormal serum alkaline phosphatase, transaminases, or bilirubin (Oettgen et al., 1970). Up to 87% develop fatty infiltration of the liver (Pratt & Johnson, 1971; Sahoo & Hart, 2003).	–
Bleomycin	10%; more common in patients older than age 70 who receive a total dose > 400 units. Toxicity is unpredictable and occasionally has occurred in young patients receiving low doses (Bristol-Myers Squibb Oncology/Immunology, 1999).	–
Busulfan	Rare; at high doses, veno-occlusive disease (VOD) may occur (Hassan, 1999). The risk of VOD may be lowered by adjusting the dose to achieve a safe systemic drug exposure (Balis et al., 1997).	–
Capecitabine	17%; 21% for patients with hepatic malignancy. At 2,500 mg/m^2 daily for two weeks, grade III or IV hyperbilirubinemia may occur. 20%–40% elevation in serum bilirubin, alkaline phosphatase, and transaminases (Chu & DeVita, 2002).	If grade II–IV elevations in bilirubin occur, interrupt capecitabine treatment immediately (Roche Laboratories, 1999).
Carmustine	Transient elevations in serum transaminases in up to 90% of patients within one week of therapy (Chu & DeVita, 2002)	Effects usually are not clinically significant (DeVita et al., 1965); however, carmustine may be associated with severe VOD when used during bone marrow transplant (BMT) (McDonald et al., 1993).
Cisplatin	Rare	Hepatotoxicity may increase with higher doses (Cavalli et al., 1978; Pollera et al., 1987).
Cyclophosphamide	Rare; less than 1% with high doses (> 120 mg/kg/day for four days). Risk increases at cumulative doses > 400–500 mg.	–
Cytarabine	–	Dose-related; elevation of transaminases and bilirubin (Katz & Cassileth, 1977; Kummar et al., 2005)
Dactinomycin	> 15%; hepatic toxicity may be dose-related. Severe hepatotoxicity is associated with the single-bolus dose schedule (Balis et al., 1997).	Elevation of serum transaminases; dose and schedule dependent
Denileukin diftitox	15%–20% experienced elevation of serum transaminases and hypoalbuminemia (albumin < 2.3 g/dl) (Chu & DeVita, 2002).	Usually seen in first course and resolved within two weeks
Doxorubicin	Rare (Perry, 1992)	Extensively metabolized in liver; reduce dose for altered hepatic function (Sifton, 2002)
Floxuridine	Intra-arterial hepatic infusion produced hepatitis in 50% of patients (Alexander et al., 2005).	90% of drug is extracted by hepatocytes (Hohn et al., 1989).
Gemcitabine	Transient elevation of serum transaminases (10%–20% develop grade III–IV), elevation of alkaline phosphatase (15%–20%), and elevation of serum bilirubin (Abratt et al., 1994)	Consider dose modification in patients with abnormal liver function because of potential for increased toxicity.

(Continued on next page)

Table 27. Hepatotoxicity of Chemotherapeutic and Biotherapeutic Drugs *(Continued)*

Medication Name	Incidence	Comments
Gemtuzumab ozogamicin	Hepatotoxicity with elevation of serum bilirubin and liver function tests (LFTs) was observed in up to 20% of patients (Chu & DeVita, 2002).	–
Ifosfamide	Transient hepatic dysfunction: rare	–
Interleukin-2	Elevated bilirubin: 40% (2% progress to grade IV) Interleukin-2 therapy is associated with elevated LFT results (23% serum glutamic-oxaloacetic transaminase increase) (Chiron Corporation, 1998).	Typically normalize within five to six days (Schwartz et al., 2002)
Melphalan	Transient hepatic elevation in LFTs at high doses used in autologous BMT	–
Methotrexate (MTX)	Transient elevation of serum transaminases. High-dose MTX combined with leucovorin rescue associated with transaminases greater than 20 times baseline and elevation of serum bilirubin up to 3 mg/dl (Locasciulli et al., 1992).	Returns to normal within 10 days (Kummar et al., 2005)
Mitoxantrone	Transient, reversible elevation of liver enzymes (Paciucci & Sklarin, 1986)	Dose modification required in patients with liver dysfunction
Paclitaxel	7%–22% (Bristol-Myers Squibb Oncology, 2003) Events usually occur at high doses or in combination therapy (Bristol-Myers Squibb Oncology, 2003); patients with liver dysfunction are at increased risk of toxicity secondary to delayed clearance. Dose reduction is recommended for these patients.	The toxicity of paclitaxel is greater for patients with elevated liver enzymes (Bristol-Myers Squibb Oncology, 2003).
Thioguanine	–	Elevation of serum bilirubin and transaminases VOD (rare)
Vincristine	Rare (Perry, 1992)	Hepatotoxicity does not tend to occur at standard doses. Consider dose modification for patients with hepatic dysfunction.
Vinorelbine	Transient elevation in LFTs (Chu & DeVita, 2002)	Metabolized in liver by cytochrome P450 microsomal system

c) Provide instruction about signs and symptoms of liver failure (e.g., jaundice, liver tenderness, changes in color of urine or stool).

d) Promote rest.

e) Encourage use of soothing lotions and cool baths to promote skin comfort. Remind patients not to scratch.

f) Suggest that patients wear lightweight, loose clothing.

g) Encourage patients to continue eating a light, high-glucose diet.

h) Reinforce the importance of having lifelong annual follow-up assessments performed by a healthcare provider familiar with their cancer history, treatment, and risk of developing late effects (Bottomley, 2004).

i) Encourage patients to have periodic LFTs and to plan appropriate follow-up.

References

Abratt, R.P., Bezwoda, W.R., Falkson, G., Goedhals, L., Hacking, D., & Rugg, T.A. (1994). Efficacy and safety profile of gemcitabine in non-small cell lung cancer: A phase II study. *Journal of Clinical Oncology, 12,* 1535–1540.

Alexander, H.R., Kemeny, N.E., & Lawrence, T.S. (2005). Metastatic cancer to the liver. In V.T. DeVita, S. Hellman, & S.A. Rosenberg (Eds.), *Cancer: Principles and practice of oncology* (7th ed., pp. 2352–2368). Philadelphia: Lippincott Williams & Wilkins.

Balis, F.M., Holcenberg, J.S., & Poplack, D.G. (1997). General principles of chemotherapy. In P.A. Pizzo & D.G. Poplack (Eds.), *Principles and practice of pediatric oncology* (3rd ed., pp. 215–272). Philadelphia: Lippincott-Raven.

Bottomley, S.J. (2004). Late effects of childhood cancer: Promoting health after childhood cancer. In N.E. Kline (Ed.), *Essentials of pediatric oncology nursing: A core curriculum* (2nd ed., pp. 290–291). Glenview, IL: Association of Pediatric Oncology Nurses.

Bristol-Myers Squibb Oncology. (2003). Blenoxane [Package insert]. Princeton, NJ: Author.

Bristol-Myers Squibb Oncology/Immunology. (1999). Taxol [Package insert]. Princeton, NJ: Author.

Capizzi, R.L., Bertino, J.R., & Handschumacher, R.E. (1970). L-asparaginase. *Annual Review of Medicine, 21,* 433–444.

Cavalli, F., Tschopp, L., Sonntag, R.W., & Zimmerman, A. (1978). A case of liver toxicity following cis-dichlorodiammineplatinum (ii) treatment. *Cancer Treatment Reports, 62,* 2125–2126.

Chiron Corporation. (1998). Proleukin [Package insert]. Emeryville, CA: Author.

Chu, E., & DeVita, V., Jr. (Eds.). (2002). *Physician's cancer chemotherapy drug manual.* Sudbury, MA: Jones and Bartlett.

DeVita, V.T., Carbone, P.P., Owens, A.H., Jr., Gold, G.I., Krant, M.J., & Edmonson, J. (1965). Clinical trials with 1, 3-bis (2-chloroethyl)-1-nitrosourea, NSC-409962. *Cancer Research, 25,* 1875–1881.

Grochow, L.B., & Baker, S.D. (1998). The relationship of age to the disposition and effects of anticancer drugs. In L.B. Grochow & M.M. Ames (Eds.), *A clinician's guide to chemotherapy pharmacokinetics and pharmacodynamics* (pp. 35–53). Baltimore: Williams & Wilkins.

Hassan, M. (1999). The role of busulfan in bone marrow transplantation. *Medical Oncology, 16,* 166–170.

Hohn, D.C., Stagg, R.J., Friedman, M.A., Hannigan, J.F., Jr., Rayner, A., Ignoffo, R.J., et al. (1989). A randomized trial of continuous intravenous versus hepatic intraarterial floxuridine in patients with colorectal cancer metastatic to the liver: The Northern California Oncology Group trial. *Journal of Clinical Oncology, 7,* 1646–1654.

Horrell, C.J. (2000). Hepatotoxicity. In D. Camp-Sorrell & R.A. Hawkins (Eds.), *Clinical manual for the oncology advanced practice nurse* (pp. 451–454). Pittsburgh, PA: Oncology Nursing Society.

Katz, M.E., & Cassileth, P.A. (1977). Hyperbilirubinemia during induction therapy of acute granulocytic leukemia. *Cancer, 40,* 1390–1397.

Kummar, S., Noronha, V., & Chu, E. (2005). Antimetabolites. In V.T. DeVita, S. Hellman, & S.A. Rosenberg (Eds.), *Cancer: Principles and practice of oncology* (7th ed., pp. 358–374). Philadelphia: Lippincott Williams & Wilkins.

Locasciulli, A., Mura, R., Fraschini, D., Gornati, G., Scovena, E., Gervasoni, A., et al. (1992). High-dose methotrexate administration and acute liver damage in children treated for acute lymphoblastic leukemia. A prospective study. *Haematologia, 77,* 49–53.

McDonald, G.B., & Tirumali, N. (1984). Intestinal and liver toxicity of antineoplastic drugs. *Western Journal of Medicine, 140,* 250–259.

Muller, H.J., & Boos, J. (1998). Use of L-asparaginase in childhood ALL. *Critical Reviews in Oncology Hematology, 28,* 108–113.

Oettgen, H.F., Stephenson, P.A., & Schwartz, M.K. (1970). Toxicity of *E. coli* L-asparaginase in man. *Cancer, 25,* 253–278.

Paciucci, P.A., & Sklarin, N.T. (1986). Mitoxantrone and hepatic toxicity. *Annals of Internal Medicine, 105,* 805–806.

Perry, M.C. (1992). Hepatotoxicity of chemotherapeutic agents. In M.C. Perry (Ed.), *The chemotherapy source book* (2nd ed., pp. 635–647). Baltimore: Williams & Wilkins.

Pollera, C.F., Ameglio, F., Nardi, M., Vitelli, G., & Marolla, P. (1987). Cisplatin-induced hepatic toxicity [Letter to the editor]. *Journal of Clinical Oncology, 5,* 318–319.

Pratt, C.B., & Johnson, W.W. (1971). Duration and severity of fatty metamorphosis of the liver following L-asparaginase therapy. *Cancer, 28,* 361–364.

Roche Laboratories. (1999). *Xeloda prescribing information.* Nutley, NJ: Author. Retrieved June 14, 2004, from http://www.rocheusa.com/products

Sahoo, S., & Hart, J. (2003). Histopathological features of L-asparaginase-induced liver disease. *Seminars in Liver Disease, 23,* 295–299.

Schwartz, R.N., Stover, L., & Dutcher, J. (2002). Managing toxicities of high-dose interleukin-2. *Oncology, 16*(11 Suppl. 13), 11–20.

Sifton, D.W. (Ed.). (2002). *Physicians' desk reference* (56th ed.). Montvale, NJ: Medical Economics.

Weiss, R.B. (2005). Miscellaneous toxicities. In V.T. DeVita, S. Hellman, & S.A. Rosenberg (Eds.), *Cancer: Principles and practice of oncology* (7th ed., pp. 2602–2614). Philadelphia: Lippincott Williams & Wilkins.

Wilkes, G.M., Ingwersen, K., & Barton-Burke, M. (2003). *2003 oncology nursing drug handbook.* Sudbury, MA: Jones and Bartlett.

I. Nephrotoxicity: Approximately one million nephrons are present in each child at birth. Not all become fully functional until adulthood. New nephrons are not formed after birth (Bergstein, 2000).
   1. Pathophysiology: Nephrotoxicity is a dose-limiting effect of some chemotherapy and biotherapy agents and can cause the following (Lydon, 1986).
      a) Direct renal cell damage (including potential damage to the glomerulus, renal blood vessels, and/or different parts of the nephron): Damage may be irreversible and lead to necrosis, especially with cisplatin and high-dose methotrexate therapy.
      b) Precipitation of metabolites in the acidic environment of the urine: As a result of rapid tumor-cell lysis, metabolite precipitation causes obstructive nephropathy, also known as tumor lysis syndrome (TLS).
         (1) TLS is an oncologic emergency and a metabolic risk for patients with large tumor burdens or tumor cell loads that are very sensitive to antineoplastic treatment modalities (e.g., acute leukemia, high-grade lymphoma, small cell lung cancer, multiple myeloma).
         (2) In addition, patients presenting with elevated lactic dehydrogenase levels are at higher risk for TLS.

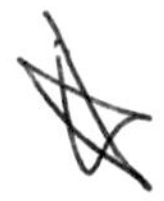

         (3) Tumor cells rapidly lyse following treatment, sending intracellular components into peripheral circulation. The results are potentially life-threatening electrolyte imbalances characterized by hyperuricemia, hyperkalemia, hyperphosphatemia, and hypocalcemia.

         (4) TLS can be life-threatening if not identified and treated early. Clinical consequences include acute renal failure, cardiac failure, and multisystem organ failure.

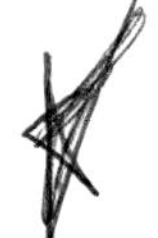

(5) The goals of preventive and treatment measures for TLS include vigorous hydration, urinary alkalinization, reduction of uric acid production with allopurinol or rasburicase, and forced diuresis (Brant, 2002; Patterson & Reams, 2001; Sanofi-Synthelabo, 2002).

c) Impaired water excretion: Treatment with certain antineoplastic agents (e.g., cyclophosphamide, ifosfamide, vinca alkaloids, cisplatin, melphalan, bortezomib) can cause a potentially emergent clinical situation known as water intoxication or the syndrome of inappropriate antidiuretic hormone (SIADH) (Flounders, 2003; Millenium Pharmaceuticals, Inc., 2003).

(1) SIADH is the inappropriate secretion of antidiuretic hormone leading to water resorption and decreased water excretion, hypervolemia, hyponatremia, and hypoosmolality.

(2) SIADH can have a rapid onset with life-threatening outcomes if the sodium level is < 105 mEq/l.

(3) SIADH can occur in regimens requiring vigorous hydration to prevent nephrotoxicity because they create a potential for water retention and severe hyponatremia.

(4) A clinical consequence is cerebral edema with neurologic signs and excess thirst as common symptoms.

(5) Treatment for SIADH relates to the presenting symptomatology and includes fluid restriction, forced diuresis, demeclocycline, and administration of hypertonic 3% saline.

d) Decreased renal perfusion and prerenal azotemia (Strohl, 2000)

(1) In patients receiving IL-2, factors contributing to nephrotoxicity include hypotension, impaired cardiac function, and decreased intravascular volume.

(2) These lead to decreased renal perfusion and prerenal azotemia.

(3) Most nephrotoxic effects of IL-2 are prerenal and fully reversible.

e) Proteinuria: With interferon and bevacizumab, the most common renal presentation is proteinuria (Genentech, Inc., 2004a).

f) Nephrotic syndrome and interstitial nephritis are rare (Genentech, Inc., 2004a; Kirkwood, 2000; Skalla, 1996).

2. Incidence (see Tables 25 and 28)
3. Risk factors

a) Age less than 12 months: Renal blood flow, glomerular filtration, and tubular function are not completely developed in children until they are 12 months old. These physiologic characteristics affect drug disposition as well as excretion and secretion rates, predisposing children to nephrotoxicity (Balis, Holcenberg, & Blaney, 2001).

b) Advancing age, during which the kidneys become slightly smaller and renal function decreases (Patterson & Reams, 2001)

c) Preexisting renal disease, which presents a direct risk (Bergstein, 2000; Patterson & Reams, 2001)

d) Connective tissue, liver, or cardiac disease, which presents an indirect risk (Patterson & Reams, 2001)

e) Poor nutrition and hydration status

f) Hypovolemia, which may increase the risk of acute renal failure (Jenkins & Rieselbach, 1982)

g) Administration of other nephrotoxic drugs (e.g., NSAIDs, aminoglycoside antibiotics, amphotericin B, cyclosporine) (Balis et al., 2001; Raymond, 1984)

h) Extravascular fluid shifts

i) Nephrectomy

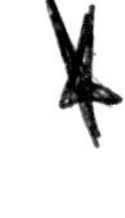

j) Pretherapy hypercalcemia or serum creatinine levels > 1.5 mg/dl

4. Clinical manifestations (Patterson & Reams, 2001): Although hypomagnesemia, hypocalcemia, hypophosphatemia, and decreased serum bicarbonate are common during IL-2 and interferon alpha therapy, the conditions are accompanied by hypoalbuminemia and are not attributable to altered renal function (Kirkwood, 2000; Schwartzentruber, 2000). Signs and symptoms listed previously for specific syndromes of TLS and SIADH include the following.

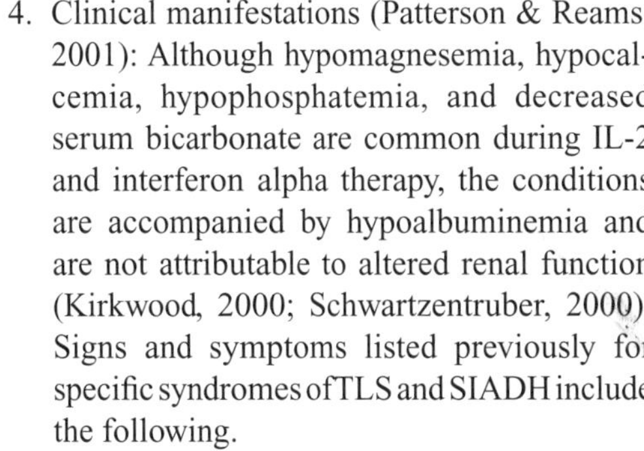

a) Oliguria

b) Increasing serum creatinine

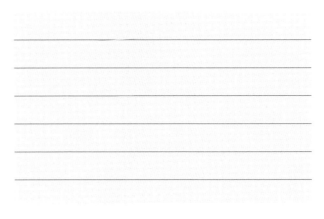

c) Declining creatinine clearance

Table 28. Nephrotoxicity of Chemotherapeutic and Biotherapeutic Drugs

Drug	Incidence	Comments
Bevacizumab	Adults: Rare Children: Unknown	Rare toxicities include proteinuria and nephrotic syndrome (Genentech, Inc., 2004a).
Bortezomib	Adults: Rare Children: Unknown	Rare toxicities include renal failure and signs of hyperuricemia, hypokalemia, hypocalcemia, and hyponatremia with possible TLS and SIADH. Also noted are rare occurrences of renal calculus, hydronephrosis, and glomerular nephritis (Millenium Pharmaceuticals, Inc., 2003).
Carmustine	Adults: Common with cumulative doses > 1,500 mg/m² (Lydon, 1986; Patterson & Reams, 2001) Children: Child-specific incidence is unavailable.	Effects include interstitial fibrosis and glomerular sclerosis (Vogelzang, 1991). The onset of renal toxicity may occur months to years after chemotherapy (Patterson & Reams, 2001).
Cisplatin	Adults: 12%–36% Adults and children: Renal sodium wasting, 10%; hypomagnesium, 1%–10% (Rossi et al., 1999)	May cause tubular injury after a single dose of 30 mg/m² IV (Evans, 1991; Lydon, 1986). Toxicity increases significantly with high-dose therapy (≥ 85 mg/m²) (Marceau et al., 1999). The most common pediatric toxicities are dose-limiting azotemia and electrolyte disturbances secondary to decreased renal blood flow, decreased glomerular filtration rate, and loss of tubular function (Balis et al., 2001).
Fludarabine	Adults: < 1% Children: Rare	Acute uric acid nephropathy can occur with acute leukemias, high-grade lymphomas, small cell lung cancer, carcinoma, and in patients with large tumor burden who have not received prophylactic allopurinol (Cheson et al., 1998).
Gemtuzumab ozogamicin	Adults: Rare, related to tumor lysis syndrome (TLS)	Rapid reduction of tumor cells can result in renal insufficiency, acute renal failure, uric acid nephropathy, acute renal failure resulting from renal tubular obstruction, and nephrolithiasis. Patients with large tumor burden are at increased risk for TLS (Wyeth Pharmaceuticals, 2004).
Ifosfamide	Adults: < 1% Children: Fanconi's syndrome, 5%; subclinical tubular dysfunction, 15% (Rossi et al., 1999)	May cause tubular damage. Incidence of damage may increase with existing renal dysfunction or prior cisplatin therapy (Vogelzang, 1991). Pediatric patients have a slightly higher incidence of tubular damage (Skinner et al., 1993). Children tend to develop proximal tubular damage as well as a condition similar to Fanconi's syndrome (Balis et al., 2001; Grochow & Baker, 1998).
Interferon	Adults: Rare, dose-related, generally reversible upon treatment cessation	Generally is the same as IL-2, but more rare (Kirkwood, 2000; Sandstrom, 1996)
Interleukin-2	Adults: Common, dose-related, transient, quickly reversible upon treatment cessation Children: Unknown	Alterations include direct renal toxicity, neurogenic bladder, and renal effects related to dehydration and metabolic or hemodynamic instability (Siegel & Puri, 1991).
Lomustine	Adults: Common with cumulative doses > 1,500 mg/m² (Lydon, 1986; Patterson & Reams, 2001) Children: Child-specific incidence is unavailable.	Effects include interstitial fibrosis and glomerular sclerosis (Vogelzang, 1991). The onset of renal toxicity may occur months to years after chemotherapy (Patterson & Reams, 2001). In children, high cumulative doses of lomustine (> 1,000 mg/m²), nitrosourea therapy longer than 15 months, and semustine therapy are associated with progressive renal atrophy (Balis et al., 2001).
Methotrexate	Adults: < 10% with high-dose therapy Children: Child-specific incidence is unavailable.	In high-dose therapy, methotrexate enters renal tubules, precipitating tubular injury (Balis et al., 1997; Crom, 1998; Lydon, 1986; Vogelzang, 1991).
Mitomycin-C	Adults: 2%–10% Children: Child-specific incidence is unavailable.	Cumulative doses > 60 mg/m² may cause hemolytic uremic syndrome (Hrozencik & Connaughton, 1988; Vogelzang, 1991). Mitomycin-C is not commonly used for children.

(Continued on next page)

Table 28. Nephrotoxicity of Chemotherapeutic and Biotherapeutic Drugs *(Continued)*		
Drug	**Incidence**	**Comments**
Rituximab	Adults: Rare, related to TLS	Same as gemtuzumab ozogamicin (Genentech, Inc., 2004b)
Streptozocin	Adults: Variable Children: Child-specific incidence is unavailable.	May cause tubular interstitial nephritis and tubular atrophy (Myerowitz et al., 1976); however, nephrotoxicity is rarely reported if the weekly dose is < 1 g/m² (Sadoff, 1979; Vogelzang, 1991). Streptozocin is not commonly used for children.

d) Elevated BUN
e) Hypomagnesemia
f) Proteinuria
g) Hematuria
h) Weight gain from fluid retention or edema

5. Laboratory values (Lydon, 1986): For pediatric patients, reference ranges are age-specific. Reference ranges differ from institution to institution. Similarly, indications to hold or delay chemotherapy for pediatric patients are based on evidence of nephrotoxicity as defined by treatment protocol. Consult institutional guidelines in regard to specific pediatric cases (Nicholson & Pesce, 2000). Note: The values cited in this section apply to adults only.
   a) BUN (Lydon, 1986)
      (1) Assess baseline and consecutive levels.
         (a) For patients not requiring vasopressors, monitor levels daily.
         (b) For inpatients requiring vasopressors, monitor levels twice daily.
         (c) For outpatients, monitor levels weekly or as clinically indicated.
      (2) Make a rough estimate of renal function. (BUN is very sensitive to hydration status and increases with the level of dehydration.)
      (3) Consider holding or reducing dose of chemotherapy with evidence of renal impairment.
   b) Serum creatinine
      (1) Assess baseline and consecutive levels. If the patient is on a research protocol, refer to protocol guidelines.
         (a) For patients not requiring vasopressors, monitor levels daily.
         (b) For inpatients requiring vasopressors, monitor levels twice daily.
         (c) For outpatients, monitor levels weekly or as clinically indicated.
      (2) Serum creatinine is a specific and sensitive indicator of renal function.
      (3) Consider holding or reducing dose of chemotherapy if serum creatinine is grade 2 toxicity (> 1.5–3.0 x upper limits of normal [ULN]) (NCI, 2003).
   c) 12-hour creatinine clearance (Lydon, 1986)
      (1) Assess baseline and consecutive levels. If the patient is on a research protocol, refer to protocol guidelines.
      (2) The 12-hour creatinine clearance can be the most sensitive test of renal function. The 12-hour test is as effective as the 24-hour test and is less costly. For pediatric patients, a test of nuclear GFR frequently is used.
      (3) Accuracy depends on collecting all urine in a specified time.
      (4) Consider holding or reducing dose of chemotherapy if creatinine clearance is decreasing or as indicated by the chemotherapy protocol.
   d) Urine cytology: Urine cytology is inaccurate if patients are cachectic (Lydon, 1986).
      (1) Assess changes in urine cytology (e.g., RBCs, WBCs, epithelial cells).
      (2) The presence of casts in urine can indicate renal tubular damage.
   e) Urine protein: Proteinuria indicates damage to the glomerular and tubular systems.
   f) Urine-specific gravity and osmolality (Lydon, 1986)
      (1) A measure of renal ability to concentrate or dilute urine
      (2) Indicates presence or absence of tubular and/or medullary damage
      (3) Is often elevated in patients who are not adequately hydrated
   g) Urine pH (Lydon, 1986)
      (1) A measure of the free hydrogen-ion concentration in urine
      (2) Expresses the strength of the urine as a dilute acid or a base solution
   h) Serum electrolytes, especially magnesium, uric acid, sodium, and potassium levels (Lydon, 1986)
      (1) Measure serum electrolytes when giving cisplatin or high-dose chemotherapy and if the patient is at risk for TLS.

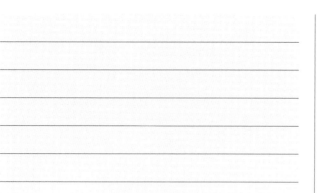

(2) Monitor serum electrolytes during biotherapy, particularly IL-2, at the following frequencies (Wilkes & Burke, 2004).
   (a) For patients not requiring vasopressors, monitor levels daily.
   (b) For patients requiring vasopressors, monitor levels as clinically indicated.

(3) Assess patient for fluid imbalance.

6. Objective physical assessment data (Strohl, 2000)
   a) Monitor intake and output.
   b) Monitor weight changes, especially weight gain and edema, daily or as clinically indicated.
   c) Monitor for changes in LOC, mental status, or behavior.

7. Collaborative management (Lydon, 1986)
   a) General strategies
      (1) Monitor renal function tests regularly.
      (2) Institute hydration of approximately three liters per day to prevent or minimize renal damage, especially with cisplatin and high-dose methotrexate regimens (Rossi, Kleta, & Ehrich, 1999). Hydration for pediatric patients is one-and-one-half to two times maintenance.
      (3) Stop or delay drug if BUN, creatinine, or electrolytes do not return to baseline.
      (4) Treat oliguria judiciously with fluid boluses.
      (5) Replace electrolytes as indicated.
   b) Follow-up recommendations (Lydon, 1986; Strohl, 2000)
      (1) Conduct periodic evaluation, including urinalysis, creatinine clearance, and serum chemistries.
      (2) If renal toxicity is severe, refer patients to a nephrologist to assess and possibly provide further workup and treatment, such as hemodialysis.

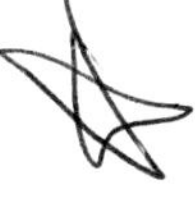

   c) Drug-specific prevention strategies (Choudhury & Ahmed, 1997; Evans, 1991; Marceau et al., 1999)
      (1) Cisplatin regimens
         (a) Administer vigorous saline hydration to minimize toxicity.
         (b) Induce diuresis with mannitol and/or a loop diuretic before or after administering cisplatin as a means of ensuring adequate urine flow. Note that an increase in cisplatin toxicities has been shown with the use of furosemide for diuresis.
         (c) Monitor renal function tests and electrolyte levels frequently.
         (d) Consider amifostine for reduction of nephrotoxicity associated with cisplatin-based regimens (ASCO, 2002; MedImmune Inc., 2003; Patterson & Reams, 2001).
            i) Amifostine is a chemoprotectant.
            ii) It is rapidly metabolized and has a very short half-life. The drug is administered intravenously over not more than 5–15 minutes and is given just prior to cisplatin after one liter of hydration has been administered.
            iii) Side effects include hypotension, nausea and vomiting, flushing, and fever/chills.
            iv) Pretreat with antiemetics, adequate hydration, monitoring of blood pressure every three to five minutes, reclining the patient during and immediately after infusion, and interrupting the amifostine infusion if blood pressure drops below the threshold level.

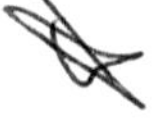

            v) Hold antihypertensives 24 hours prior to amifostine administration.
      (2) High-dose methotrexate regimens
         (a) Alkalinize the urine by giving sodium bicarbonate orally or by IV. Assess urine pH; urine pH should be at minimum ≥ 7.0 (Wilkes & Burke, 2004).
         (b) It is essential to administer leucovorin at scheduled times (first dose usually 24 hours after methotrexate). Subsequent doses are given at six-hour intervals and continue until methotrexate level is within

acceptable range. Leucovorin bypasses the folic acid antagonizing effect of methotrexate, decreasing the overall toxicities of methotrexate.

(c) Avoid taking folic acid, aspirin, penicillins, and sulfonylureas (e.g., glipizide) 48 hours before and after methotrexate (Wilkes & Burke, 2004).

(d) Discontinue treatment with NSAIDs, clotimoxazole, and trimethoprim and sulfamethoxazole until the methotrexate level has decreased (Wilkes & Burke, 2004).

(e) Reduce subsequent doses based on degree of toxicity.

(3) For patients receiving IL-2 and interferon (Sandstrom, 1996)

(a) Encourage the patient to drink two to three liters of noncaffeinated fluid daily.

(b) Monitor output.

(4) Other regimens (Cheson, Frame, Vena, Quashu, & Sorensen, 1998)

(a) Anticipate TLS in patients with tumors that have high growth fractions (e.g., Burkitt's and other high-grade lymphomas, acute and chronic leukemias).

(b) Administer allopurinol or rasburicase to decrease uric acid level, which can rapidly lead to acute uric acid nephropathy and renal failure if untreated.

8. Patient and family education (Lydon, 1986; Strohl, 2000)

a) Ensure that patients understand the reasons for changes in urine output, electrolyte depletion, and increasing creatinine and BUN.

b) Inform patients that nephrotoxicity is a risk associated with certain cytotoxic agents. Provide reassurance that impaired renal function usually is temporary and reversible.

c) Reinforce the importance of complying with preventive measures.

d) Reinforce the importance of collecting urine at 12 and 24 hours for creatinine clearance.

e) Encourage patients to increase fluid intake; intake should be two to three liters of noncaffeinated fluid daily.

f) Ensure that patients understand the need to comply with instructions to alkalinize urine and complete leucovorin rescue, allopurinol therapy, and/or amifostine treatment.

g) Explain the reason for weight gain during specific therapies and the need for diuresis after therapy is completed.

h) Instruct patients to avoid the use of drugs that potentiate renal dysfunction.

i) Ensure that patients know to notify the healthcare team if

(1) They are unable to make urine for more than 12 hours.

(2) Urine becomes very dark or concentrated.

(3) They produce only very small amounts of urine.

References

American Society of Clinical Oncology. (2002). *2002 update of recommendations for the use of chemotherapy and radiotherapy protectants: Clinical practice guidelines of the American Society of Clinical Oncology.* Retrieved January 13, 2005, from http://www.asco.org/ac/1,1003,_12-002306,00.asp

Balis, F.M., Holcenberg, J.S., & Blaney, S.M. (2001). General principles of chemotherapy. In P.A. Pizzo & D.G. Poplack (Eds.), *Principles and practice of pediatric oncology* (4th ed., pp. 237–308). Philadelphia: Lippincott Williams & Wilkins.

Bergstein, J.M. (2000). Glomerular disease and renal failure. In R.E. Berhman, R.M. Kliegman, & H.B. Jenson (Eds.), *Nelson textbook of pediatrics* (16th ed., pp. 1573–1576, 1604–1612). Philadelphia: Saunders.

Brant, J. (2002). Rasburicase: An innovative new treatment for hyperuricemia associated with tumor lysis syndrome. *Clinical Journal of Oncology Nursing, 6,* 12–16.

Cheson, D.D., Frame, J.N., Vena, D., Quashu, N., & Sorensen, J.M. (1998). Tumor lysis syndrome: An uncommon complication of fludarabine therapy of chronic lymphocytic leukemia. *Journal of Clinical Oncology, 16,* 2313–2320.

Choudhury, D., & Ahmed, Z. (1997). Drug-induced nephrotoxicity. *Medical Clinics of North America, 81,* 705–717.

Crom, W.R. (1998). Methotrexate. In L.B. Grochow & M.M. Ames (Eds.), *A clinician's guide to chemotherapy pharmacokinetics and pharmacodynamics* (pp. 311–330). Baltimore: Williams & Wilkins.

Evans, S. (1991). Nursing measures in the prevention and treatment of renal cell damage associated with cisplatin administration. *Cancer Nursing, 14,* 91–97.

Flounders, J. (2003). Syndrome of inappropriate antidiuretic hormone. *Oncology Nursing Forum, 30,* E63–E70. Retrieved March 25, 2004, from http://www.ons.org/publications/journals/ONF/Volume30/Issue3/3003381.asp

Genentech, Inc. (2004a). Avastin [Package insert]. Retrieved March 25, 2004, from http://www.gene.com/gene/products/information/oncology/avastin/insert.jsp

Genentech, Inc. (2004b). Rituxan [Package insert]. Retrieved January 18, 2005, from http://www.gene.com/gene/products/information/oncology/rituxan/index.jsp

Grochow, L.B., & Baker, S.D. (1998). The relationship of age to the disposition and effects of anticancer drugs. In L.B. Grochow & M.M. Ames (Eds.), *A clinician's guide to chemotherapy pharmacokinetics and pharmacodynamics* (pp. 35–54). Baltimore: Williams & Wilkins.

Hrozencik, S.P., & Connaughton, M.J. (1988). Cancer-associated hemolytic uremic syndrome. *Oncology Nursing Forum, 15,* 755–759.

Jenkins, P.G., & Rieselbach, R.E. (1982). Acute renal failure: Diagnosis, clinical spectrum, and management. In R.E. Rieselbach & M.B. Garnick (Eds.), *Cancer and the kidney* (pp. 103–179). Philadelphia: Lea & Febiger.

Kirkwood, J.M. (2000). Interferon-alpha and -beta: Clinical applications. In S.A. Rosenberg (Ed.), *Principles and practice of the biologic therapy of cancer* (pp. 224–251). Philadelphia: Lippincott Williams & Wilkins.

Lydon, J. (1986). Nephrotoxicity of cancer treatment. *Oncology Nursing Forum, 13*(2), 68–77.

Marceau, D., Poirer, M., Masson, E., & Beaulieu, E. (1999, May). *High incidence of nephrotoxicity with cisplatin therapy despite adequate hydration: Risk factor correlation.* Abstract from the Annual Meeting of the American Society of Clinical Oncology, Atlanta, GA.

MedImmune Inc. (2003). Ethyol [Package insert]. Retrieved January 18, 2005, from http://www.medimmune.com/products/ethyol/index.asp

Millenium Pharmaceuticals, Inc. (2003). Velcade [Package insert]. Retrieved March 18, 2004, from http://www.mlnm.com/clinicians/oncology/velcade/index.asp

Myerowitz, R.L., Sartiano, G.P., & Cavallo, T. (1976). Nephrotoxic and cytoproliferative effects of streptozotocin. *Cancer, 38,* 1550–1555.

National Cancer Institute. (2003). *Common terminology criteria for adverse events* (version 3.0). Retrieved January 18, 2005, from http://ctep.info.nih.gov/reporting/ctc.html

Nicholson, J.F., & Pesce, M.A. (2000). Reference ranges for laboratory tests and procedures. In R.E. Berhman, R.M. Kliegman, & H.B. Jenson (Eds.), *Nelson textbook of pediatrics* (16th ed., pp. 2181–2234). Philadelphia: Saunders.

Patterson, W.P., & Reams, G.P. (2001). Renal and electrolyte abnormalities due to chemotherapy. In M.C. Perry (Ed.), *The chemotherapy source book* (3rd ed., pp. 494–503). Philadelphia: Lippincott Williams & Wilkins.

Raymond, J.R. (1984). Nephrotoxicities and antineoplastic and immunosuppressive agents. *Current Problems in Cancer, 8*(16), 1–32.

Rossi, R., Kleta, R., & Ehrich, J.H.H. (1999). Renal involvement in children with malignancies. *Pediatric Nephrology, 13,* 153–162.

Sadoff, L. (1979). Nephrotoxicity of streptozotocin (NSC85998). *Cancer Chemotherapy Reports, 54,* 457–459.

Sandstrom, S.K. (1996). Nursing management of patients receiving biological therapy. *Seminars in Oncology Nursing, 12,* 152–162.

Sanofi-Synthelabo. (2002). ELITEK [Package insert]. Retrieved August 29, 2004, from http://www.sanofi-synthelabo.us/products/pi_elitek/pi_elitek.html

Schwartzentruber, D.J. (2000). Interleukin-2: Clinical applications: Principles of administration and management of side effects. In S.A. Rosenberg (Ed.), *Principles and practice of the biologic therapy of cancer* (3rd ed., pp. 32–50). Philadelphia: Lippincott Williams & Wilkins.

Siegel, J.P., & Puri, R.K. (1991). Interleukin-2 toxicity. *Journal of Clinical Oncology, 9,* 694–704.

Skalla, K. (1996). The interferons. *Seminars in Oncology Nursing, 12,* 97–105.

Skinner, R., Sharkey, I.M., Pearson, A.D., & Craft, A.W. (1993). Ifosfamide, mesna, and nephrotoxicity in children. *Journal of Clinical Oncology, 11,* 173–190.

Strohl, R. (2000). Hemorrhagic cystitis. In D. Camp-Sorrell & R.A. Hawkins (Eds.), *Clinical manual for the oncology advanced practice nurse* (pp. 547–549). Pittsburgh, PA: Oncology Nursing Society.

Vogelzang, N.J. (1991). Nephrotoxicity from chemotherapy: Prevention and management. *Oncology, 5*(10), 97–102.

Wilkes, G.M., & Burke, M.B. (2004). *2004 oncology nursing drug handbook*. Sudbury, MA: Jones and Bartlett.

Wyeth Pharmaceuticals. (2004). Mylotarg [Package insert]. Retrieved January 18, 2005, from http://www.wyeth.com/products/wpp_products/full_pharma_az.asp

J. Neurotoxicity

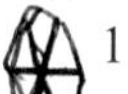

1. Pathophysiology
   a) Neurotoxicity can arise as direct or indirect damage to the CNS, peripheral nervous system, cranial nerves (CNs), or any combination of the three (Gilbert, 2000; Voss & Wilkes, 1999).

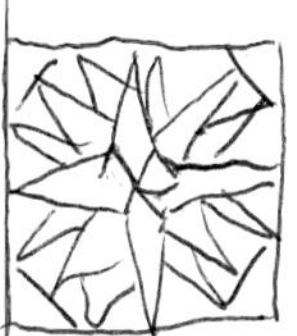

      (1) CN deficits: These deficits result from damage to one of the 12 cranial nerves arising from the brain stem. The result depends on which nerve is damaged (Cassidy & Misset, 2002; Meehan & Johnson, 1992; Voss & Wilkes, 1999). Examples of cranial nerve deficits include the following.
         (a) Olfactory (CN I): Loss or decrease of smell
         (b) Optic (CN II): Loss of visual acuity, optic atrophy, altered visual field
         (c) Oculomotor (CN III): Ptosis, dilated pupils, altered ocular muscle function, nystagmus
         (d) Trochlear (CN IV): Altered ocular muscle function causing nystagmus
         (e) Trigeminal (CN V): Numbness, poor blink reflex, weakened chewing
         (f) Abducens (CN VI): Altered ocular muscle function causing nystagmus
         (g) Facial (CN VII): Facial paralysis, drooping mouth, sagging lower eyelid, flat nasolabial fold
         (h) Acoustic (CN VIII): Sensory neuronal hearing loss, vertigo, ataxia, nausea and/or vomiting
         (i) Glossopharyngeal (CN IX): Altered sense of taste, altered throat sensation
         (j) Vagus (CN X): Hoarseness, altered gag reflex, altered swallowing function
         (k) Spinal accessory (CN XI): Tilting of head, weakness of shoulder muscles
         (l) Hypoglossal (CN XII): Abnormal tongue movement

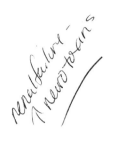

(2) Peripheral deficits: These deficits result from damage to sensory and motor nerves outside the CNS, including the autonomic nerves. Functional deficit is related to type of nerve affected. Peripheral nerves also are subdivided into small fiber (predominantly sensory and autonomic) and large fiber (predominantly motor) nerves (Almadrones, Armstrong, Gilbert, & Schwartz, 2002; Marrs & Newton, 2003; Vallat & Vallat-Decouvelaere, 2001). Examples of peripheral deficits include the following.

(a) Sensory nerve fibers

i) Large fiber: Symmetrical decreased perception of touch and position sense

ii) Small fiber: Symmetrical decreased sense of temperature and pain (paresthesias)

iii) Pain sense may be increased (dysesthesias, hyperesthesias) or decreased (paresthesias).

iv) Sensory deficit usually begins in distal extremities and moves proximally in a classic stocking-glove distribution.

(b) Motor nerve fibers: Symmetrical generalized motor weakness that may affect balance, strength, activity level, foot or wrist drop, myalgias, and muscle cramping (Armstrong, Almadrones, & Gilbert, 2005)

(c) Decreased or absent deep-tendon reflexes

(d) Autonomic nerves: Constipation, paralytic ileus (rare), urinary retention, incontinence, erectile dysfunction, orthostatic hypotension

(3) CNS deficits: These deficits have multiple causes (e.g., metabolic imbalances, intracranial hemorrhage or infection related to chemotherapy-induced coagulopathy or myelosuppression, IT or intra-arterial administration, high-dose therapy). Deficits depend on the area of brain or brain stem affected (Armstrong, Rust, & Kohtz, 1997; Gilbert, 2000).

(a) Acute or chronic encephalopathy: Somnolence and lethargy, confusion, disorientation, memory loss, cognitive dysfunction, seizures (rare)

(b) Cerebellar dysfunction: Truncal, limb, and gait ataxia; dysarthria (staggered gait and postural imbalance); difficulty speaking; slow or irregular speech; nystagmus

b) Some biologic agents are thought to have a direct effect on neuroendocrine secretions, mediation via neurotransmitters, and cytokine pathways, resulting in altered mental status (Trask, Esper, Riba, & Redman, 2000; Valentine, Meyers, Kling, Richelson, & Hauser, 1998).

c) IL-2 and its receptors directly affect the brain and its function. IL-2 increases the permeability of the blood-brain barrier (Licinio, Kling, & Hauser, 1998).

d) Thalidomide's mechanism of action is unclear, but it is thought to inhibit angiogenesis and is associated with symmetric paresthesias (Tariman, 2003).

2. Incidence

a) Neurotoxicity related to chemotherapy: Exact incidence is unknown, but incidence is increasing with greater use of high-dose chemotherapy, the use of more than one neurotoxic agent at a time or sequentially, and with increased detection because of objective and subjective assessment (Armstrong & Gilbert, 2002; Cavalletti & Zanna, 2002; Postma & Heimans, 2000). Incidence of peripheral neuropathy usually increases temporarily after discontinuation of cisplatin but may be permanent (Posner, 2001).

b) Neurotoxicity related to biotherapy

(1) Neurotoxicity occurs in 0%–70% of patients receiving interferon (Trask et al., 2000).

(2) Neurotoxicities associated with biologic response modifiers commonly are related to dosage, duration, route of administration, and underlying disease (Trask et al., 2000; Valentine et al., 1998). Symptoms rarely are severe and are reversible.

(3) The proteasome inhibitor bortezomib is associated with sensory peripheral neuropathy in 31% of patients (Richardson et al., 2003).

3. Risk factors
   a) Regimens including high-dose methotrexate, high-dose cytarabine, vinblastine, vinorelbine, ifosfamide, vincristine, vindesine, cisplatin, carboplatin, paclitaxel, docetaxel, oxaliplatin, altretamine, procarbazine, thalidomide, bortezomib, 5-FU, or steroids (Armstrong & Gilbert, 2002; Richardson et al., 2003; Tariman, 2003; Voss & Wilkes, 1999; Wilkes, 2002; Wilson, 2000)
   b) Intracarotid or IT chemotherapy
   c) Concomitant cranial radiation therapy
   d) Age
      (1) Cerebellar neurotoxicity of cytarabine increases with increasing age. However, cytarabine neurotoxicity varies with dose and route of administration (Voss & Wilkes, 1999).
      (2) Children are at higher risk for ototoxicity than are adults because children's inner ears are not fully developed.
      (3) Compared to adults, children are at higher risk for neurotoxicity resulting from cranial radiation. Children younger than age three are particularly susceptible.
      (4) Elderly and pediatric patients receiving biologic agents are at increased risk for neurotoxicity (Wheeler, 1997).
   e) Cumulative doses of vinca alkaloids, especially vincristine, and platinum analogs, especially cisplatin and taxanes: Cause peripheral neuropathies
   f) Renal failure or renal impairment
   g) Concurrent or subsequent administration of diuretics or aminoglycoside antibiotics: May increase cisplatin-induced sensory neuropathy and ototoxicity and may increase cerebellar damage from cytarabine administration (Gilbert, 2000)
   h) Steroid use: Commonly causes muscle weakness, anxiety, and "steroid psychosis." Symptoms also may include headache, confusion, insomnia, seizures, and coma. Doses of steroids should be tapered immediately upon detection of neurologic changes (Furlong, 1993).
   i) Preexisting neuropathy caused by concomitant medical conditions (e.g., diabetes, vitamin B_{12} deficiency, thyroid dysfunction, cachexia, Charcot-Marie-Tooth disease, hearing loss) (Armstrong & Gilbert, 2002)
   j) History of heavy alcohol consumption (Voss & Wilkes, 1999)
   k) Medications that alter mood (e.g., procarbazine, asparaginase, ifosfamide)
   l) A variety of supportive-care medications, especially antiemetics, pain medications, and antidepressants

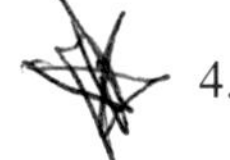

4. Assessment
   a) Obtain a thorough history and review of systems prior to administration of chemotherapy or biotherapy, including current medications.
   b) Identify patients who are at increased risk for neurotoxicity based on risk factors.
   c) Perform a brief neurologic examination prior to each chemotherapy/biotherapy treatment and subsequent medical visit that includes evaluation of sensory and motor function, gait, range of motion, CN function, and reflexes (Brant, 1998; Seidel, Ball, Dains, & Benedict, 1999). Manifestations include
      (1) Cranial nerve deficits as described in Section 1.*a)*
      (2) Peripheral neuropathy as described in Section 1.*b)*
      (3) CNS deficits as described in Section 1.*c)*
   d) Administer self-report questionnaires that assess neurologic function and quality of life at baseline and subsequent visits (Almadrones, McGuire, Walczak, Florio, & Tian, 2004; Cella, Peterman, Hudgens, Webster, & Socinski, 2003; Greimel et al., 2003; Postma & Heimans, 2000).
   e) Assess hearing with audiogram prior to ototoxic chemotherapy (e.g., cisplatin, carboplatin).
   f) Assess patient and family coping.
   g) Assess patients' environment to ensure safety at the impaired level of function.
5. Collaborative management: See Table 29.
   a) Use assessment guidelines for early detection and treatment.

Table 29. Neurotoxicity of Chemotherapeutic Drugs

Toxicity/Symptoms	Grade	General Risk Factors	Chemotherapy Agent/Risk Factors/Symptoms	Mechanism of Damage	Protective/ Management Measures
Cerebellar • Unsteady gait • Nystagmus • Ataxia • Dizziness • Seizures • Hemiparesis • Confusion • Coma Autonomic • Ileus • Constipation • Impotence • Urinary retention • Postural hypotension Peripheral/cranial • Facial palsies • Diplopia • Paresthesia of hands and feet • Muscle atrophy • Foot drop • Loss of deep tendon reflexes • Areflexia • Sensory loss • Sensory perception loss • Hoarseness	Neurocerebellar 0 = None 1 = Sight incoordination dysdiadokinesis 2 = Intention tremor dysmetria, slurred speech 3 = Locomotor ataxia 4 = Cerebellar necrosis Neurocortical 0 = None 1 = Mild somnolence or agitation 2 = Moderate somnolence or agitation 3 = Severe somnolence or agitation 4 = Coma, seizures, psychosis Neurosensory 0 = None 1 = Mild paresthesias, loss of deep tendon reflexes 2 = Mild or moderate objective sensory loss, moderate paresthesias Neuromotor 0 = None 1 = Subjective weakness 2 = Mild objective weakness 3 = Objective weakness with impairment of function 4 = Paralysis	• Dosage • Cranial radiation • Intrathecal administration • Age • Central nervous system (CNS) depressants (i.e., antiemetics, tranquilizers, and sedatives) • History of diabetes, chronic alcohol abuse	Ifosfamide • High doses • Cerebellar and cranial dysfunction Vincristine • Dose related, > 2 mg/m² of unit dose • Hepatic dysfunction • Autonomic, peripheral dysfunction Cisplatin • Dose related • Renal dysfunction • Dehydration • Autonomic, peripheral dysfunction • Concurrent treatment with vincristine or etoposide Methotrexate • High dose (> 1 g/m²) • Cerebellar dysfunction • Concurrent cranial radiation therapy • Intrathecal dose • Increased effect with cytarabine, daunorubicin, salicylates, sulfonamides, vinblastine, vincristine Cytarabine • High doses (> 2 g/m²) • Cerebellar and peripheral effects 5-fluorouracil • Cerebellar dysfunction • Dose and schedule related Taxanes • Peripheral neuropathies • Myalgias/arthralgia	• Accumulation of drug metabolite (chloroacetaldehyde) with direct CNS effect • Disrupts microtubules in the neural tissues • Damages large fibers, resulting in sensory change • Damage/loss of inner hair cells in the organ of Corti • Demyelination of nerve fibers	• Place on bowel regimen. • Oral diazepam 5 mg every six hours at the time of treatment, to manage muscle spasms • Eliminate furosemide. • Avoid concurrent administration of aminoglycosides. • Audiometric testing for high risk • Withhold therapy for severe toxicity (i.e., muscle weakness or pain). • Neurologic recovery, start drug at 50% dose reduction. • Monitor neurologic signs and symptoms. • Monitor electrolytes. • Institute safety measures. • Administer amifostine with cisplatin.

Note. From "Chemotherapy: Toxicity Management" (p. 477), by D. Camp-Sorrell in C.H. Yarbro, M.H. Frogge, M. Goodman, and S.L. Groenwald (Eds.), *Cancer Nursing: Principles and Practice* (5th ed.), 2000, Sudbury, MA: Jones and Bartlett. Copyright 2000 by Jones and Bartlett. Reprinted with permission.

b) Reduce drug dose, discontinue drug, or switch to a less-neurotoxic drug as ordered when neurologic deficits are noted (Rose & Smereker, 2003; Vasey, 2002).
c) No proven pharmacologic intervention currently is available for neurotoxicity prevention. Clinical trials using amifostine and glutamine have been equivocal (Moore et al., 2003; Vahdat et al., 2001).
d) Manage concomitant medical conditions known to cause and increase chemotherapy-related neurotoxicity.
e) Provide supplemental nutrition and treat vitamin deficiency, if needed.
f) Administer analgesics and consider topical analgesics available over-the-counter (Huebscher, 2000; Smith, Whedon, & Bookbinder, 2002).
g) Administer tricyclic antidepressants (e.g., amitriptyline, imipramine, nortriptyline) or anticonvulsants (e.g., gabapentin, phenytoin, carbamazepine) (Smith et al., 2002; Voss & Wilkes, 1999).
h) Consider consultation with neurologist, occupation, physical, or speech therapist, or audiologist.
i) Consider nonpharmacologic management (e.g., exercise, relaxation techniques—yoga, meditation, deep breathing, guided imagery) (Richardson, Sandman, & Vela, 2001; Voss & Wilkes, 1999).

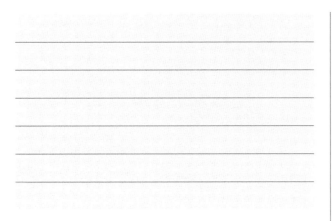

6. Patient and family education
   a) Instruct patients and significant others that neurotoxicity is a possible side effect of selected cytotoxic agents.
   b) Emphasize patient safety issues and provide educational materials (Almadrones & Arcot, 1999).
   c) Provide information regarding signs and symptoms of neurotoxicity, and instruct patients to report these symptoms to the physician and/or nurse if they occur.
   d) Provide information about the potential side effects of medications that could cause or change neurologic symptoms.
   e) Educate patients and significant others regarding any needed referrals, support organizations, adaptations, and rehabilitative strategies.
   f) Provide education regarding avoidance of behaviors (e.g., alcohol consumption) or medication that may alter neurologic status (Sandstrom, 1996).
   g) For pediatric patients, provide information to parents regarding school re-entry and intervention.

References

Almadrones, L., & Arcot, R. (1999). Patient guide to peripheral neuropathy. *Oncology Nursing Forum, 26,* 1359–1360.

Almadrones, L., Armstrong, T., Gilbert, M., & Schwartz, R. (2002). *Chemotherapy-induced neurotoxicity* [Monograph]. Philadelphia: Phillips Group Oncology Communications.

Almadrones, L., McGuire, D., Walczak, J.R., Florio, C., & Tian, C. (2004). Psychometric evaluation of two scales assessing functional status and peripheral neuropathy associated with chemotherapy for ovarian cancer: A Gynecologic Oncology Group study. *Oncology Nursing Forum, 31,* 615–623.

Armstrong, T., Almadrones, L., & Gilbert, M.R. (2005). Chemotherapy-induced peripheral neuropathy. *Oncology Nursing Forum, 32,* 305–311.

Armstrong, T., & Gilbert, M. (2002). Chemotherapy-induced peripheral neuropathy. In W.T. Fetner (Ed.), *The female patient* (pp. 27–30). Chatham, NJ: Quadrant HealthCom.

Armstrong, T., Rust, D., & Kohtz, J.R. (1997). Neurologic, pulmonary, and cutaneous toxicities of high-dose chemotherapy. *Oncology Nursing Forum, 24*(Suppl. 1), 23–33.

Brant, J.M. (1998). Cancer-related neuropathic pain. *Nurse Practitioner Forum, 9,* 154–162.

Cassidy, J., & Misset, J.L. (2002). Oxaliplatin-related side effects: Characteristics and management. *Seminars in Oncology, 29*(Suppl. 15), 11–20.

Cavalletti, G., & Zanna, C. (2002). Current status and future prospects for the treatment of chemotherapy-induced peripheral neurotoxicity. *European Journal of Cancer, 38,* 1832–1837.

Cella, D., Peterman, A., Hudgens, S., Webster, K., & Socinski, M. (2003). Measuring the side effects of taxane therapy in oncology. *Cancer, 98,* 822–831.

Furlong, T.E. (1993). Neurologic complications of immunosuppressive cancer therapy. *Oncology Nursing Forum, 20,* 1337–1352.

Gilbert, M.R. (2000). Neurologic complications. In M.D. Abeloff, J.O. Armitage, A.S. Lichter, & J.E. Neiderhuber (Eds.), *Clinical oncology* (2nd ed., pp. 89–105). New York: Churchill Livingstone.

Greimel, E., Bottomley, A., Cull, A., Waldenstrom, A., Arraras, L., Chauvenet, L., et al. (2003). An international field study of the reliability and validity of a disease-specific questionnaire module (the QLQ-OV28) in assessing the quality of life of patients with ovarian cancer. *European Journal of Cancer, 39,* 1402–1408.

Huebscher, R. (2000). Peripheral neuropathy: Alternative and complementary options. *Nurse Practitioner Forum, 11,* 73–77.

Licinio, J., Kling, M., & Hauser, P. (1998). Cytokines and brain function: Relevance to interferon—An induced mood and cognitive changes. *Seminars in Oncology, 25*(Suppl. 1), 30–38.

Marrs, J., & Newton, S. (2003). Updating your peripheral neuropathy "Know-how." *Clinical Journal of Oncology Nursing, 7,* 299–303.

Meehan, J., & Johnson, B. (1992). The neurotoxicity of antineoplastic agents. *Current Issues in Cancer Nursing Practice Updates, 1*(8), 1–11.

Moore, D.H., Donnelly, J., McGuire, W.P., Almadrones, L., Cella, D., Herzog, T.J., et al. (2003). Limited access trial using amifostine for protection against cisplatin and three-hour paclitaxel-induced peripheral neurotoxicity: A phase II study of the Gynecologic Oncology Group. *Journal of Clinical Oncology, 21,* 4207–4213.

Posner, J.B. (2001). Neurotoxicity caused by chemotherapeutic agents. In D. Dale & D. Federman (Eds.), *Scientific American medicine* (pp. 1–14). New York: WebMD.

Postma, T.J., & Heimans, J.J. (2000). Grading of chemotherapy-induced peripheral neuropathy. *Annals of Oncology, 11,* 509–513.

Richardson, J.K., Sandman, D., & Vela, S. (2001). A focused exercise regimen improves clinical measures of balance in patients with peripheral neuropathy. *Archives of Physical Medicine and Rehabilitation, 82,* 205–209.

Richardson, P.G., Barlogie, B., Berenson, J., Singhal, S., Jagannath, S., Irwin, D., et al. (2003). A phase 2 study of bortezomib in relapsed, refractory myeloma. *New England Journal of Medicine, 348,* 2609–2617.

Rose, P.G., & Smereker, M. (2003). Improvement of paclitaxel-induced neuropathy by substitution of docetaxel for paclitaxel. *Gynecologic Oncology, 91,* 423–425.

Sandstrom, S.K. (1996). Nursing management of patients receiving biological therapy. *Seminars in Oncology Nursing, 12,* 152–162.

Seidel, H.M., Ball, J.W., Dains, J.E., & Benedict, G.W. (1999). *Mosby's guide to physical examination* (4th ed., pp. 755–804). St. Louis, MO: Mosby.

Smith, E.L., Whedon, M.B., & Bookbinder, M. (2002). Quality improvement of painful peripheral neuropathy. *Seminars in Oncology Nursing, 18,* 36–43.

Tariman, J.D. (2003). Thalidomide: Current therapeutic uses and management of its toxicities. *Clinical Journal of Oncology Nursing, 7,* 143–147.

Trask, P., Esper, P., Riba, M., & Redman, B. (2000). Psychiatric side effects of interferon therapy: Prevalence, proposed mechanism, and future directions. *Journal of Clinical Oncology, 18,* 2316–2326.

Vahdat, L., Papadopoulos, K., Lange, D., Leuin, S., Kaufman, E., Donovan, D., et al. (2001). Reduction of paclitaxel-induced peripheral neuropathy with glutamine. *Clinical Cancer Research, 7,* 1192–1197.

Valentine, A., Meyers, C.A., Kling, M.A., Richelson, E., & Hauser, P. (1998). Mood and cognitive side effects of interferon-α therapy. *Seminars in Oncology, 25*(Suppl. 1), 39–47.

Vallat, J.M., & Vallat-Decouvelaere, A.V. (2001). Nerve biopsy: Current indications and results. In D. Cross (Ed.), *Peripheral neuropathy: A practical approach to diagnosis and management* (pp. 20–42). Philadelphia: Lippincott Williams & Wilkins.

Vasey, P.A. (2002). Survival and longer-term toxicity results of the SCOTROC study: Docetaxel-carboplatin vs. paclitaxel-carboplatin in epithelial ovarian cancer [Abstract]. *Proceedings of the American Society of Clinical Oncology, 21,* Abstract No. 804.

Voss, M.A.B., & Wilkes, G.M. (1999). Neurotoxicities. *American Journal of Nursing, 99*(Suppl. 4), 20–23.

Wheeler, V. (1997). Biotherapy. In M.H. Frogge, C.H. Yarbro, M. Goodman, & S.L. Groenwald (Eds.), *Cancer nursing: Principles and practice* (4th ed., pp. 426–458). Sudbury, MA: Jones and Bartlett.

Wilkes, G.M. (2002). New therapeutic options in colon cancer: Focus on oxaliplatin. *Clinical Journal of Oncology Nursing, 3,* 1–12.

Wilson, R. (2000). Optimizing nutrition for patients with cancer. *Clinical Journal of Oncology Nursing, 4,* 23–27.

K. Pancreatitis: Inflammation of the pancreas
   1. Pathophysiology (Hruban & Wilentz, 2005)
      a) Pancreatitis is a group of disorders ranging from mild, transient changes to life-threatening inflammatory process and irreversible loss of function.
      b) Causes are secondary to ductal obstruction (e.g., cholelithiasis), acinar cell injury (e.g., drugs, viruses), or defective intracellular transport (e.g., alcohol).
   2. Risk factors (Ellsworth-Wolk, 1998; Hruban & Wilentz, 2005)
      a) Chemotherapy drugs, including asparaginase and mercaptopurine (Hruban & Wilentz, 2005)
      b) Hypertriglyceridemia
      c) TLS
      d) Placement of an intrahepatic catheter
      e) Alcohol abuse
      f) Illicit drug use
      g) Cholelithiasis
      h) Pediatrics: Post–BMT
   3. Clinical manifestations (Steinberg, 1997)
      a) Epigastric, periumbilical, or left/right upper abdominal pain
      b) Pain radiating to the back
      c) Fever, tachycardia
      d) Severe nausea and vomiting
      e) Signs and symptoms of shock with severe or acute pancreatitis
      f) Hypoactive bowel sounds, ileus
      g) Elevated serum amylase, lipase, triglycerides, and LFTs
      h) Frequently elevated WBC count
   4. Assessment: Physical examination must be performed to find and document the preceding clinical manifestations.
   5. Collaborative management (Horrell, 2000)
      a) Hold or discontinue any agent that may be the cause of the condition.
      b) Implement nothing-by-mouth (NPO) orders and place an NG tube to rest the gut during the acute phase of pancreatitis.
      c) If NPO more than three to five days, consider TPN to prevent malnutrition.

d) Administer vigorous hydration with electrolyte replacement (e.g., calcium, potassium, magnesium) as indicated.

e) Monitor serum lipase, amylase, and electrolyte levels and LFTs.

f) Provide effective pain control.

g) Anticipate orders for diagnostic imaging of the abdomen (e.g., ultrasound, CT scan).

h) Administer antibiotic therapy.

i) Ensure bedrest.

j) Monitor vital signs, including oxygen saturation, level of consciousness, and condition carefully for signs of shock or electrolyte imbalance.

k) When food is reintroduced, provide a lipid-restricted diet

6. Patient and family education (Horrell, 2000)

a) Instruct patients to use analgesics for pain control.

b) Implement effective oral and nasal care while NPO with an NG tube.

c) Ensure that patients know the importance of adherence to dietary and pharmacologic recommendations.

d) Ensure that patients and significant others can recognize the early symptoms of pancreatitis, and instruct them to seek medical intervention when these appear.

References

Ellsworth-Wolk, J. (1998). Acute pancreatitis. In C.C. Chernecky & B.J. Berger (Eds.), *Advanced and critical care oncology nursing: Managing primary complications* (pp. 26–38). Philadelphia: Saunders.

Horrell, C.J. (2000). Pancreatitis. In D. Camp-Sorrell & R.A. Hawkins (Eds.), *Clinical manual for the oncology advanced practice nurse* (pp. 461–464). Pittsburgh, PA: Oncology Nursing Society.

Hruban, R.H., & Wilentz, R.E. (2005). The pancreas. In V. Kumar, A.K. Abbas, & N. Fausto (Eds.), *Robbins & Cotran pathologic basis of disease* (7th ed., pp. 939–953). Philadelphia: Elsevier.

Steinberg, W.M. (1997). Diagnosis and management of acute pancreatitis. *Cleveland Clinical Journal of Medicine, 64,* 182–186.

L. Alterations in sexuality and reproductive function: Systemic effects of cytotoxic therapy can affect fertility, body image, and sexual functioning. Chemotherapy may cause either temporary or permanent gonadal failure as well as changes in body image (see Table 30). Wilmoth (1998) provided an excellent review of the effects of cancer therapy on sexuality and intimate relationships and the role of the oncology nurse in the provision of high-quality, holistic care. Issues of sexuality may be especially difficult for adolescents because they may not experience normal pubertal changes (Dragone, 1996).

1. Pathophysiology: Gonadal tissues are sensitive to the effects of cytotoxic drugs. Many, but

Table 30. Chemotherapeutic Agents Affecting Sexual or Reproductive Function

Agent	Complication
Alkylating agents • Altretamine • Busulfan • Chlorambucil • Cisplatin • Cyclophosphamide • Ifosfamide • Melphalan • Nitrogen mustard	Amenorrhea, oligospermia, azoospermia, decreased libido, ovarian dysfunction, erectile dysfunction
Antimetabolites • Cytosine arabinoside • Fludarabine phosphate • 5-fluorouracil • Methotrexate	As for alkylating agents
Antitumor antibiotics • Dactinomycin • Daunorubicin	As for alkylating agents
Plant products	
• Vinblastine	Decreased libido, ovarian dysfunction, erectile dysfunction
• Vincristine	Retrograde ejaculation, erectile dysfunction
Miscellaneous agents	
• Aminoglutethimide	Irregular menses, acne
• Androgens	Masculinization (women)
• Antiandrogens	Decreased libido, impotence
• Antiestrogens	Gynecomastia, impotence
• Corticosteroids	Transient impotence
• Estrogens	Gynecomastia, acne
• Goserelin acetate	Impotence
• Interferons	Amenorrhea, pelvic pain
• Procarbazine	As for alkylating agents
• Progestins	Menstrual abnormalities, change in libido, masculinization (women)

Note. From "Sexual and Reproductive Dysfunction" (p. 839), by L.U. Krebs in C.H. Yarbro, M.H. Frogge, M. Goodman, and S.L. Groenwald (Eds.), *Cancer Nursing: Principles and Practice* (5th ed.), 2000, Sudbury, MA: Jones and Bartlett. Copyright 2000 by Jones and Bartlett. Reprinted with permission.

not all, chemotherapy regimens present a risk of infertility. Many chemotherapy drugs are known teratogens (Ganz, Litwin, & Myerowitz, 2001).

a) In females: Chemotherapy affects the structurally and functionally interdependent granulosa cells (cells that produce sex hormones) and the oocyte (Sklar, 1999).

(1) Alkylating agents can cause primary ovarian failure, resulting in amenorrhea, decreased estradiol, and elevated gonadotropin levels.

(2) Ovarian suppression in premenopausal women may result in symptoms of menopause (e.g., hot flashes, vaginal dryness, dyspareunia).

(a) Women close to or older than age 40 have a higher risk of permanent menopause following chemotherapy than do younger women.

(b) Possible consequences of estrogen deficiency may be short-term, intermediate, or long-term.

i) Short-term (less than two years): Vasomotor instability resulting in "hot flashes" and depression

ii) Intermediate: Urogenital atrophy

iii) Long-term (more than 10 years): Increased risk of cerebrovascular accident, and/or osteoporosis. The recent findings from the Women's Health Initiative Study dispel the longstanding belief that hormone replacement therapy (HRT) protects women from coronary artery disease (Writing Group for the Women's Health Initiative Investigators, 2002).

b) In males

(1) Effects on germ cells (which produce sperm): Alkylating agents can cause azoospermia (absence of sperm in semen).

(2) Effects on Leydig cells: Leydig cells are relatively resistant to chemotherapy, maintaining testosterone levels at normal or near-normal levels (Mulder, 1999).

2. Incidence

a) Sexual dysfunction

(1) Following chemotherapy, 40%–100% of patients report some evidence of sexual dysfunction (Schover, 1997).

(2) Sexual dysfunction frequently is underreported because medical personnel do not routinely assess it, and patients may be reluctant to broach this sensitive subject. The topic is especially difficult for older children and adolescents to discuss with the healthcare team and their families.

(3) Loss of libido is universal. Many men maintain the ability to have erections and ejaculations despite antiandrogen therapy (Ganz et al., 2001).

b) Reproductive dysfunction: Varies according to the agent and dose (e.g., more than 9 g cyclophosphamide produces azoospermia) (Fairley, Barrie, & Johnson, 1972).

(1) In females

(a) The closer a woman is to being age 40 or older, the greater the likelihood that she will experience permanent cessation of menses after chemotherapy.

(b) Compared to women older than age 35, women younger than 35 can tolerate much higher doses of chemotherapy without becoming infertile (McInnes & Schilsky, 1996).

(c) Eighty percent of women younger than age 25 experience normal menses after chemotherapy.

(d) The majority of long-term female survivors of childhood ALL reach menarche at the expected time (normal timeframe for menarche is 10.5–15 years). Women were found to have normal levels of gonadal steroids and gonadotropins as well as an adequate increase in basal body temperature after intensified treatment for ALL, indicating intact follicle function and ovulation (Larsen, Muller, Schmiegelow, Rechnitzer, & Andersen, 2003).

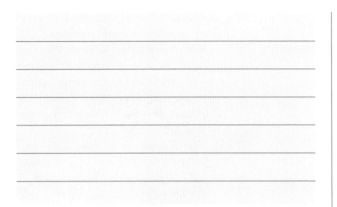

(e) The majority of women treated for Hodgkin disease with combination chemotherapy (including alkylating agents) prepuberty or at puberty have intact ovarian function (Hudson & Donaldson, 1997; McInnes & Schilsky, 1996).
(f) Young women treated with alkylating agents alone demonstrate normalization of follicle-stimulating hormone (FSH) levels over time, but a minority experience irreversible ovarian failure that requires treatment with HRT. A few of these women are at risk for premature menopause (Chiarelli, Marrett, & Darlington, 1999; Sklar, 1999).
(g) Early menopause can be anticipated when primary and secondary amenorrhea result immediately after therapy, especially if treatment involved alkylating agents and/or direct radiation of the ovaries (Byrne, 1999).
(h) Women who receive high-dose myeloablative therapy with alkylating agents prior to BMT are at high risk for irreversible ovarian failure (Sklar, 1999).

(2) In males
(a) Azoospermia or oligospermia commonly is present at the time of diagnosis in men with testicular cancer or Hodgkin disease, whereas men with non-Hodgkin lymphoma commonly have normal pretreatment sperm counts and motility (McInnes & Schilsky, 1996). Awareness of pretreatment abnormalities is important in order to differentiate disease-related sexual problems from treatment-related problems.
(b) Testicular damage is primarily dependent upon the total dose of drug administered, whereas the specific drug and the age of the patient are less important. The primary damage to testicular function appears to be depletion of the germinal epithelium lining the seminiferous tubules. This damage leads to testicular atrophy with subsequent impaired spermatogenesis.
(c) Alkylating agents are the drugs that cause the greatest alteration in male sexuality and fertility. Cumulative doses of greater than 400 mg/m^2 of cisplatin are associated with permanent azoospermia.
(d) Recovery of spermatogenesis appears to be related to the patient's age, the total dose received, the type of drug, and the time since therapy. A general guideline is that if fertility is to be recovered, sperm counts should return to normal within three years after completing therapy (McInnes & Schilsky, 1996).

(3) In children
(a) The age of the child at the time of chemotherapy affects the incidence of dysfunction. Younger children may be at less risk of infertility than are older children; however, children treated with cranial radiation therapy before age six (whether for brain tumors or childhood leukemia) may have a higher risk for infertility than those older than age six (Byrne, 1999). Age at treatment does not seem to be a factor in determining the reproductive effect of alkylating agents (Sklar, 1999). Pubertal males are at highest risk of toxicity because of the high rate of activity in developing gonads (in general, the more metabolically active the cell line, the greater the effect chemotherapeutic agents have on the line). Prepubertal males, in whom gametogenesis is not fully active, are not as resistant to the side effects of chemotherapy as was once believed (Heikens, Behrendt, Adriaanse, & Berghout, 1996; Hieb, Ogle, & Hobbie, 2004).

(b) Delayed puberty and primary amenorrhea are observed with ovarian failure that occurs prior to the onset of puberty. Arrested puberty, secondary amenorrhea, and menopausal symptoms generally are observed if ovarian failure resolves during or after pubertal maturation (Sklar, 1999).

(c) Germ-cell damage and infertility following treatment for childhood Hodgkin disease is generally longstanding and probably permanent in the majority of cases (Heikens et al., 1996; Papadakis et al., 1999).

(4) In connection with specific agents

(a) Mechlorethamine (nitrogen mustard), procarbazine, and cyclophosphamide are the most common agents implicated in gonadal dysfunction. The incidence is as high as 80%–90%, with minimal prospect for recovery (Heikens et al., 1996; Kulkarni et al., 1997).

(b) The combination of doxorubicin, bleomycin, vinblastine, and dacarbazine (the ABVD chemotherapy regimen)—when used without an alkylating agent—is associated with a 30%–55% incidence of gonadal dysfunction. The resulting azoospermia often is temporary and reversible (Kulkarni et al., 1997).

(c) Combination therapies that include etoposide and alkylating agents (e.g., procarbazine, mechlorethamine, cyclophosphamide) cause elevated FSH levels and/or azoospermia or oligospermia in 30%–40% of pubertal and postpubertal males with stage I to stage IIa Hodgkin disease. Testicular function may be normal if the same patients are treated with etoposide and nonalkylating agents (e.g., vincristine, prednisone, doxorubicin) (Gerres, Bramswig, Schlegel, Jurgens, & Schellong, 1998).

3. Risk factors (Krebs, 2000)

a) Type of malignancy and its effect on the reproductive organs and other body systems (e.g., endocrine system irregularities of the hypothalamic-pituitary axis)

b) Treatment with specific chemotherapy agents (see Table 30)

c) Concurrent medication with sedatives, antihypertensives, antidepressants, and opioids

d) Other treatment modalities (e.g., surgery or radiation to the testes or cranium)

e) Age: See Incidence.

f) Developmental stage: See Incidence.

g) Prior surgical procedures

h) History of radiation therapy to the pelvis

i) Hormonal therapy

j) Fatigue

k) Depression and/or psychosocial stressors

l) Chronic diseases (e.g., diabetes)

m) Pain

4. Manifestations

a) Sexual dysfunction (Gossfield & Cullen, 1997; Krebs, 2000)

(1) In females

(a) Decreased libido

(b) Sleep disturbances

(c) Hot flashes

(d) Irritability

(e) Poor or distorted self-image (McInnes & Schilsky, 1996), concerns about attractiveness to partner, difficulties with relationships, concerns about reproductive capability, social isolation, and/or anxiety

(f) Changes in body and/or appearance

(g) Dyspareunia

(h) Difficulty reaching orgasm

(i) Changes in cognitive function

(2) In males (McInnes & Schilsky, 1996)

(a) Decreased libido

(b) Poor or distorted self-image related to changes in body and/or appearance; concerns about attractiveness to partner, difficulties with relationships, concerns about reproductive capacity, social isolation, and/or anxiety

(c) Mild, intermediate, or severe erectile dysfunction
(d) Difficulty maintaining an erection
(e) Premature ejaculation
(f) Difficulty reaching orgasm

b) Reproductive dysfunction
(1) In females (Byrne, 1999; Gossfield & Cullen, 1997)
(a) Delayed or arrested pubertal development and menarche (Use the Tanner staging of breast and genital development, regularity of menses, and endocrine variables to assess development.)
(b) Temporary or permanent amenorrhea, other menstrual irregularities, difficulty becoming pregnant
(c) Early menopause and accompanying symptoms
(d) Ovarian fibrosis and sterility
(e) Abnormal levels of luteinizing hormone (LH), FSH, and estradiol
(2) In males (Heikens et al., 1996; Hieb et al., 2004)
(a) Delayed or arrested pubertal development (Use the Tanner staging of body hair, endocrine variables, and, if appropriate, penis and testicle size, testicular volume, and semen analysis to assess development.)
(b) Azoospermia
(c) Oligospermia (may last up to three years or never return to pretreatment levels)
(d) Abnormal hormone levels
i) Leydig-cell dysfunction is indicated by decreased production of testosterone and an increase in FSH and LH (Hieb et al., 2004).
ii) Germ-cell dysfunction is associated with increased FSH and normal LH and testosterone levels (Hieb et al., 2004).

5. Management of chemotherapy-induced menopause: Swan (1998) reported that whether menopause was chemotherapy-induced or natural, subjects demonstrated reduced quality of life if menopausal. Carpenter, Johnson, Wagner, and Andrykowski (2002) reported that the hot flashes experienced by breast cancer survivors were significantly more frequent, more severe, more distressing, and of greater duration than those experienced by healthy women. The breast cancer survivors with severe hot flashes reported significantly greater mood disturbance; higher negative affect; more interference with daily activities, including sleep, concentration, and sexuality; and poorer overall quality of life in comparison to the healthy controls (Carpenter et al.). Poniatowski and Grimm (2003) reported that women experiencing menopause most commonly had hot flashes, fatigue and tiredness, anxiety/nervousness, and sleep disturbances. The most severe symptoms were sleep disturbances and anxiety/nervousness.

a) Hormonal agents: HRT, which refers to noncontraceptive hormone treatment with estrogen or estrogen in combination with progestins, currently is the most prevalent and effective intervention for managing symptoms associated with estrogen deficiency (Pritchard, 2001). However, for women who have had breast or endometrial cancers, HRT typically is not recommended because of controversial evidence about the relationship between estrogen and/or progesterone and breast cancer recurrence and mortality (Collaborative Group on Hormonal Factors in Breast Cancer, 1997; O'Meara et al., 2001; Ursin et al., 2002; Vikas & Sood, 2001). Furthermore, recent findings have contraindicated the longstanding belief that HRT prevents cardiovascular disease (Writing Group for the Women's Health Initiative Investigators, 2002). Controversial and inconclusive findings about the risks and benefits of HRT continue to complicate a woman's decision to accept this type of therapy. Graf and Geller (2003) provided a recent review of alternative treatments to HRT.
(1) Estrogen vaginal cream is effective for vaginal dryness and may eliminate dyspareunia. Some systemic absorption may result (it is estimated to be approximately 25% that of a comparable oral dose).

(2) Medroxyprogesterone and low-dose (20 mg) megestrol acetate have been successful in relieving hot flashes (Loprinzi et al., 1994). Side effects may affect acceptability and compliance. Breast cancer survivors should be cautious because of the potential risks associated with low doses of a progesterone-like substance (Pritchard, 2001). Whether megestrol acetate has a negative, positive, or neutral effect on breast cancer cell growth or recurrence currently is unknown (Quella et al., 2000).

b) Nonhormonal agents: The agents that follow may relieve menopausal symptoms in some patients.

(1) Topical agents: Water-soluble topical agents are available to improve vaginal lubrication. Patients report that newer topical agents, such as Replens® and Astroglide® lubricants, are superior to K-Y® Jelly. Replens appears to increase vaginal moisture and elasticity and returns vaginal pH to the premenopausal state (Nachtigall, 1994).

(2) Antihypertensives: Low-dose clonidine (0.1 mg/day), administered either orally or by transdermal patch, reduces the frequency and severity of vasomotor symptoms (Goldberg et al., 1992). Dose escalation may improve symptom control but may result in dizziness, nausea, dry mouth, and headache.

(3) Vitamins

(a) Vitamin E sometimes is used by women for the treatment of menopausal symptoms, although studies have shown, at best, a marginal clinical benefit (Sloan et al., 2001). Recommended dose is 200–800 mg/day.

(b) Vitamin B_6 at 200–250 mg daily has been anecdotally reported to have some clinical benefit in the treatment of menopausal symptoms, although no research is available to support its use at this time.

(4) Antidepressants: Loprinzi et al. (2000) were the first to study the use of venlafaxine to reduce hot flashes and found that at 75 mg daily, it reduced hot flashes by 61% as compared to a 27% reduction with placebo. More recent studies of the selective serotonin reuptake inhibitors (SSRIs) paroxetine and fluoxetine have shown them to be more effective than placebo in reducing hot flash frequency and severity (Loprinzi et al., 2002; Sloan et al., 2001; Stearns et al., 2000). Although the antidepressants produced side effects (e.g., dry mouth, nausea, constipation, fatigue), the majority of the patients enrolled in these studies elected to continue on the antidepressants, indicating that the benefits of hot flash reduction outweighed the side-effect profile (Loprinzi et al, 1998).

(5) Herbal therapies commonly are used by women to reduce menopausal symptoms. Some popular remedies include soy, evening primrose, black cohosh, angelica (dong quai), ginseng, and licorice root. Currently, no research evidence exists to suggest that these herbal therapies reduce menopausal symptoms in women.

(6) Diet modifications, including increased soy and flax intake, may ameliorate menopausal symptoms. These foods contain phytoestrogens that affect estrogen levels. The impact of soy and flax on women with breast and endometrial cancer is unknown.

(7) Relaxation techniques; exercise; cold compresses to the neck; layering of clothing; avoiding alcohol, caffeine, and spicy foods; and reducing intake of refined sugar may improve symptomatic control of hot flashes.

6. Interventions for adult and older pediatric males

a) Monitor serum FSH and testosterone levels. This is especially important for men who were treated for Hodgkin disease in childhood or early adolescence. Reports indicate that the testosterone levels and bone mineral density of these men decreases over time. Therefore, ongoing evaluation of Leydig-cell function is necessary in this population.

b) Obtain semen analysis to evaluate fertility.

c) Use testosterone replacement if indicated. Kaempher, Wiley, Hoffman, and Rhodes (1985) and Schilsky and Erlichman (1982) reported on the success of testosterone replacement. Positive effects include maintenance of bone and muscle mass in older patients (Kaiser, 1992). Testosterone treatment may be used to prompt secondary sex characteristics, promote growth and normal body composition and bone density, and enhance the well-being of pubertal patients (Hieb et al., 2004; Mulder, 1999).

d) Refer patients to an endocrinologist if necessary. Thyroid dysfunction and chronic illness can affect reproductive function.

e) Assess medication history. Many medications may interfere with sexual functioning in men.

f) Consider making a referral to a urologist. Medications and devices are available to treat erectile dysfunction.

7. Nursing management of sexual alterations: The PLISSIT Model (Annon, 1976) consists of four stages of intervention and is frequently used for sexual counseling. Schwartz and Plawecki (2002) used this model in a recent review of the consequences of chemotherapy on the sexuality of patients with lung cancer. The four stages are as follows.

a) Permission (P): Ask patients about their sexual or reproductive concerns. This "normalizes" patients' concerns and opens the door for further dialogue.

b) Limited information (LI): Provide specific factual information to clarify concerns and misconceptions and dispel myths.

c) Specific suggestions (SS): Provide specific suggestions based on the patients' concerns. These may include strategies for improving symptom control and enhancing sexual expression.

d) Intensive therapy (IT): If the three earlier steps are insufficient to manage the patients' concerns, consider referral to a qualified sex therapist.

8. Patient and family education

a) Provide patients with information regarding contraception to prevent pregnancy during chemotherapy treatment. Oral contraceptives used by an older girl or female adolescent will suppress ovarian function, making the ovaries more resistant to the effects of chemotherapeutic agents and conserving oocytes (Hieb et al., 2004; McInnes & Schilsky, 1996). Discuss at what time after treatment pregnancy might be appropriate (Hieb et al.).

b) Explore fertility options prior to initiation of cancer treatment. Nurses have a role as listeners, advocates, educators, and providers of support as patients consider their options.

(1) Options for female patients: Female patients should be referred to a reproductive gynecologist to explore potential options, but the potential delay in initiating treatment may make this unfeasible. Options include in vitro fertilization; gamete intrafallopian transfer; use of donor oocytes, a surrogate gestational carrier, or a surrogate mother; cryopreservation and embryo donation; embryo banking; adoption; and child-free living (Gossfield & Cullen, 1997; Krebs, 2000).

(2) Options for male patients: Semen cryopreservation provides men an opportunity to father a child even when their sperm count is less than adequate. Even adolescent males who have just achieved puberty may produce sperm that can be cryopreserved for the purpose of reproduction. When appropriate, discuss sperm banking with adolescent males and their parents (Muller et al., 2000). Patient and family education should include information about cryopreservation. The desire to collect sperm for cryopreservation should not significantly delay treatment.

c) Provide patients with information about peer support groups that may be helpful in dealing with issues of sexuality and body image.

d) Reinforce the importance of having an annual follow-up examination conducted by a healthcare provider familiar with the patient's cancer history, treatment, and risk of developing late effects.

References

Annon, J. (1976). The PLISSIT model: A proposed conceptual scheme for behavioral treatment of sexual problems. *Journal of Sex Education Therapy, 2,* 1–15.

Byrne, J. (1999). Infertility and premature menopause in childhood cancer survivors. *Medical and Pediatric Oncology, 33,* 24–28.

Carpenter, J.S., Johnson, D.H., Wagner, L.J., & Andrykowski, M.A. (2002). Hot flashes and related outcomes in breast cancer survivors and matched comparison women [Online exclusive]. *Oncology Nursing Forum, 29*(3), E16–E25.

Chiarelli, A.M., Marrett, L.D., & Darlington, G. (1999). Early menopause and infertility in females after treatment for childhood cancer diagnosed in 1964–1988 in Ontario, Canada. *American Journal of Epidemiology, 150,* 245–253.

Collaborative Group on Hormonal Factors in Breast Cancer. (1997). Breast cancer and hormone replacement therapy: Collaborative reanalysis of data from 51 epidemiological studies of 52,705 women with breast cancer and 108,411 women without breast cancer. *Lancet, 350,* 1047–1059.

Dragonc, M.A. (1996). Cancer. In P.L. Jackson & J.A. Vessey (Eds.), *Primary care of the child with a chronic condition* (pp. 193–227). St. Louis, MO: Mosby.

Fairley, K.F., Barrie, J.U., & Johnson, W. (1972). Sterility and testicular atrophy related to chemotherapy. *Lancet, 1,* 568–569.

Ganz, P.A., Litwin, M.S., & Meyerowitz, B.E. (2001). Sexual problems. In V.T. DeVita, S. Hellman, & S.A. Rosenberg (Eds.), *Cancer: Principles and practice of oncology* (6th ed., pp. 3032–3049). Philadelphia: Lippincott Williams & Wilkins.

Gerres, L., Bramswig, J.H., Schlegel, W., Jurgens, H., & Schellong, G. (1998). The effects of etoposide on testicular function in boys treated for Hodgkin's disease. *Cancer, 83,* 2217–2222.

Goldberg, R.M., Loprinzi, C.L., Gerstner, J., Miser, A., O'Fallon, J., Mailliard, J., et al. (1992). Prospective trial of transdermal clonidine in breast cancer patients suffering from tamoxifen-induced hot flashes: A Mayo Clinic and North Central Cancer Center Treatment Group trial [Abstract]. *Proceedings of the American Society of Clinical Oncology, 11,* 378.

Gossfield, L.M., & Cullen, M.L. (1997). Sexuality and fertility issues. In G.J. Moore (Ed.), *Women and cancer: A gynecologic oncology nursing perspective* (pp. 540–578). Sudbury, MA: Jones and Bartlett.

Graf, M.C., & Geller, P.A. (2003). Treating hot flashes in breast cancer survivors: A review of alternative treatments to hormone replacement therapy. *Clinical Journal of Oncology Nursing, 7,* 637–640.

Heikens, J., Behrendt, H., Adriaanse, R., & Berghout, A. (1996). Irreversible gonadal damage in male survivors of pediatric Hodgkin's disease. *Cancer, 78,* 2020–2024.

Hieb, B.A., Ogle, S.K., & Hobbie, W. (2004). Reproductive system: Testes. In N.E. Kline (Ed.), *Essential of pediatric oncology nursing: A core curriculum* (2nd ed., pp. 278–279). Glenview, IL: Association of Pediatric Oncology Nurses.

Hudson, M.M., & Donaldson, S.S. (1997). Hodgkin's disease. *Pediatric Clinics of North America, 44,* 891–906.

Kaempfer, S.H., Wiley, F.M., Hoffman, D.J., & Rhodes, E. (1985). Fertility considerations and procreative alternatives in cancer care. *Seminars in Oncology Nursing, 1,* 25–34.

Kaiser, F.E. (1992). Sexual function and the older patient. *Oncology, 6*(Suppl. 2), 112–118.

Krebs, L.U. (2000). Sexual and reproductive dysfunction. In C.H. Yarbro, M.H. Frogge, M. Goodman, & S.L. Groenwald (Eds.), *Cancer nursing: Principles and practice* (5th ed., pp. 831–854). Sudbury, MA: Jones and Bartlett.

Kulkarni, S.S., Sastry, P.S.R.K., Saikia, T.K., Parikh, P.M., Gogal, R., & Advani, S.H. (1997). Gonadal function following ABVD therapy for Hodgkin's disease. *American Journal of Clinical Oncology, 20,* 354–357.

Larsen, E.C., Muller, J., Schmiegelow, K., Rechnitzer, C., & Andersen, A.N. (2003). Reduced ovarian function in long-term survivors of radiation and chemotherapy-treated. *Journal of Clinical Endocrinology and Metabolism, 88,* 5307–5314.

Loprinzi, C.L., Kugler, J.W., Sloan, J.A., Mailliard, J.A., LaVasseur, B.I., Barton, D.L., et al. (2000). Venlafaxine in management of hot flashes in survivors of breast cancer: A randomized controlled trial. *Lancet, 356,* 2059–2063.

Loprinzi, C.L., Michalak, J.C., Quella, S.K., O'Fallon, J.R., Hatfield, A.K., Nelimark, R.A., et al. (1994). Megestrol acetate for the prevention of hot flashes. *New England Journal of Medicine, 331,* 347–352.

Loprinzi, C.L., Pisansky, T.M., Fonseca, R., Sloan, J.A., Zahansky, K.M., Quella, S.K., et al. (1998). Pilot evaluation of venlafaxine hydrochloride for the therapy of hot flashes in cancer survivors. *Journal of Clinical Oncology, 16,* 2377–2381.

Loprinzi, C.L., Sloan, J.A., Perez, E.A., Quella, S.K., Stella, P.J., Mailliard, J.A., et al. (2002). Phase III evaluation of fluoxetine for treatment of hot flashes. *Journal of Clinical Oncology, 20,* 1578–1583.

McInnes, S., & Schilsky, R.L. (1996). Infertility following cancer chemotherapy. In B.A. Chabner & D.L. Longo (Eds.), *Cancer chemotherapy and biotherapy* (pp. 31–44). Philadelphia: Lippincott-Raven.

Mulder, J.E. (1999). Benefits and risks of hormone replacement therapy in young adult cancer survivors with gonadal failure. *Medical and Pediatric Oncology, 33,* 46–52.

Muller, J., Sonksen, J., Sommer, P., Schmiegelow, M., Petersen, P.M., Heilman, C., et al. (2000). Cryopreservation of semen from pubertal boys with cancer. *Medical and Pediatric Oncology, 34,* 191–194.

Nachtigall, L.E. (1994). Comparative study: Replens versus local estrogen in menopausal women. *Fertility Sterility, 61,* 178–180.

O'Meara, E.S., Rossing, M.A., Daling, J.R., Elmore, J.G., Barlow, W.E., & Weiss, N.S. (2001). Hormone replacement therapy after a diagnosis of breast cancer in relation to recurrence and mortality. *Journal of the National Cancer Institute, 93,* 754–761.

Papadakis, V., Vlachopapadopoulou, E., Van Syckle, K., Ganshaw, L., Kalmanti, M., Tan, C., et al. (1999). Gonadal function in your patients successfully treated for Hodgkin's disease. *Medical and Pediatric Oncology, 32,* 366–372.

Poniatowski, B., & Grimm, P. (2003, May). *Chemotherapy-induced menopausal symptoms in women aged 21–45 years of age.* Poster presented at the Oncology Nursing Society 28th Annual Congress, Denver, CO.

Pritchard, K.I. (2001). The role of hormone replacement therapy in women with a previous diagnosis of breast cancer and a review of possible alternatives. *Oncologist, 6,* 353–362.

Quella, S.K., Loprinzi, C.L., Sloan, J.A., Vaught, N.L., DeKrey, W.L., Fischer, T., et al. (2000). Long-term use of megestrol acetate by cancer survivors for the treatment of hot flashes. *Cancer, 82,* 1784–1788.

Schilsky, R.L., & Erlichman, C. (1982). Late complications of chemotherapy: Infertility and carcinogenesis. In B. Chabner (Ed.), *Pharmacologic principles of cancer treatment* (pp. 109–128). Philadelphia: Saunders.

Schover, L.R. (1997). *Sexuality and fertility after cancer.* New York: Wiley.

Schwartz, S., & Plawecki, H.M. (2002). Consequences of chemotherapy on the sexuality of patients with lung cancer. *Clinical Journal of Oncology Nursing, 6,* 212–216.

Sklar, C. (1999). Reproductive physiology and treatment-related loss of sex hormone production. *Medical and Pediatric Oncology, 33,* 2–8.

Sloan, J.A., Loprinzi, C.L., Novotny, P.J., Barton, D.L., LaVasseur, B.I., & Windschitl, H. (2001). Methodological lessons learned from hot flash studies. *Journal of Clinical Oncology, 19,* 4280–4290.

Stearns, V., Isaacs, C., Rowland, J., Crawford, J., Ellis, M.J., Kramer, R., et al. (2000). A pilot trial assessing the efficacy of paroxetine hydrochloride (Paxil) in controlling hot flashes in breast cancer survivors. *Annals of Oncology, 11,* 11–22.

Swan, D.K. (1998, May). *The effects of chemotherapy induced menopause versus natural menopause and age on breast cancer survivors' quality of life.* Paper presented at the Oncology Nursing Society 23rd Annual Congress, San Francisco, CA.

Ursin, G., Tseng, C.C., Paganini-Hill, A., Enger, S., Wan, P.C., Formenti, S., et al. (2002). Does menopausal hormone replacement therapy interact with known factors to increase risk of breast cancer? *Journal of Clinical Oncology, 20,* 699–706.

Vikas, M., & Sood, A.K. (2001). Hormone replacement therapy and cancer risk. *Current Opinions in Oncology, 13,* 384–389.

Wilmoth, M.C. (1998). Sexuality. In C. Burke (Ed.), *Psychosocial dimensions of oncology nursing care* (pp. 103–125). Pittsburgh, PA: Oncology Nursing Society.

Writing Group for the Women's Health Initiative Investigators. (2002). Risks and benefits of estrogen plus progestin in healthy postmenopausal women. *JAMA, 288,* 321–333.

M. Cutaneous toxicity: Patients receiving chemotherapy may experience a variety of cutaneous complications (Goodman, 2004). Table 31 details the most common cutaneous complications following chemotherapy administration.
   1. Pathophysiology: Exact mechanism is unknown.
   2. Incidence: Frequency varies according to reaction.
   3. Assessment: See Table 31 for a description of complications and comments regarding the care of these patients.

Reference

Goodman, M. (2004). Skin and nail bed changes. In C.H. Yarbro, M.H. Frogge, & M. Goodman (Eds.), *Cancer symptom management* (3rd ed., pp. 319–330). Sudbury, MA: Jones and Bartlett.

N. Ocular toxicity
   1. Pathophysiology
      a) The causes of ocular toxicity are varied and not fully understood. They may include the following.
         (1) Damage to the eye or eye structures related directly to treatment (e.g., distribution of cytotoxic drugs in tears, direct vascular injury during intracarotid administration) (Fraunfelder & Fraunfelder, 2001)
         (2) Secondary to the treatment process (e.g., eye irritation caused by loss of eyelashes in the presence of neutropenia)
         (3) Secondary to the concurrent disease process
         (4) Metastases to the eyes or CNS
         (5) Caused by factors unrelated to cytotoxic therapy
      b) A broad spectrum of disorders has been documented, including inflammatory conditions (e.g., uveitis, conjunctivitis, keratitis, blepharitis, iritis), development of retinal opacities, cataract formation, lid and lacrimation disorders, optic neuritis, and other neurologic injuries (Fraunfelder & Fraunfelder, 2001).
      c) Ocular effects are becoming more common because of the use of more aggressive regimens as well as new agents and new drug combinations (al-Tweigeri, Nabholtz, & Mackey, 1996).
      d) Because of the frequent use of combination therapy, determining which specific drug is causing complications may be difficult (Fraunfelder & Fraunfelder, 2001).
      e) Patients may experience toxicity-related visual impairment during chemotherapy and up to two weeks after chemotherapy (Kende, Sirkin, Thomas, & Freeman, 1979). Neurologic damage including effects to the eye have occurred up to 43 days following chemotherapy (Warrell & Berman, 1986).
      f) Ocular changes may go unnoticed until damage is irreversible.
      g) Ocular signs and symptoms may precede the development of peripheral neuropathies and thus may be an important marker of neurologic status (Burns, 2001).
      h) The presence of ocular signs or symptoms may predict development of GVHD in patients who have received allogeneic BMT (Kim et al., 2002).
      i) Ocular changes may be incorrectly attributed to the aging process.
   2. Incidence: Incidence varies according to drug classification, dose, and route of administration (see Table 32).
   3. Risk factors: Causal relationships between agents and ocular toxicities are difficult to establish. Risk factors are equally difficult to establish.
   4. Clinical manifestations: See Table 32.
   5. Assessment: Ask patients about any history of eye disturbance. In addition, assess the following (Bickley, 2003).
      a) Eyelid: Observe and palpate for signs of erythema and edema. Assess for signs of exudates, crusting, and presence of ptosis. Observe condition of lashes.
      b) Conjunctiva: Invert eyelids and observe for hyperemia (engorgement of tissue by blood caused by blockage), edema, and discharge.
      c) Cornea: Observe for smooth appearance and clarity. Test corneal reflex by gently touching a cotton swab to corneal surface.
      d) Iris and pupil: Observe iris and pupil. Margins should be clearly identified. Note pain and photophobia.

Table 31. Cutaneous Reactions to Chemotherapy and Biotherapy

Cutaneous Reaction	Description	Associated Chemotherapy	Comments
Transient erythema or urticaria	Usually occurs within hours of chemotherapy and disappears within a few hours. May be generalized or local at the site of chemotherapy or along the vein.	• Doxorubicin can cause an erythematous flare with pruritus at the IV site and along the vein. • Mechlorethamine can cause erythema and urticaria. • Cytarabine can cause transient erythema. • Bleomycin causes erythema over pressure points and hyperpigmentation. • Cyclophosphamide causes generalized urticaria. • Chlorambucil, methotrexate, melphalan, and thiotepa can cause urticaria and angioedema. • Asparaginase can cause urticaria, fever, chills, and hypotension (skin testing is advised). • Aldesleukin can cause a diffuse erythematous reaction that may progress into a pruritic papular rash. • Interferon alfa-2a and interferon alfa-2b can cause a dry, scaling skin or pruritic maculopapular reaction. • Filgrastim can cause transient erythematous eruptions and pruritus.	When combining chemotherapy and biologic response modifiers, it is important to note the occurrence of cutaneous reactions with each new agent to determine the offending agent. The drug may need to be discontinued if the reaction is severe or associated with systemic reactions such as a generalized rash.
Erythema multiforme	Generally presents as a macular papular erythematous lesion that may progress to vesicles. Can even progress to Stevens-Johnson syndrome and toxic epidermal necrolysis.	Occurs with high-dose therapy, including hydroxyurea, mechlorethamine, busulfan, etoposide, chlorambucil, procarbazine, bleomycin, methotrexate, cytarabine, and 5-FU. Symptoms also can occur with phenytoin sodium, carbamazepine, allopurinol, and various antibiotics.	Record description, presentation, and severity (consult a grading scale). Consult with physician regarding possible etiology. Consider discontinuing offending agent. Examine areas of tissue breakdown and attend to comfort measures with skin care and pain management strategies.
Acneform eruptions	Generally presents as a diffuse erythema over the face and body, progressing to follicular papules and pustules resembling acne.	Dactinomycin, high-dose methotrexate, and cyclosporine are generally the causative agents. Long-term steroids can also cause papules and pustules over shoulders, chest, back, and upper arms.	Causative agent should be discontinued. Area should be kept clean with a gentle soap to avoid infection. Area heals usually within five days. Macular hyperpigmentation may persist.
Pruritus or itching	May be localized or generalized.	Asparaginase, cisplatin, carboplatin, cytarabine, etoposide, teniposide, Interferon alfa-2a and interferon alfa-2b, doxorubicin, melphalan, and daunorubicin can all cause a rash. Gemcitabine has been associated with a perianal pruritus.	Symptoms may be worsened with dehydration. Patients should be encouraged to drink 8–10 glasses of fluid per day and minimize salt and alcohol intake. Skin care includes the use of mild soaps such as Aveeno® Oatmeal bath, Neutrogena®, Ivory®, and Basis® soaps. Apply moisturizing lotions such as Aquaphor®, Lubriderm®, Alpha-Keri®, or Nivea® following the bath.

(Continued on next page)

Table 31. Cutaneous Reactions to Chemotherapy and Biotherapy *(Continued)*

Cutaneous Reaction	Description	Associated Chemotherapy	Comments
Hyperpigmentation	Occurs most commonly in persons of Mediterranean descent. The drugs are thought to stimulate the melanocytes to produce more melanin. Darkening may occur within 2–3 weeks of chemotherapy and persist for months following the completion of therapy. Hyperpigmentation may involve the nail beds, oral mucosa, tongue, palms and soles, along veins, and may be generalized to involve the skin.	Occurs most commonly with doxorubicin, carmustine, busulfan, mechlorethamine, bleomycin, cyclophosphamide, 5-FU, hydroxyurea, melphalan, and etoposide.	Because this is not a serious consequence of chemotherapy, the drug treatment would not be interrupted. Flagellate streaks caused by nails scratching the skin have been reported with parenteral and intrapleural administration of bleomycin.
Acral erythema	Generally presents as dysesthesia with tingling in the hands and feet progressing to pain. After 4 or 5 days of intense edematous erythema and even fissures of the palms, soles, and digital joints, progressing to desquamation and reepithelialization occurs. Resolves 5–7 days after therapy is discontinued.	May be the presenting symptom of GVHD. Symptoms may be worsened by cyclosporine or trimethoprim-sulfamethoxazole. Symptoms are associated with high-dose cytarabine, cyclophosphamide, docetaxel, doxorubicin, liposomal doxorubicin, hydroxyurea, methotrexate, mercaptopurine, mitoxantrone, paclitaxel, and vinorelbine.	The etiology is not clear but may be related to concentration of the drug in the eccrine glands of the palms and soles. Applying cold compresses and elevating the hands and feet during drug administration may minimize incidence and degree of toxicity. Skin care and comfort measures are instituted as soon as symptoms are evident.
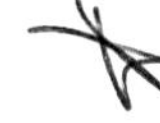 Hand-foot syndrome	First appears as mild redness on the palms and soles with tingling sensations in the hands, usually at the fingertips. Symptoms progress to a more intense burning pain and tenderness. Palms and soles appear edematous and patients may have difficulty walking or grasping objects. Ulceration may occur if therapy is not stopped.	Occurs most commonly with infusional therapy of 5-FU and/or doxorubicin. Capecitabine therapy is commonly associated with hand-foot syndrome because it is given orally and is a prodrug of 5-FU. Liposomal encapsulated doxorubicin (Doxil®) also is associated with hand-foot syndrome. Xeloda PO-	Incidence and severity of symptoms is related to protracted exposure of cells to the drug. Early recognition and cessation of drug administration is critical to symptom management.
Telangiectasis	Veins appear as eruptions under the skin.	Radiation may cause telangiectasis and is thought to be related to the destruction of the capillary bed. Topical carmustine and mechlorethamine cause vessel fragility and destruction.	Telangiectases are not harmful but can be disturbing for the patient depending on where they are located. Generally considered a permanent change in the vessel, but can fade over time.
Photosensitivity	Reaction appears as an erythematous response to ultraviolet radiation. Skin will appear red with erythema, edema, with or without vesicles.	Occurs most often with high-dose methotrexate following sun exposure. Other agents associated with photosensitivity include 5-FU, dactinomycin, doxorubicin, bleomycin, dacarbazine, hydroxyurea, and vinblastine.	Patients are instructed to wear a wide brim hat, cover their extremities while in the sun, and to avoid the direct rays of the sun between 10 am and 3 pm. They should wear a sunscreen with an SPF of at least 15.

Note. From "Skin and Nail Bed Changes" (pp. 320–321), by M. Goodman in C.H. Yarbro, M.H. Frogge, and M. Goodman (Eds.), *Cancer Symptom Management* (3rd ed.), 2004, Sudbury, MA: Jones and Bartlett. Copyright 2004 by Jones and Bartlett. Reprinted with permission.

Table 32. Ocular Toxicities Associated With Chemotherapy and Biotherapy

Classification	Agent	Ocular Toxicity	Comments
Alkylating agents	Busulfan	Longstanding reports of cataract formation (Burns, 2001); rare cases of keratoconjunctivitis sicca (Sidi et al., 1977)	Toxic effects are believed to act on proliferating lens epithelial cells (Burns, 2001).
	Carboplatin	*IV:* Rare cases of blurred vision, eye pain (al-Tweigeri et al., 1996); reports of maculopathy and optic neuropathy with transient cortical blindness when given to patients with renal dysfunction (O'Brien et al., 1992) *Intracarotid:* Reports of severe ocular and orbital toxicity in ipsilateral eye following intracarotid injection (Watanabe et al., 2002)	–
	Chlorambucil	Keratitis, diplopia, bilateral papilledema, retinal hemorrhages (al-Tweigeri et al., 1996; Burns, 2001)	Ocular toxicity is rare (Burns, 2001).
	Cisplatin	*IV:* Blurred vision, altered color perception, papilledema, decreased visual acuity, retrobulbar neuritis, transient cortical blindness (Becher et al., 1980) *Intracarotid:* Ipsilateral visual loss (15%–60%) from retinal and/or optic nerve ischemia; possibly prevented by infusion distal to ophthalmic artery (Burns et al., 1990)	–
	Cyclophosphamide	Blurred vision (reversible), keratoconjunctivitis sicca, pinpoint pupils (Jack & Hicks, 1981; Kende et al., 1979)	–
	Ifosfamide	Blurred vision (reversible), conjunctivitis (Choonara et al., 1987)	–
	Mechlorethamine	*Intracarotid:* Rare reports of ipsilateral necrotizing uveitis and necrotizing vasculitis of choroids (Burns, 2001)	No reports of ocular toxicity with IV administration (Burns, 2001)
	Nitrosoureas Carmustine Lomustine	*IV:* Rare reports of delayed blurred vision and loss of depth perception (Burns, 2001) *Intracarotid:* Severe, ipsilateral occurrences including arterial narrowing, disc edema, and intraretinal hemorrhages (Greenberg et al., 1984; Shingleton et al., 1982)	–
Antibiotics	Doxorubicin	Conjunctivitis, increased lacrimation (Curran & Luce, 1989); increased lacrimation occurs in up to 25% of patients receiving doxorubicin (Blum, 1975).	Serious ocular side effects are rare (Burns, 2001).
	Mitomycin-C	*IV:* Blurred vision (al-Tweigeri et al., 1996) *Topical:* Keratoconjunctivitis (Burns, 2001)	–
	Mitoxantrone	Conjunctivitis, discoloration of sclera (Fraunfelder & Fraunfelder, 2001)	Drug is secreted in tears (Fraunfelder & Fraunfelder, 2001).
Antimetabolites	Capecitabine	Ocular irritation, decreased vision, corneal deposits (Walkhom et al., 2000)	Ocular effects are seen in 10%–15% of patients (Fraunfelder & Fraunfelder, 2001).

(Continued on next page)

Table 32. Ocular Toxicities Associated With Chemotherapy and Biotherapy *(Continued)*

Classification	Agent	Ocular Toxicity	Comments
Antimetabolites *(cont.)*	Cytarabine	*IV:* Keratitis (40%–100%), blurred vision with evidence of bilateral conjunctival hyperemia, ocular pain, photophobia, and foreign body sensation at high doses (al-Tweigeri et al., 1996; Burns, 2001); case reports of corneal toxicity with low-dose of cytarabine (Lochhead et al., 2003) *Intrathecal:* Optic neuropathy leading to severe visual loss (may be potentiated by cranial radiation therapy) (Hopen et al., 1981; Margileth et al., 1977)	Starting glucocorticoid eye drops prior to cytarabine therapy minimizes risk (al-Tweigeri et al., 1996). The use of artificial tears rather than glucocorticoid eye drops may be equally effective because of dilution of intraocular drug concentrations (Higa et al., 1991).
	Pentostatin	Keratitis, conjunctivitis (Burns, 2001)	Mild to moderate, transient in nature (Burns, 2001)
	5-fluorouracil	25%–35% of patients have ocular side effects (Fraunfelder & Fraunfelder, 2001), including conjunctivitis (Christophidis et al., 1979); excessive lacrimation (Hamersley et al., 1973); tear duct fibrosis (Haidak et al., 1978); blepharitis (Fraunfelder & Fraunfelder, 2001).	Loprinzi et al. (1994) studied the use of ice packs to decrease ocular irritation.
	Fludarabine	Decreased visual acuity (most common presenting sign before development of progressive encephalopathy); rare cases of diplopia, photophobia, and optic neuritis (al-Tweigeri et al., 1996; Chun et al., 1986; Warrell & Berman, 1986)	Effects are dose-dependent (Burns, 2001).
	Methotrexate	*IV:* Blepharitis, conjunctival hyperemia, increased lacrimation, periorbital edema, photophobia *IT:* With concurrent radiation, case report of bilateral ophthalmoplegia with exotropia; optic nerve atrophy *Intraarterial:* Retinal changes in ipsilateral eye (Fraunfelder & Fraunfelder, 2001)	Up to 25% of patients may develop ocular toxicity (al-Tweigeri et al., 1996); toxicity is more common with higher doses (Burns, 2001). Drug is found in tears (Fraunfelder & Fraunfelder, 2001).
Biotherapy agents	Granulocyte–colony-stimulating factor (G-CSF) Granulocyte macrophage–colony-stimulating factor (GM-CSF)	Case report of acute iritis in healthy stem cell donor taking G-CSF (Parkkali et al., 1996); marginal keratitis and mild uveitis in healthy stem cell donor following both G-CSF and GM-CSF (Esmaeli et al., 2002).	–
	Interferon alpha Interferon beta Interferon gamma	Retinopathy, primarily retinal hemorrhages; cotton wool spots (Esmaeli, Koller, et al., 2001)	Incidence is 50% or higher (Kawano et al., 1996). Risk is increased in patients with hypertension or diabetes and those receiving higher doses (Fraunfelder & Fraunfelder, 2001).
	Interleukin-2	Neuro-ophthalmic effects including scotoma, diplopia, transient blindness, visual hallucinations (Fraunfelder & Fraunfelder, 2001)	–
	Retinoid	Blepharoconjunctivitis, corneal opacities, papilledema, pseudotumor cerebri, night blindness (al-Tweigeri et al., 1996)	Avoid concurrent use of tetracyclines and drugs causing intracranial hypertension (Fraunfelder & Fraunfelder, 2004).

(Continued on next page)

Table 32. Ocular Toxicities Associated With Chemotherapy and Biotherapy *(Continued)*

Classification	Agent	Ocular Toxicity	Comments
Miscellaneous agents	Bisphosphonates	Conjunctivitis, uveitis, scleritis (Fraunfelder & Fraunfelder, 2004)	Bisphosphonates must be discontinued for symptoms to resolve (Fraunfelder & Fraunfelder, 2004).
	Corticosteroids	Posterior subcapsular cataracts, glaucoma, retinal hemorrhage (Loredo et al., 1972), opportunistic eye infections	–
	Cyclosporine A	Optic neuropathy (Mejico et al., 2000), blurred vision, retinopathy, case reports of cortical blindness (Burns, 2001)	–
	Tacrolimus (FK506)	Optic neuropathy (Mejico et al., 2000); rare cortical blindness (Burns, 2001)	–
	Tamoxifen	Cataracts and decreased color vision; increased risk with doses greater than 20 mg/day (Fraunfelder & Fraunfelder, 2001; Gorin et al., 1998)	A baseline ophthalmic exam is recommended within the first year (Gorin et al., 1998).
Taxanes	Docetaxel	Epiphora, canalicular stenosis (Esmaeli, Valero, et al., 2001); successful treatment with bicanalicular silicone intubation (Ahmadi & Esmaeli, 2001)	Drug is secreted in tears (Esmaeli et al., 2002).
	Paclitaxel	Scintillating scotomas or "shooting lights" occur in 20% of cases; resolved spontaneously (Capri et al., 1994).	Scotomas usually occur toward the end of three-hour infusion (Fraunfelder & Fraunfelder, 2001).
Vinca alkaloids	Etoposide	*Intracarotid:* Optic neuritis, transient cortical blindness (Lauer et al., 1999)	Given in combination with carboplatin (Lauer et al., 1999)
	Vinblastine	Extraocular muscle palsies (Fraunfelder & Fraunfelder, 2001)	–
	Vincristine	Cranial nerve palsies, optic neuropathy, case reports of transient cortical blindness (Burns, 2001)	80% of toxicity is reversible (Fraunfelder & Fraunfelder, 2001).

e) Lacrimation: Note dryness, foreign-body sensation, and excessive tearing.

f) Visual disturbances: Assess acuity using near-vision card held at arm's length; patients who wear glasses or contact lenses should remove them. Note visual changes, unilateral or bilateral involvement, and precipitating and relieving factors.

g) Cranial nerves: Observe ocular alignment, light reflex, and extraocular muscles by having the patient follow finger movements in six planes.

6. Collaborative management

a) Refer to an ophthalmologist for further evaluation and treatment (Burns, 2001).

b) Instruct patient to use pharmacologic management as appropriate (e.g., antibiotics, steroids, artificial tears).

c) Prevent further damage: Discontinue causative agent, promote symptom management.

d) Surgical interventions may be necessary (e.g., cataract surgery, dilatation for punctual stenosis, enucleation).

7. Patient and family education

a) Teach patients self-examination techniques; emphasize the importance of close monitoring and prompt reporting of any structural changes in eyelids or eyelashes, as well as changes in vision.

b) Emphasize the importance of careful hygiene and handwashing techniques to minimize cross-contamination.

c) Demonstrate the proper use of eye drops and lubricants.

d) Encourage patients to schedule regular eye examinations.

References

Ahmadi, M.A., & Esmaeli, B. (2001). Surgical treatment of canalicular stenosis in patients receiving docetaxel weekly. *Archives of Ophthalmology, 119,* 1802–1804.

al-Tweigeri, T., Nabholtz, J., & Mackey, J.R. (1996). Ocular toxicity and cancer chemotherapy. *Cancer, 78,* 1359–1373.

Becher, R., Schütt, P., Osieka, R., & Schmidt, C.G. (1980). Peripheral neuropathy and ophthalmologic toxicity after treatment with cis-dichlorodiammineplatinum II. *Journal of Cancer Research and Clinical Oncology, 96,* 219–221.

Bickley, L.S. (2003). Techniques of examination. In L.S. Bickley & P.G. Szilagyi (Eds.), *Bates' guide to physical examination and history taking* (8th ed., pp. 115–208). Philadelphia: Lippincott Williams & Wilkins.

Blum, R. (1975). An overview of studies with Adriamycin in the United States. *Cancer Chemotherapy Reports, 6,* 247–251.

Burns, L.J. (2001). Ocular side effects of chemotherapy. In M.C. Perry (Ed.), *The chemotherapy source book* (3rd ed., pp. 452–458). Philadelphia: Lippincott Williams & Wilkins.

Capri, G., Munzone, E., Tarenzi, E., Fulfaro, F., Gianni, L., Caraceni, A., et al. (1994). Optic nerve disturbances: A new form of paclitaxel neurotoxicity. *Journal of the National Cancer Institute, 86,* 1099–1100.

Choonara, I.A., Overend, M., & Bailey, C.C. (1987). Blurring of vision due to ifosfamide. *Cancer Chemotherapy Pharmacology, 20,* 349.

Christophidis, N., Vajda, F.J.E., Lucas, I., & Louis, W.J. (1979). Ocular side effects with 5-fluorouracil. *Australian and New Zealand Journal of Medicine, 9,* 143–144.

Chun, H.G., Leyland-Jones, B.R., Caryk, S.M., & Hoth, D.F. (1986). Central nervous system toxicity of fludarabine phosphate. *Cancer Treatment Reports, 70,* 1225–1228.

Curran, C.F., & Luce, J.K. (1989). Ocular adverse reactions associated with Adriamycin. *American Journal of Ophthalmology, 108,* 709–711.

Esmaeli, B., Ahmadi, M.A., Kim, S., Onan, H., Korbling, M., & Anderlini, P. (2002). Marginal keratitis associated with administration of filgrastim and sargramostim in a healthy peripheral blood progenitor cell donor. *Cornea, 21,* 621–622.

Esmaeli, B., Koller, C., Papadopoulos, N., & Romaguera, J. (2001). Interferon-induced retinopathy in asymptomatic cancer patients. *Ophthalmology, 108,* 858–860.

Esmaeli, B., Valero, V., Ahmadi, M.A., & Booser, D. (2001). Canalicular stenosis secondary to docetaxel: A newly recognized side effect. *Ophthalmology, 108,* 994–995.

Fraunfelder, F.T., & Fraunfelder, F.W. (2001). Oncolytic agents. In F.T. Fraunfelder & F.W. Fraunfelder (Eds.), *Drug-induced ocular side effects* (5th ed., pp. 435–480). Boston: Butterworth-Heinemann.

Fraunfelder, F.W., & Fraunfelder, F.T. (2004). Adverse ocular drug reactions recently identified by the National Registry of Drug-Induced Ocular Side Effects. *Ophthalmology, 111,* 1275–1279.

Gorin, M.B., Day, R., Costantino, J.P., Fisher, B., Redmond, C.K., Wickerham, L., et al. (1998). Long-term tamoxifen citrate use and potential ocular toxicity. *American Journal of Ophthalmology, 125,* 493–501.

Greenberg, H.S., Ensiminger, W.D., Chandler, W.F., Layton, P.B., Junck, L., Knake, J., et al. (1984). Intra-arterial BCNU chemotherapy for treatment of malignant gliomas of the central nervous system. *Journal of Neurosurgery, 61,* 423–429.

Haidak, D.J., Hurwitz, B., & Yeung, K.Y. (1978). Tear-duct fibrosis (dacryostenosis) due to 5-fluorouracil. *Annals of Internal Medicine, 88,* 657.

Hamersley, J., Luce, J.K., Florentz, T.R., Burkholder, M.M., & Pepper, J.J. (1973). Excessive lacrimation from fluorouracil treatment. *JAMA, 225,* 747–748.

Higa, G.M., Gockerman, J.P., & Hunt, A.L. (1991). The use of prophylactic eye drops during high-dose cytosine arabinoside therapy. *Cancer, 68,* 1691–1693.

Hopen, G., Mondino, B.J., Johnson, B.L., & Chervenick, P.A. (1981). Corneal toxicity with systemic cytarabine. *American Journal of Ophthalmology, 91,* 500–504.

Jack, M.K., & Hicks, J.D. (1981). Ocular complications in high-dose chemoradiotherapy and marrow transplantation. *Annals of Ophthalmology, 13,* 709–711.

Kawano, T., Shigehira, M., Uto, H., Nakama, T., Kato, J., Hayashi, K., et al. (1996). Retinal complications during interferon therapy for chronic hepatitis C. *The American Journal of Gastroenterology, 91,* 309–313.

Kende, G., Sirkin, S.R., Thomas, P.R., & Freeman, A.I. (1979). Blurring of vision: A previously undescribed complication of cyclophosphamide therapy. *Cancer, 44,* 69–71.

Kim, R.Y., Anderlini, P., Naderi, A.A., Rivera, P., Ahmadi, M.A., & Esmaeli, B. (2002). Scleritis as the initial clinical manifestation of graft-versus-host disease after allogenic bone marrow transplantation, *American Journal of Ophthalmology, 133,* 843–845.

Lauer, A.K., Wobig, J.L., Shults, W.T., Neuwelt, E.A., & Wilson, M.W. (1999). Severe ocular and orbital toxicity after intracarotid etoposide phosphate and carboplatin therapy. *American Journal of Ophthalmology, 127,* 230–233.

Lochhead, J., Salmon, J.F., & Bron, A.J. (2003). Cytarabine-induced corneal toxicity. *Eye, 17,* 677–678.

Loprinzi, C.L., Wender, D.B., Veeder, M.H., O'Fallon, J.R., Vaught, N.L., Dose, A.M., et al. (1994). Inhibition of 5-fluorouracil-induced ocular irritation by ocular ice packs. *Cancer, 74,* 945–948.

Loredo, A., Rodriquez, R.S., & Murillo, L. (1972). Cataract after short-term corticosteroids treatment. *New England Journal of Medicine, 186,* 160.

Margileth, D.A., Poplack, D.G., Pizzo, P.A., & Levanthal, B.G. (1977). Blindness during remission in two patients with acute lymphoblastic leukemia: A possible complication of multimodality therapy. *Cancer, 39,* 58–61.

Mejico, L.J., Bergloeff, J., & Miller, N.R. (2000). New therapies with potential neuro-ophthalmologic toxicity. *Current Opinion in Ophthalmology, 11,* 389–394.

O'Brien, M.E., Tonge, K., Blake, P., Moskovic, E., & Wiltshaw, E. (1992). Blindness associated with high-dose carboplatin. *Lancet, 339,* 558.

Parkkali, T., Volin, L., Siren, M.K., & Ruutu, T. (1996). Acute iritis induced by granulocyte colony-stimulating factor used for mobilization in a volunteer unrelated peripheral blood progenitor cell donor. *Bone Marrow Transplantation, 17,* 433–434.

Shimamura, Y., Chikama, M., Tanimoto, T., Kawakami, Y., & Tsutsumi, A. (1990). Optic nerve degeneration caused by supraopthalmic carotid artery infusion with cisplatin and ACNU. *Journal of Neurosurgery, 72,* 285–288.

Shingleton, B.J., Bienfang, D.C., Albert, D.M., Ensminger, W.D., Chandler, W.F., & Greenberg, H.S. (1982). Ocular toxicity associated with high-dose carmustine. *Archives of Ophthalmology, 100,* 1766–1772.

Sidi, Y., Douer, D., & Pinkhas, J. (1977). Sicca syndrome in a patient with toxic reaction to busulfan. *JAMA, 238,* 1951.

Walkhom, B., Fraunfelder, F.T., & Henner, W.D. (2000). Severe ocular irritation and corneal deposits associated with capecitabine use. *New England Journal of Medicine, 343,* 740–741.

Warrell, R.P., & Berman, E. (1986). Phase I and II study of fludarabine phosphate in leukemia: Therapeutic efficacy with delayed central nervous system toxicity. *Journal of Clinical Oncology, 4,* 74–79.

Watanabe, W., Kuwabara, R., Nakahara, T., Hamasaki, O., Sakamoto, I., Okada, K., et al. (2002). Severe ocular and orbital toxicity after intracarotid injection of carboplatin for recurrent glioblastomas. *Archives of Clinical Experimental Ophthalmology, 240,* 1033–1035.

O. Secondary malignancies

1. Pathophysiology: See Table 33.

a) Chemotherapeutic agents used to treat malignancies induce secondary neoplasms and depend on the following.

(1) Primary diagnosis

(a) Ovarian cancer

(b) Pediatric cancers

(c) Hodgkin disease

(d) BMT recipients treated with both chemotherapy and TBI

(e) Lymphoma

(f) Testicular cancer

(g) Questions arise if the secondary cancer is related to the diagnosis, radiation therapy, or chemotherapy, especially with Hodgkin disease and testicular cancer (Children's Oncology Group [COG], 2004; Erlichman & Moore, 2001; Nelson, 2005).

(2) Dosage

(a) Duration of treatment

(b) Weak evidence exists, however, that combining modalities of chemotherapy and radiation increases the risk of secondary leukemia, but there is a clear connection with the development of solid tumors (Boice, 2001; Dreyer, Blatt, & Bleyer, 2002; Erlichman & Moore, 2001).

b) The cancer-producing capacity of chemotherapeutic agents varies (Boice, 2001; COG, 2004; Erlichman & Moore, 2001; Monteleone & Meadows, 2004; Nelson, 2005).

(1) The epipodophyllotoxins, anthracyclines, and alkylating agents are strongly tied to secondary leukemias.

(2) Antimetabolites and vinca alkaloids do not appear to be related to secondary malignancies.

(3) Several interrelated systems are involved in the development of secondary treatment-related cancers.

(a) DNA intercalation

(b) DNA alkylation

(c) DNA-topoisomerase II inhibition

(d) Mitotic inhibition

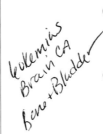

(e) Cellular metabolism interference (Boice, 2001)

c) Secondary malignancies occur months to years after treatment for primary cancer and may be associated with the following.

(1) Increased survival from improvements in therapy and long latency periods for human carcinogenic expression (Erlichman & Moore, 2001)

(2) Survivors of childhood cancer have a 10- to 20-fold risk of developing a secondary malignancy when compared to others in their age group (Dreyer et al., 2002).

(3) Recurrence of the primary tumor is the most prevalent cause of death, followed by death from a secondary malignancy (Boice, 2001; Dreyer et al., 2002; Erlichman & Moore, 2001).

(4) ALL is the most common malignancy of childhood and has a low occurrence of secondary cancers. Patients treated for T-cell ALL who received epipodophyllotoxins are an outlying high-risk group (Dreyer et al., 2002).

(5) Occurrence of secondary brain tumors in previously treated ALL patients is less than 2%, but it remains the largest category of secondary cancers in this group. Predisposing factors include 2,400 cGy cranial irradiation, TBI, treatment with 6-mercaptopurine, and age younger than five years when treated (Dreyer et al., 2002).

d) Acute nonlymphocytic leukemia is the most often noted secondary malignancy (Boice, 2001; Dreyer et al., 2002).

(1) Myelodysplastic syndromes also are seen.

(2) Alkylating agents are closely associated with the development of acute nonlymphocytic leukemia.

(3) Up to 20% of newly diagnosed leukemias may be a result of treatment for a prior malignancy.

Table 33. Secondary Malignancies Related to Chemotherapy

Secondary Malignancy	Primary Malignancy Factors	Occurrence	Risk Factors
Leukemia	Breast	At 10 years: 0.7%	Melphalan-based adjuvant therapy, high-dose cyclophosphamide (Boice, 2001)
	Gastrointestinal (colon, gastric, rectal)	Unknown	Mitoxantrone (Carli et al., 2000; Saso et al., 2000), lomustine (Boice et al., 1983)
	Hodgkin disease (stage not a factor)	Up to 10 years after treatment: 2%–10% occurrence	Mechlorethamine; vincristine; mechlorethamine, vincristine, procarbazine, prednisone (MOPP) combination (Boice, 2001; Boivin et al., 1995; Tucker et al., 1988)
	Small cell lung	Actuarial risk of 44 at 2.5 years	Nitrosoureas, procarbazine, and alkylating agents given over long duration (Boice, 2001)
	Non-small cell lung	No specific time to occurrence	Etoposide, busulfan, procarbazine, nitrosoureas (Boice, 2001; Chak et al., 1984; Stott et al., 1977)
	Multiple myeloma	17% at 50 months	Alkylating agents (Boice, 2001)
	Non-Hodgkin lymphoma	Cumulative risk at 15 years is 17% if combined with low-dose radiation.	Chlorambucil, mechlorethamine, cyclophosphamide, vincristine, prednimustine, combined chemotherapy and radiation therapy
	Ovarian	Five to six years after treatment ends	Alkylating agents, including cyclophosphamide, and melphalan (Greene et al., 1986)
	Polycythemia vera[a]	No specific time to occurrence	Chlorambucil
	Testicular	Five years: 0.6% actuarial risk	Etoposide > 2 g/m^2 weekly or twice weekly and in combination with cyclophosphamide and alkylating agents (Boice, 2001)
	Pediatric solid tumors	10–37 months after treatment ends	High-dose alkylating agents in combination with doxorubicin, etoposide, or epipodophyllotoxins (Boice, 2001)
Non-Hodgkin lymphoma	Hodgkin disease	No specific time to occurrence	Relationship is unclear (Boice, 2001).
Endometrial	Breast	Within eight years after starting treatment	Tamoxifen (Erlichman & Moore, 2001)
Bladder	Various cancers[b]	No specific time to occurrence	Cyclophosphamide (Travis et al., 1995; Wall & Clausen, 1975)
Brain	Acute lymphocytic leukemia	6–29 years after treatment ends	Cranial irradiation in combination with antimetabolites (Boyett et al., 1999)
Breast	Hodgkin disease	10–20 years after treatment, ends in females younger than age 30 treated with mantle-field irradiation; 14 times that of the general population	Mantle radiation therapy and chemotherapy (Dreyer et al., 2002)
Respiratory and intrathoracic (including lung)	Hodgkin disease	Five years; risk increases with time	Thoracic radiation therapy and chemotherapy (Boivin et al., 1995; Van Leeuwen et al., 1994)
Thyroid	Hodgkin disease	18 times that of the general population	Radiation (Dreyer et al., 2002)

(Continued on next page)

Table 33. Secondary Malignancies Related to Chemotherapy *(Continued)*

Secondary Malignancy	Primary Malignancy Factors	Occurrence	Risk Factors
Gastrointestinal	Testicular	Relative risk: 1.27–2.1	Radiation therapy within 10–20 years (Erlichman & Moore, 2001)
Osteosarcoma	Hereditary retinoblastoma	Up to 20 years after treatment	Alkylating agents with or without radiation (Boice, 2001)
	Soft-tissue tumors, neuroblastoma, Ewing's sarcoma	Mean latency more than 15 years	Radiation therapy (Dreyer et al., 2001)

[a] Has potential to transform to leukemia as disease-related phenomenon (Berk et al., 1981)
[b] Strong dose-response relationship reported

(4) Therapy-related acute nonlymphocytic leukemia and myelodysplastic syndromes often are fatal.

(5) Secondary leukemias may develop months after the cessation of treatment, and the risk for developing a secondary leukemia remains elevated for up to 10 years before decreasing.

(6) Abnormalities of chromosomes 5 and 7 may predict the evolution of acute nonlymphocytic leukemia.

(7) A short but concentrated treatment may be less likely to induce a secondary cancer than a protracted less-potent treatment regimen (Boice, 2001).

(8) Age and gender play a role in the development of secondary cancers.
   - *(a)* Females are at higher risk for the development of leukemia and secondary malignancies in general than are males (Beatty et al., 1995; Boice, 2001).
   - *(b)* Adolescents appear to be more susceptible than younger children, and adults beyond their fourth decade carry a substantially higher risk, four times or more that of younger adults (Boice, 2001).

(9) Secondary leukemia related to epipodophyllotoxin administered in combination with alkylating agents or cisplatin is associated with a short latency period and 11q23 and 21q22 abnormalities (Boice, 2001).

(10) Newer treatments not using nitrosoureas, procarbazine, and melphalan may be less prone to carcinogenesis.

(11) Bone and bladder cancer are the only solid tumors clearly associated with prior use of antineoplastic agents (Boice, 2001).

e) Causes

(1) Single-agent chemotherapy
   - *(a)* Alkylating agents (melphalan, cyclophosphamide)
   - *(b)* Epipodophyllotoxins (etoposide, teniposide)
   - *(c)* Mitoxantrone
   - *(d)* Anthracyclines (doxorubicin) (Dreyer et al., 2002; Neglia, Friedman, & Yasui, 2001).

(2) Combination chemotherapy
   - *(a)* MOPP (mechlorethamine, vincristine, procarbazine, prednisone)
   - *(b)* ABVD (doxorubicin, bleomycin, vinblastine, dacarbazine)
   - *(c)* MVPP (mechlorethamine, vinblastine, procarbazine, prednisone) (Boice, 2001)

(3) Combination chemotherapy and radiation therapy
   - *(a)* The most recent review of the literature ascertains that although large doses of radiation may induce leukemia, localized doses result in cellular death rather than transformation (Boice, 2001).
   - *(b)* Leukemia caused by radiation therapy is rare and has been associated with treatment for Hodgkin disease in a limited number of cases (Beatty et al., 1995; Boice, 2001; Dreyer et al., 2002).
   - *(c)* The synergistic effect of radiation on the cancer-producing effect of antineoplastic agents seems small. "The most recent evidence . . . indicates that extensive radiotherapy and chemotherapy are associated with a leukemia risk that is similar to that observed with chemotherapy alone" (Boice, 2001, p. 528).

(d) Solid tumors, unlike leukemia, are more often linked to radiation than chemotherapy (Boice, 2001; Dreyer et al., 2002; Neglia et al., 2001). Breast, bone, and soft tissue cancers are the most frequently occurring.

i) Patients younger than age 30 who received mantle radiation have an increased risk for breast cancer.

ii) The risk is significantly increased if the patient was 10–15 years of age when treated (Dreyer et al., 2002).

(4) Hormonal therapy: Tamoxifen is associated with the secondary development of endometrial cancer (Braithwaite et al., 2003; Senkus-Konefka, Konefka, & Jassem, 2004).

2. Incidence

a) The risk for secondary malignancy is frequently reported as absolute risk over the comparison population (e.g., 3 more cancers per 100 patients).

b) The risk for secondary leukemia in most cases is vertiginous for a decade following treatment before beginning to decline (Boice, 2001).

c) Few solid tumors other than bone and bladder have been credibly associated with chemotherapeutic agents (Boice, 2001).

d) The estimated cumulative risk of secondary malignancy among survivors of childhood malignancies, 20 years following primary treatment, varies between 3% and 10% and is 5 to 20 times greater than expected in the general population (National Cancer Policy Board, 2003).

e) Radiation therapy is associated with the development of thyroid cancer, melanoma and other skin cancers, brain tumors, and bone and soft tissue sarcomas. Increased incidence of thyroid cancer has been noted following radiotherapy for childhood malignancies (Inskip, 2001). Thyroid cancer in survivors of Hodgkin disease is 18 times that seen in normal populace, and a limited number of cases of thyroid cancer and adenomas have been associated with radiation to the cranium (Dreyer et al., 2002).

f) The vulnerability for the development of solid tumors may escalate with time, but it is believed to be a slow increase as has been shown with 20–30-year follow-up studies. The average time span for the development of a secondary cancer following radiation therapy is 15 years, but this may not be long enough for childhood survivors to develop adult cancers even when an escalated risk exists (Dreyer et al., 2002).

g) Breast cancer is the most frequently observed solid tumor in women who were treated for pediatric Hodgkin disease (Crom, Hudson, Hinds, Gattuso, & Tye, 2000). The Late Effects Study Group estimated a 15.4% increase in the occurrence of breast cancer in female survivors of childhood Hodgkin disease, which becomes 35% by the fourth decade (Erlichman & Moore, 2001). The age of the patient at the time of radiation exposure and the radiation dose influence the risk of breast cancer. Women treated during puberty and those who received doses exceeding 2,000 cGy appear to be at greatest risk (Crom et al.; Erlichman & Moore). Because of this increased risk, female survivors of pediatric Hodgkin disease should undergo regular breast screenings starting before age 40 (Crom et al.).

h) Long-term survivors of certain childhood cancers are at high risk for the development of secondary cancers if they were treated with now-obsolete high doses of radiation, epipodophyllotoxins, or alkylating agents. These cancers include Wilms' tumor (genetic type), retinoblastoma, and Hodgkin disease (Dreyer et al., 2001).

3. Risk factors

a) Genetic predisposition

(1) Patients with von Recklinghausen's neurofibromatosis or Li-Fraumeni family cancer syndrome, which contributed to the development of their original cancer, are at increased risk for a secondary cancer (Dreyer et al., 2002).

(2) Gender and age are possible mitigating factors in the development of secondary cancers (Boice, 2001).

b) Type of therapy
   (1) Proof is beginning to emerge that newer and briefer drug regimens depending less on melphalan, procarbazine, and nitrosoureas induce fewer instances of leukemia. On the other end of the spectrum are epipodophyllotoxins, which, when given with alkylating agents, induce early-occurring leukemias. Cisplatin alone or in combination with alkylating agents can induce leukemia (Boice, 2001).
   (2) Acute nonlymphocytic leukemia has been decisively associated with the alkylating agents cyclophosphamide and mechlorethamine, two alkylating agents commonly used in combination chemotherapy regimens. The multiple drug regimen ABVD has rarely been associated with secondary cases of acute nonlymphocytic leukemia (Dreyer et al., 2002).
   (3) Duration of therapy may play a role in the development of secondary cancers. It is believed that treatment plans of short term but high dose exposure are less carcinogenic than lengthy exposures of low-dose agents (Erlichman & Moore, 2001).
   (4) Radiation, in differentiation from chemotherapy, has been more closely associated as a causative factor in the development of solid tumors. Most of these tumors develop within radiation ports and are cancers of the breast, thyroid, and skin or sarcomas of the bone or soft tissues. The average latency period is approximately 10 to more than 16 years (Dreyer et al., 2002).

4. Collaborative management (Hudson, 2000; Monteleone & Meadows, 2004)
   a) Follow up with a primary care physician who is fully informed about the patient's history of cancer, his "baseline" physical examination, and the need for recommended cancer screenings
   b) Irradiated skin and soft tissues should be thoroughly evaluated and continually reassessed.
   c) Survivors should follow adult cancer screening recommendations.
      (1) This is especially important for childhood cancer survivors who have an additional risk for developing adult cancers prematurely.
      (2) Women who have been treated with mantle irradiation should begin breast self-examination on a monthly basis at the time of puberty, and a medical breast examination should be performed every six months for women between the ages of 20 and 40. At age 25, a baseline mammogram should be obtained and repeated every third year until the age of 40. Beginning at age 40, mammograms should be done annually (Hudson, 2000).

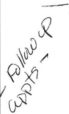

5. Patient and family education (Bottomley, 2004; Monteleone & Meadows, 2004; Nelson, 2005)
   a) Provide information about the treatment and potential late effects related to disease and treatment received.
   b) Explain the risks of secondary malignancy, the typical time to onset, signs and symptoms of secondary cancers, and the importance of follow-up visits.

6. Professional education
   a) Educate primary care professionals who may be working with these patients after they are no longer followed by an oncologist.
   b) Ensure that healthcare providers have the same information about secondary malignancies as the patients do and that they are aware of recommended follow-up.

References

Beatty, O., Hudson, M.M., Greenwald, C., Luo, X., Fang, L., Wilimas, J.A., et al. (1995). Subsequent malignancies in children and adolescents after treatment for Hodgkin's disease. *Journal of Clinical Oncology, 13,* 603–609.

Berk, P.D., Goldberg, J.D., Silverstein, M.N., Weinfeld, A., Donovan, P.B., Ellis, J.T., et al. (1981). Increased incidence of acute leukemia in polycythemia vera associated with chlorambucil therapy. *New England Journal of Medicine, 304,* 441–447.

Boice, J.A. (2001). Second malignancies after chemotherapy. In M.C. Perry (Ed.), *The chemotherapy source book* (pp. 526–536). Philadelphia: Lippincott Williams & Wilkins.

Boice, J.D., Jr., Greene, M.H., Killen, J.Y., Jr., Ellenberg, S.S., Keehn, R.J., McFadden, E., et al. (1983). Leukemia and preleukemia after adjuvant treatment of gastrointestinal cancer with semustine (methyl-CCNU). *New England Journal of Medicine, 309,* 1079–1084.

Boivin, J., Hutchinson, G.B., Zauber, A., Bernstein, L., Davis, F., Michel, R., et al. (1995). Incidence of second cancers in patients treated for Hodgkin's disease. *Journal of the National Cancer Institute, 87,* 732–741.

Bottomley, S.J. (2004). Promoting health after childhood cancer. In N.E. Kline (Ed.), *Essentials of pediatric oncology nursing: A core curriculum* (pp. 290–291). Glenview, IL: Association of Pediatric Oncology Nursing.

Boyett, J.M., Evans, W.E., Felix, C.A., Hancock, M.L., Kun, L.E., Pui, G.H., et al. (1999). High incidence of secondary brain tumours after radiotherapy and antimetabolites. *Lancet, 354,* 34–39.

Braithwaite, R.S., Chlebowski, R.T., Lau, J., George, S., Hess, R., & Col, N.F. (2003). Meta-analysis of vascular and neoplastic events associated with tamoxifen. *Journal of General Internal Medicine, 18,* 937–947.

Carli, P.M., Sgro, C., Parchin-Geneste, N., Isambert, N., Mugneret, F., Girodon, F., et al. (2000). Increase therapy-related leukemia secondary to breast cancer. *Leukemia, 14,* 1014–1017.

Chak, L.Y., Sikic, B.I., Tucker, M.A., Horns, R.C., Jr., & Cox, R.S. (1984). Increased incidence of acute nonlymphocytic leukemia following therapy in patients with small cell carcinoma of the lung. *Journal of Clinical Oncology, 2,* 385–390.

Children's Oncology Group. (2004). *Long-term follow-up guidelines for survivors of childhood, adolescent, and young adult cancers.* Retrieved March 24, 2005, from http://www.childrensoncologygroup.org

Crom, D., Hudson, M., Hinds, P., Gattuso, J., & Tyc, V. (2000). [Perceived vulnerability among survivors of Hodgkin's disease.] Unpublished data. Memphis, TN: St. Jude Children's Research Hospital.

Dreyer, Z.E., Blatt, J., & Bleyer, A. (2002). Late effects of childhood cancer and its treatment. In P.A. Pizzo & D.G. Poplack (Eds.), *Principles and practice of pediatric oncology* (4th ed., pp. 1431–1461). Philadelphia: Lippincott Williams & Wilkins.

Erlichman, C., & Moore, M. (2001). Carcinogenesis: A late complication of cancer chemotherapy. In B.A. Chabner & D.L. Longo (Eds.), *Cancer chemotherapy and biotherapy: Principles and practice* (pp. 67–84). Philadelphia: Lippincott Williams & Wilkins.

Greene, M.H., Harris, E.L., Gershenson, D.M., Malkasian, G.D., Jr., Melton, L.J., III, Dembo, A.J., et al. (1986). Melphalan may be a more potent leukemogen than cyclophosphamide. *Annals of Internal Medicine, 105,* 360–367.

Hudson, M.M. (2000). Long-term follow-up after childhood cancer. In G. Steen & A. Mirro (Eds.), *Childhood cancer: A handbook from St. Jude Children's Research Hospital* (pp. 513–515). Cambridge, MA: Perseus.

Inskip, P.D. (2001). Thyroid cancer after radiotherapy for childhood cancer. *Medical and Pediatric Oncology, 36,* 568–573.

Monteleone, P.M., & Meadows, A.T. (2004). *Late effects of childhood cancer and treatment.* Retrieved March 24, 2005, from http://www.emedicine.com/ped/topic2591.htm//section~second_malignancies

National Cancer Policy Board. (2003). *Childhood cancer survivorship: Improving care and quality of life.* Washington, DC: Author.

Neglia, J.P., Friedman, D.L., & Yasui, Y. (2001). Second malignant neoplasms in five-year survivors of childhood cancer: Childhood cancer survivor study. *Journal of the National Cancer Institute, 93,* 618–629.

Nelson, M.B. (2005). Late effects of chemotherapy. In N.E. Kline, D.E. Echtenkamp, R. Norville, & M. Silva (Eds.), *Pediatric chemotherapy and biotherapy curriculum* (pp. 143–150). Glenview, IL: Association of Pediatric Oncology Nurses.

Saso, R., Kulkarni, S., Mitchell, P., Treleaven, J., Swansbury, G.J., Mehta, J., et al. (2000). Secondary myelodysplastic syndrome/acute myeloid leukaemia following mitoxantrone-based therapy for breast cancer. *British Journal of Cancer, 83,* 91–94.

Senkus-Konefka, E., Konefka, T., & Jassem, J. (2004). The effects of tamoxifen on the female genital tract. *Cancer Treatment Review, 30,* 291–301.

Stott, H., Fox, W., Girling, D.J., Stephens, R.J., & Galton, D.A. (1977). Acute leukemia after busulphan. *BMJ, 2,* 1513–1517.

Travis, L.B., Curtis, R., Glimelius, B., Holowaty, E., Van Leeuwen, F., Lynch, C., et al. (1995). Bladder and kidney cancer following cyclophosphamide therapy for non-Hodgkin's lymphoma. *Journal of the National Cancer Institute, 87,* 524–530.

Tucker, M.A., Coleman, C.N., Cox, R.S., Varghese, A., & Rosenberg, S.A. (1988). Risk of second cancers after treatment for Hodgkin's disease. *New England Journal of Medicine, 318,* 76–81.

Van Leeuwen, F.E., Klokman, W.J., Hagenbeek, A., Noyon, R., van den Belt-Dusebout, A.W., van Kerkhoff, E., et al. (1994). Second cancer risk following Hodgkin's disease: A 20-year follow-up study. *Journal of Clinical Oncology, 12,* 312–325.

Wall, R.L., & Clausen, K.P. (1975). Carcinoma of the urinary bladder in patients receiving cyclophosphamide. *New England Journal of Medicine, 293,* 271–273.

IX. Post-Treatment Care

Because of advances in cancer care, experts estimate that, soon, 1 in 900 people ages 15–45 will be a survivor of childhood cancer (Dreyer, Blatt, & Bleyer, 2002). The increasing number of childhood cancer survivors over the past decade has brought to light the special needs and issues that survivors must face. Nurses have an important role in the continuing care of survivors. This role includes monitoring, assessing, and treating children and adult survivors for the effects of treatment that emerge long after the completion of therapy, as well as teaching survivors about leading a healthful lifestyle and how to minimize the late effects for which the survivors may be at risk.

The survival rates for many childhood cancers have been improving at a remarkable pace, such that the overall cure rate for pediatric malignancies is now greater than 75% (Dreyer et al., 2002). Currently, there are an estimated 270,000 survivors of childhood cancer in the United States. As of 1997, about 1 in 640 adults ages 20–39 is a childhood cancer survivor (National Cancer Policy Board, 2003). With the development of curative therapy for most pediatric malignancies, the result is a growing population of survivors with potential side effects related to treatment and their disease.

A. General principles (Hudson, 2000)
   1. After completion of therapy, care must include both surveillance for disease recurrence and monitoring for chronic or late effects of the disease or treatment. The intervals between follow-up visits may vary, but follow-up visits must continue at least annually for life.
   2. Information about "late effects" is an emerging body of knowledge that is growing larger as the number of survivors and duration of survival increase.
      a) Clinicians must be open to discovering effects as the understanding of effects evolves.
      b) Specialty clinics are available for patients or as resources for community clinicians (Keene, Hobbie, & Ruccione, 2000).
   3. Chronic or late effects may be exacerbated by (Boice, 2001)
      a) Drugs or drugs administered
      b) Length of treatment
      c) Total amount of drug received over time
      d) Age
      e) Radiation.
   4. Age is an important factor in regard to the development, extent, and effect of post-treatment conditions (Dreyer et al., 2002).
      a) Developing organs may be especially vulnerable to the effects of medication and radiation.
      b) Older people may be unable to compensate for lost function.
   5. The severity of late effects is directly related to the size of chemotherapy doses.
   6. Early recognition of problems and appropriate interventions may minimize long-term problems.

B. Classification of effects
   1. Timing
      a) Early effects: Effects that occur during treatment or immediately after treatment
      b) Late effects: Effects that occur more than six months to one year after completion of treatment
   2. Course
      a) Recovering
      b) Stable
      c) Progressive
   3. Types of effects
      a) Physical effects: See Table 34.
      b) Psychosocial: Psychosocial effects may increase with physical late effects of disease or treatment. Psychosocial effects may influence the following (Donohoe, 2000; Wiard & Jogal, 2000).
         (1) Development: Emotional adjustment, maturity, and independence
         (2) Relationships: Socialization, partnerships, marriage, and parenting
         (3) Political or social issues: Employment, insurability, and educational assistance

C. Nursing assessment (Hudson, 2000)
   1. Take a history. Include information about the following.
      a) Chemotherapy, surgery, and radiation received
      b) Toxicities noted during therapy
      c) Physical and psychosocial systems
      d) Preexisting diseases that may exacerbate effects or contribute to synergistic effects
   2. Perform a physical exam. Pay special attention to actual and potential problems noted in the history. Record patients' height, weight, pulse, respiration rate, and blood pressure.

Table 34. Late Effects Associated With Childhood Cancer Treatments

Organ System	Risk Factors	Potential Late Effects	Evaluation/Interventions
Central nervous system—cognitive	Methotrexate (high-dose IV or IT) ARA-C (IT or high-dose intervention)	Learning disabilities Leukoencephalopathy	Arrange for the following. • Neurocognitive testing • Psychoeducational assistance • A CT or an MRI scan (at baseline and when there are symptoms) • An EEG • An audiogram • Vision screening • A neurologic consultation as indicated • Educational and vocational testing • Referral to school liaison program
Central nervous system—peripheral neuropathy	Vincristine Vinblastine Etoposide Cisplatin	Generalized weakness Tingling and numbness Foot drop Paresthesias Areflexia	Arrange for a thorough neurologic examination on an annual basis. Encourage the patient to protect the affected area from exposure to extreme temperature. Arrange for physical/occupational therapy. Provide a referral to pain team (for neuropathic pain management).
Ophthalmology	Steroids	Cataracts	Recommend an annual ophthalmoscopic exam. Assess for a decreased red reflex. Patient may require cataract extraction.
Ears/hearing	Carboplatin Cisplatin—cumulative dose $\geq$ 360 mg/m^2	Sensorineural high-frequency hearing loss Tinnitus Vertigo	Perform baseline audiogram BAER and then one every two to three years and at every three and five years if abnormal; follow every year until stable, then every three years. Examine the canal. Recommend preferential seating in school, amplification, and hearing aids, as indicated. Patient may require speech therapy, as indicated. Consult with an ENT, an audiologist, and a neurologist, as indicated.
Dental	Vincristine Dactinomycin Methotrexate Mercaptopurine Cyclophosphamide Procarbazine Mechlorethamine	Abnormal tooth and root development, thinning or shortening Dental caries	Recommend orthodontic evaluations as indicated. Provide periodontal prophylaxis. Obtain radiographic studies of irradiated bone every three to five years. Recommend dental examination and hygiene every six months. Promote regular fluoride applications.

(Continued on next page)

Table 34. Late Effects Associated With Childhood Cancer Treatments *(Continued)*

Organ System	Risk Factors	Potential Late Effects	Evaluation/Interventions
Cardiovascular	Anthracyclines > 300 mg/m^2 > 200 mg/m^2 with radiation therapy to the thorax (including chest, mantle, mediastinal, whole lung, and spinal) Other chemotherapy, primarily high-dose cyclophosphamide Radiation > 3,000 cGy to mediastinum, or whole lung or mantle > 2,500 cGy when given with anthracyclines > 3,000 cGy to spine Total body irradiation Female gender Black race Younger than age five at treatment	Arrythmias Cardiomyopathy Pericardial damage	Obtain MUGA/echo, EKG, and chest x-ray (baseline and then < 300 mg/m^2: every five years; < 300 mg/m^2 plus radiation to the heart: every two years; ≥ 300–400 mg/m^2: every two years; ≥ 300 mg/m^2 plus radiation to the heart: yearly; ≥ 400 mg/m^2: yearly. Refer to a cardiologist, as indicated. Use Holter monitor and have exercise testing done as clinically indicated. Patient may require cardiac medication. Provide anticipatory guidance for symptoms of cardiac dysfunction and the side effects of cardiac medications. End-stage cardiomyopathy may require a heart transplant. Additional evaluation recommended for patients who receive > 300 mg/m^2 in the following situations. • Pregnancy • Prior to initiation of exercise (especially isometric programs)
Respiratory	Bleomycin Busulfan Chlorambucil Mitomycin Methotrexate Cytarabine Carmustine Lomustine Vinca alkaloids, alkylating agents Increased with radiation dose ≥ 4,000 cGy Combination of radiation and radiation-sensitizing chemotherapy	Pneumonitis Fibrosis	Obtain a chest x-ray (baseline, then every two to five years, if normal). Perform pulmonary function tests, including diffusion capacity (baseline, then every three to five years if normal and prior to anesthesia). Perform a CT scan, which may help to define lung volumes. Perform a ventilation quotient scan, as indicated. Prescribe pneumococcal and influenza virus vaccines annually. Refer patient to a pulmonologist, as needed. Provide education regarding healthy behaviors, avoidance or cessation of smoking, and maintaining physical conditioning. Treat the patient's symptoms with corticosteroids, bronchodilators, expectorants, antibiotics, oxygen, and bedrest, as needed. Provide anticipatory guidance for those who have received bleomycin regarding the risk of pulmonary failure with high levels of oxygen (avoid scuba diving).
Gastrointestinal	Doxorubicin Dactinomycin; radiation therapy enhances methotrexate and 6-mercaptopurine	Fibrosis, strictures, obstruction Enteritis Adhesions Ulcers	Obtain height and weight on an annual basis. Obtain stool guaiac on an annual basis, and perform annual rectal examination after the age of 40 years. Obtain a CBC with mean corpuscular value on an annual basis. Obtain blood chemistries on an annual basis. Provide anticipatory guidance regarding dietary modification, as needed. Refer to or consult a gastroenterologist, as needed. Dilate the fibrotic or obstructed area. Obtain radiographic studies, as indicated. Educate the patient regarding medication administration and side effects, as needed. Educate the patient regarding a high-fiber diet.

(Continued on next page)

Table 34. Late Effects Associated With Childhood Cancer Treatments *(Continued)*

Organ System	Risk Factors	Potential Late Effects	Evaluation/Interventions
Hepatic	Dactinomycin, radiotherapy enhancer, methotrexate, 6-mercaptopurine	Fibrosis	Refer to or consult a gastroenterologist, as needed. Obtain the following. • Chemistry panel on an annual basis • Baseline hepatitis panel • Abdominal ultrasound or liver biopsy, as indicated to assess for hepatitis Patient may require dietary management for fibrosis. Hepatitis may require treatment with interferon. End-stage liver disease may require a liver transplant. Educate patient about healthy behaviors as well as avoiding alcohol or other hepatotoxic drugs. Educate patient regarding medication administration and side effects, as indicated.
Genitourinary	Cisplatin Ifosfamide Cyclophosphamide Supportive therapies Aminoglycosides Cyclosporine Amphotericin	Glomerular dysfunction (cisplatin) Tubular dysfunction (cisplatin and ifosfamide) Fibrosis, hypoplasia, or secondary malignancy of bladder (cyclophosphamide, ifosfamide) Hemorrhagic cystitis, (cyclophosphamide, ifosfamide)	Perform an annual examination with close attention to the patient's blood pressure, height, and weight. Obtain a urinalysis, BUN, creatinine, hemoglobin/hematocrit, creatinine clearance, or GFR (yearly). Consult a nephrologist or urologist as indicated for patients with hypertension, proteinuria, culture-negative hematuria, or progressive renal insufficiency. Patient may require low-protein, low-salt dietary modifications. Monitor serum sodium, potassium chloride, carbon dioxide, calcium, magnesium phosphorus (for those at risk for tubular dysfunction) (baseline; if normal, repeat every five years). Supplement magnesium and phosphorus as indicated. End-stage kidney disease may require dialysis or a kidney transplant. Patient may require medication for hypertension as indicated. Educate the patient regarding kidney health after a nephrectomy, recommend that the patient avoid contact sports and maintain hydration, and encourage the patient to wear a Medic Alert® bracelet. Provide anticipatory guidance related to potential problems with incontinence and infertility, as needed. Counsel/educate patient regarding prompt reporting of dysuria or gross hematuria.

(Continued on next page)

Table 34. Late Effects Associated With Childhood Cancer Treatments *(Continued)*

Organ System	Risk Factors	Potential Late Effects	Evaluation/Interventions
Reproductive—Testes	Alkylating agents (procarbazine, cisplatin, cyclophosphamide, ifosfamide, nitrosoureas [carmustine, lomustine], busulfan, mechlorethamine, melphalan, chlorambucil) Surgery (orchiectomy or peritoneal node dissection) Age (pubertal males have the highest risk for toxicity) Thyroid dysfunction	Oligospermia or azoospermia Ejaculatory or other dysfunction Infertility Hypogonadism	Assess pubertal history. Assess Tanner stage annually. Determine testicular size (volume and turgor). Obtain LH, FSH, and testosterone levels for delayed pubertal development and when it is clinically indicated. Obtain thyroxine and TSH levels. Refer to or consult with an endocrinologist when necessary. Perform semen analysis, as needed. Obtain a bone age film, as indicated. Obtain analysis of sperm at maturity and when clinically indicated. Provide anticipatory guidance regarding symptoms of testosterone deficiency or germ cell damage. Consult an endocrinologist when it is indicated. Provide fertility counseling. Educate the patient regarding performing testicular exams on himself. Provide education regarding hormone replacement therapy and side effects, if indicated. Educate the patient regarding prevention of osteoporosis and atherosclerosis.
Reproductive—Ovaries	Alkylating agents (procarbazine, nitrosoureas [carmustine, lomustine], busulfan, ifosfamide, cyclophosphamide, mechlorethamine, melphalan, chlorambucil)	Delayed menarche Delayed or arrested pubertal development Oligomenorrhea or amenorrhea after puberty Infertility Early menopause	Assess pubertal history. Assess Tanner stage annually. Obtain LH, FSH, and estradiol levels for delayed pubertal development and when it is clinically indicated. Obtain thyroxine and TSH levels. Obtain menstrual and pregnancy history. Obtain a bone age film, as indicated. Obtain an ultrasound of the ovaries, as indicated. Recommend measurement of basal body temperature. Consult with an endocrinologist when indicated. Provide anticipatory guidance regarding the symptoms of estrogen deficiency and early menopause. Provide fertility counseling and education regarding alternate strategies for parenting. Patient may require hormone replacement. Provide education regarding hormone replacement therapy and prevention of osteoporosis and atherosclerosis. Counsel women at risk for early menopause regarding fertility options.

(Continued on next page)

Table 34. Late Effects Associated With Childhood Cancer Treatments *(Continued)*

Organ System	Risk Factors	Potential Late Effects	Evaluation/Interventions
Musculoskeletal/growth	Steroids Vinca alkaloids Methotrexate	Muscle weakness Avascular necrosis	Make a careful comparison and measurement of irradiated and unirradiated areas. Obtain a bone age film as indicated. Obtain and plot on growth chart the patient's height, weight, and sitting height measurements annually. Perform radiographic studies of the irradiated area (baseline, yearly during rapid growth, and if normal, then every five years). Refer to or consult an orthopedist as clinically indicated. Encourage a routine physical exercise program for both range of motion and strengthening. Educate the patient about the importance of weight control and exercise. Provide anticipatory guidance regarding realistic expectations about potential growth and function of the affected area and educate regarding osteoporosis prevention with calcium and vitamin D. Treat exacerbating or predisposing conditions (e.g., hypogonadism).
Hematopoietic and immunologic	Chemotherapy • High doses for extended periods • Etoposide, teniposide • Alkylating agents—melphalan or nitrogen mustard	Hypoplastic or aplastic bone Frequent, recurrent infection Decreased immunoglobulin levels Overwhelming bacterial infection Acute myeloid leukemia	Obtain a CBC with differential. Perform a bone marrow aspiration as indicated. Obtain immunoglobulin levels as indicated. Obtain T cell studies as indicated. Consult with an immunologist when it is indicated. Encourage annual evaluations. Provide recommendations for asplenic individuals. • Prophylactic penicillin • Pneumococcal vaccine, meningococcal, *H. influenza* • Prompt treatment with symptoms of fever, chills, or infection Encourage patient to wear Medic Alert bracelet noting asplenia. Test for HIV.

BAER—brain stem auditory evoked response; BUN—blood urea nitrogen; CBC—complete blood count; CT—computed tomography; EEG—electroencephalogram; EKG—electrocardiogram; ENT—ear, nose, and throat (specialist); FSH—follicle-stimulating hormone; GFR—glomerular filtration rate; HIV—human immunodeficiency virus; IT—intrathecal; IV—intravenous; LH—luteinizing hormone; MRI—magnetic resonance imaging; MUGA—multiple-gated acquisition; TSH—thyroid-stimulating hormone

Note. From "Late Effects of Childhood Cancer: Definition and Overview" (pp. 261–266), by S.J. Bottomley in N.E. Kline (Ed.), *Essentials of Pediatric Oncology Nursing: A Core Curriculum* (2nd ed.), 2004, Glenview, IL: Association of Pediatric Oncology Nurses. Copyright 2004 by the Association of Pediatric Oncology Nurses. Adapted with permission.

3. Record the results of laboratory tests. At minimum, tests performed should be
   a) CBC, blood chemistry panel, urinalysis (Urinalysis should be performed at least yearly, or more often if results are abnormal.)
   b) Any tests that suggest history, physical examination, or previous treatment are necessary.
4. Perform imaging studies as indicated (e.g., chest x-ray).
5. Administer function testing as indicated (e.g., pulmonary function tests, echocardiogram).

D. Collaborative management (Hudson, 2000)
1. Coordinate follow-up visits with an oncologist, or refer patients to their primary physician.
2. Identify problems suggested by the history, physical exam, or test results. Develop a plan for medical intervention, follow-up, or referral.
3. Coordinate consultation or referral to specialists if problems require management.
4. Provide patient and family education.
   a) Teach the importance of maintaining a treatment record and health diary.
   b) Remind patients and significant others of the need to continue follow-up for life.
   c) Provide a summary sheet, and educate patients and significant others about the potential problems related to cancer therapy.
   d) Encourage health-promoting practices, such as limiting fat intake and alcohol use, exercising regularly, and avoiding tobacco.
   e) Teach proper medication administration and the signs of potential side effects.
5. Help patients to manage problems by identifying available resources.

References

Boice, J.A. (2001). Second malignancies after chemotherapy. In M.C. Perry (Ed.), *The chemotherapy source book* (pp. 1–24). Philadelphia: Lippincott Williams & Wilkins.

Donohoe, M. (2000). Social concerns of children with cancer. In G. Steen & J. Mirro (Eds.), *Childhood cancer: A handbook from St. Jude Children's Research Hospital* (pp. 471–476). Cambridge, MA: Perseus Publishing.

Dreyer, Z.E., Blatt, J., & Bleyer, A. (2002). Late effects of childhood cancer and its treatment. In P.A. Pizzo & D.G. Poplack (Eds.), *Principles and practice of pediatric oncology* (4th ed., pp. 1431–1461). Philadelphia: Lippincott Williams & Wilkins.

Hudson, M.M. (2000). Long term follow-up after childhood cancer. In G. Steen & J. Mirro (Eds.), *Childhood cancer: A handbook from St. Jude Children's Research Hospital* (pp. 505–515). Cambridge, MA: Perseus Publishing.

Keene, N., Hobbie, W., & Ruccione, K. (2000). *Childhood cancer survivors: A practical guide to your future*. Sebastopol, CA: O'Reilly & Associates.

National Cancer Policy Board. (2003). *Childhood cancer survivorship: Improving care and quality of life*. Washington, DC: Author.

Wiard, S., & Jogal, S. (2000). The psychosocial impact of cancer. In G. Steen & J. Mirro (Eds.), *Childhood cancer: A handbook from St. Jude Children's Research Hospital* (pp. 461–469). Cambridge, MA: Perseus Publishing.

X. The Clinical Practicum

A. Course description: The clinical practicum allows the nurse to apply the knowledge gained in the didactic component to direct patient-care situations. Emphasis is placed on the clinical skills that a nurse must demonstrate prior to being considered competent to administer chemotherapy and biotherapy (see Appendices 5 and 6).

B. Course objectives: At the completion of the clinical practicum, the nurse will be able to
1. Demonstrate proficiency regarding the safe preparation, storage, transport, handling, administration, and disposal of chemotherapy drugs and equipment.
2. Identify appropriate physical and laboratory assessments for specific chemotherapy agents.
3. Demonstrate skill in venipuncture, including vein selection, distention, and sterile technique.
4. Demonstrate skill in the care and use of various VADs.
5. Identify patient and family education needs in relation to specific chemotherapy agents.
6. Identify acute local or systemic reactions as a result of extravasation or anaphylaxis in association with specific chemotherapy drugs and appropriate interventions.
7. Demonstrate proficiency in the safe administration of chemotherapy and disposal of chemotherapy wastes and equipment.
8. Verbalize knowledge of institutional policies and procedures regarding chemotherapy administration.
9. Document pertinent information in the medical record.

C. Clinical activities
1. The nurse should be supervised by a qualified preceptor to ensure safe practice.
2. The preceptor and the nurse should establish specific objectives at the beginning of the clinical practicum. Ideally, the nurse and the preceptor should select a specific population of patients, and the nurse should assume responsibility for planning the care for these patients with supervision by the preceptor.
3. The length of time spent in the supervised clinical practicum should be individualized, depending on the nurse's ability and skill in meeting the specific objectives and institutional standards.
4. After the nurse becomes proficient and independent in administering nonvesicants, progression to vesicant administration can occur.
5. The nurse should verbalize to the preceptor potential adverse reactions, side effects, toxicities, and measures to prevent and/or manage these reactions.
6. Various clinical settings can be used for the nurse to demonstrate knowledge of chemotherapy administration. It may not be realistic for all settings or agencies to provide chemotherapy education and training. Other recommendations include
   a) Contracting with major institutions to credential nurses for specific needs (e.g., vesicant, nonvesicant, IV push, short infusion, continuous infusion)
   b) Creating a simulated lab to substitute for the clinical component when patients are not available.

D. Evaluation: An evaluation tool based on the practicum course objectives should be used to determine
1. The nurse's knowledge of chemotherapy drugs and the associated nursing implications
2. The nurse's knowledge of the necessary technical skills required for the administration of chemotherapy agents (e.g., venipuncture, VAD access and management, indwelling catheter management)
3. The nurse's knowledge of patient and family education, which should be initiated based on the chemotherapy administered
4. The nurse's knowledge of steps to be taken in the event of an untoward response following chemotherapy administration (e.g., anaphylaxis, hypersensitivity reaction, extravasation)
5. Following successful completion of the clinical practicum, the nurse should complete a skills inventory to demonstrate his or her ability to perform the four criteria described above. This can be done in a simulated setting (e.g., skills lab) or as a precepted experience in the clinical setting. It is recommended that the learner administer at least three chemotherapy agents under the supervision of trained personnel. Two should be administered by an IV push—the first should be a nonvesicant agent, the second should be a vesicant agent. Annual education is recommended, and the content should, at a minimum, emphasize any new information available.

Appendix 1. Nursing Flow Sheet[a]

Name____________________ **Age**________ **Diagnosis** ________________

Allergies ______________________________

Medical problems ____________________________

Date					
RN signature					
Type of visit					
VAD					
VAD flush					
Comments					
Vesicant location 1–5 R/L					
Reactions					
Mucositis 0–3					
Infection					
Rx					
Resolved					
Alopecia 0–3					
Bleeding Y/N					
Comments					
Diarrhea # episodes/24 hours					
Rx					
Constipation # BM/d/wk					
Normal/abnormal (N/ABNL)					
Rx					
Bladder symptoms 0–5					
Rx					
Relief Y/N					
Pain Y/N					
Sites					
Intensity 0–10					
Characteristics					
Analgesics					
Relief 0–10					
Relief adequate Y/N					
Comments					

[a]As used at Yale New Haven Hospital, New Haven, CT

(Continued on next page)

Appendix 1. Nursing Flow Sheet[a] *(Continued)*

Date					
Insomnia Y/N					
Rx					
Rx effective Y/N					
Fatigue 0–10					
Nausea severity 0–3					
Vomiting # episodes/24 hours					
Duration					
Antiemetic relief					
Comments					
Appetite 0–4					
Diet 1–5					
Supplements, amount/24 hours					
Altered taste Y/N					
Other					
Cough Y/N					
Productive Y/N					
Rx					
Relief 1,2					
SOB 0–3					
O_2 specify					
Sexual difficulties 0–3					
Mobility 1–4					
Motor weakness 0–3					
Neuropathy 0–3					
Comments					
Anxiety 0–3					
Coping effectiveness Y/N					
Rx					
Counseling Y/N					
Homecare agency (specify)					
VNA/hospice					
HHA/homemaker					
Social services					
Patient education 1–7					
Education materials					
Other					

(Continued on next page)

Appendix 1. Nursing Flow Sheet[a] *(Continued)*

Nursing Flow Sheet Key	
Date	
RN Signature	
Type of visit	P = Phone C = Clinic
VAD	P = Port H = Hickman
VAD flush	Check, specify heparin amount.
Comments	Note difficulty drawing blood, etc.
Vesicant location	1–5, see diagram R = right/L = left
Reactions	Describe discomfort, burning, urticaria localized, follows vein path, entire extremity, phlebitis, extravasation (requires note), necrosis
Mucositis	0 = Absent 1 = Soreness 2 = Ulcerations, can eat 3 = Ulcerations, can't eat
Infection	Specify candida, herpes, bacteria, other.
Rx	Medication
Resolved	Check
Alopecia	0 = None 1 = Thinning 2 = 50% loss 3 = Complete hair loss
Bleeding	Y = Yes N = No
Comments	Specify sites
Diarrhea episodes	#/24 hours
Rx	Medication
Relief	Y = Yes N = No
Constipation	# BM/day/week
Normal/Abnormal	Above pattern normal for patient or not
Rx	Medication
Relief	Y = Yes N = No
Bladder side effects	0 = None 1 = Dysuria 2 = Frequency 3 = Hematuria 4 = Incontinence 5 = Oliguria
Rx	Medication
Relief	Y = Yes N = No
Pain	Y = Yes N = No
Sites	
Intensity	0 = No pain–10 = worst pain imaginable
Characteristics	C = Constant I = Intermittent
Analgesics	Medication, schedule
Relief	0 = No relief–10 = Complete relief
Relief adequate	Y = Yes N = No

Antecubital Space

2	Ventral Proximal Forearm	Dorsal Proximal Forearm	4
1	Ventral Distal Forearm	Dorsal Distal Forearm	3
		Dorsum of Hand	5

(Continued on next page)

Appendix 1. Nursing Flow Sheet[a] *(Continued)*

Nursing Flow Sheet Key	
Insomnia	Y = Yes N = No
Rx	Medication
Rx effective	Y = Yes N = No
Fatigue	0 = Quite rested–10 = Completely exhausted
Nausea severity	0 = None 1 = Mild 2 = Moderate 3 = Severe
Vomiting episodes	# vomiting episodes/24 hrs.
Duration	# hrs. after chemo vomiting started/stopped (e.g.,+3/+18)
Antiemetic relief	1 = Adequate 2 = Inadequate
Comments	
Appetite	0 = None 1 = 25% normal 2 = 50% normal 3 = 75% normal 4 = 100%
Diet	1 = Solids 2 = Liquids 3 = Soft 4 = 1,2 + Supplements 5 = Supplements
Supplements	Specify type and amount/24 hrs.
Altered taste	Y = Yes N = No
Comments	
Cough	Y = Yes N = No
Productive	Y = Yes N = No
Rx	Medication
Relief	1 = Adequate 2 = Inadequate
SOB	0 = None 1 = Mild 2 = Moderate 3 = Severe
O_2	Specify liter flow.
Sexual difficulties	0 = None 1 = Mild dysfunction 2 = Moderate dysfunction 3 = Severe limitations
Mobility	1 = Ambulatory 2 = Ambulatory with assist 3 = Wheel chair 4 = Bedridden
Motor weakness	0 = None 1 = Mild 2 = Moderate 3 = Severe
Neuropathy	0 = None 1 = Paresthesias, numbness/tingling feet and/or fingers 2 = Slapping gait, ataxia 3 = Visual, auditory disturbances
Comments	Location, etiology of muscle weakness, etc.
Anxiety	0 = None 1 = Mild 2 = Moderate 3 = Severe
Coping effectiveness	Y = Yes N = No
Rx	Medication
Counseling	Y = Yes N = No
Homecare agency	Specify name of agency, date initiated and discharged.
VNA/hospice	Check
HHA/homemaker	Check, note hrs./day or week
Social services	Check
Patient education	1 = Chemo side effects 2 = Symptom management 3 = Emergency 4 = Homecare resources 5 = Community 6 = Coping 7 = Specify
Education materials	Pamphlets or brochures given, videos used, etc.
Other	Other (e.g., complaints, problems, appliances [ostomies, trach, etc.])

Note. From "A Nursing Flow Sheet for Documentation of Ambulatory Oncology," by J.M. Moore and M.T. Knobf, 1991, *Oncology Nursing Forum, 18,* pp. 933–939. Copyright 1991 by the Oncology Nursing Society. Reprinted with permission.

Appendix 2. Chemotherapy Flow Sheet[a]

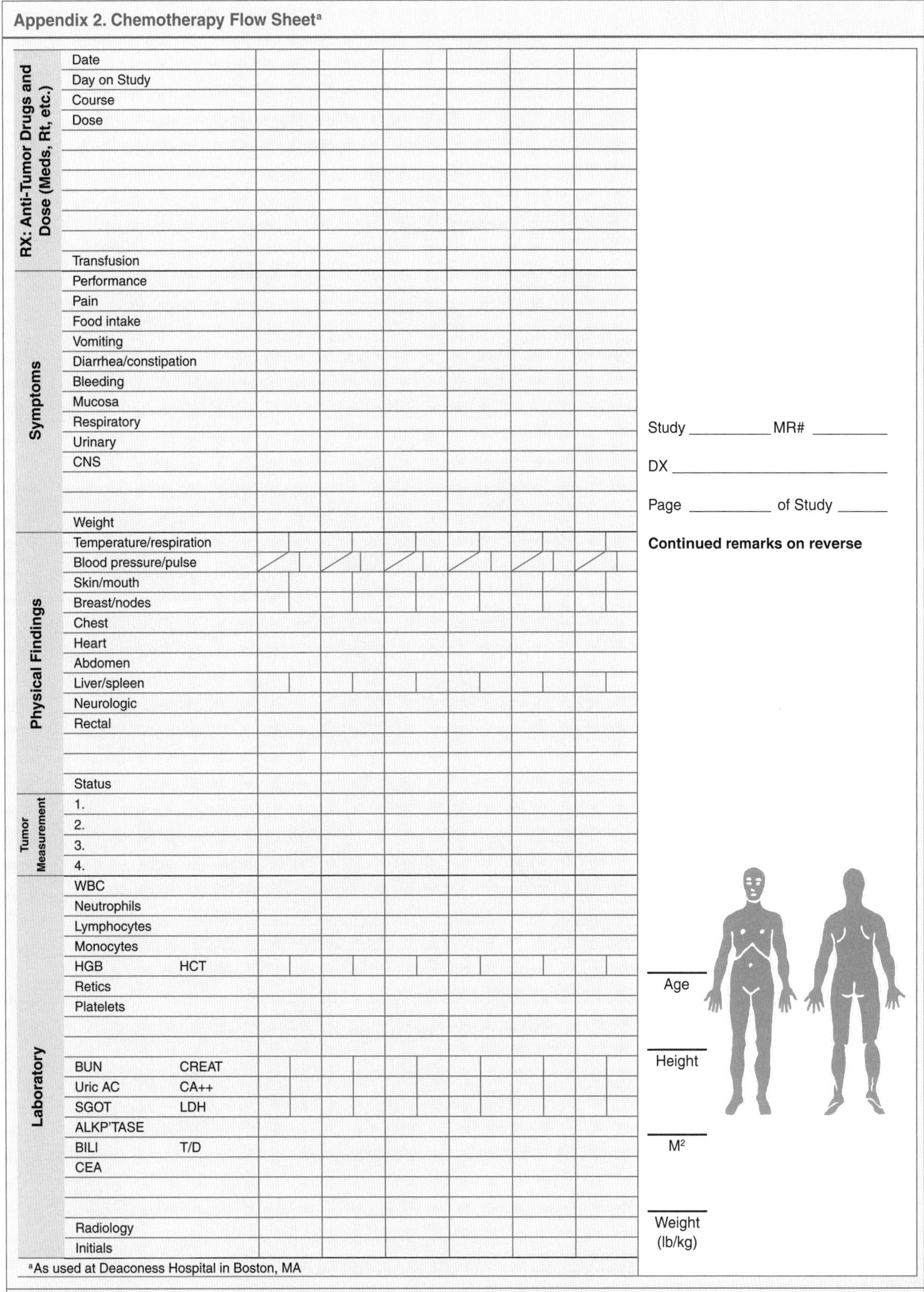

RX: Anti-Tumor Drugs and Dose (Meds, Rt, etc.)	Date						
	Day on Study						
	Course						
	Dose						
	Transfusion						
Symptoms	Performance						
	Pain						
	Food intake						
	Vomiting						
	Diarrhea/constipation						
	Bleeding						
	Mucosa						
	Respiratory						
	Urinary						
	CNS						
	Weight						
Physical Findings	Temperature/respiration						
	Blood pressure/pulse						
	Skin/mouth						
	Breast/nodes						
	Chest						
	Heart						
	Abdomen						
	Liver/spleen						
	Neurologic						
	Rectal						
	Status						
Tumor Measurement	1.						
	2.						
	3.						
	4.						
Laboratory	WBC						
	Neutrophils						
	Lymphocytes						
	Monocytes						
	HGB HCT						
	Retics						
	Platelets						
	BUN CREAT						
	Uric AC CA++						
	SGOT LDH						
	ALKP'TASE						
	BILI T/D						
	CEA						
	Radiology						
	Initials						

Study __________ MR# __________

DX ____________________________

Page __________ of Study ______

Continued remarks on reverse

______ Age

______ Height

______ M^2

______ Weight (lb/kg)

[a]As used at Deaconess Hospital in Boston, MA

(Continued on next page)

Appendix 2. Chemotherapy Flow Sheet[a] *(Continued)*

Administration	Date						
	IV site						
	Needle type and size						
	Adverse reaction						
	Treatment schedule: drug and adminstration method						
Patient Teaching	Instructions per institutional instruction sheet for:						
	1. Nausea/vomiting						
	2. Myelosuppression						
	3. Mouth						
	Self-care measures per institutional standards						
Nursing Observations/Assessments/Management	Acknowledgment of initial teaching (patient signature)						
	Nurse:						

Key: I = Initial teaching R = Reviewed W = Written materials P = See progress note N/A = Not applicable S = Side effects verbalized or reported

RN			RN			RN			RN
RN			RN			RN			RN

Note. From "Flowsheet Documentation of Chemotherapy Administration and Patient Teaching," by M. Lynch and L. Yanes, 1991, *Oncology Nursing Forum, 18,* pp. 777–783.

Appendix 3. Safe Management of Chemotherapy in the Home

You are receiving chemotherapy to treat your cancer. You must take special precautions to prevent the chemotherapy from coming into accidental contact with others. This document teaches you and your family how to avoid exposure to chemotherapy and how to handle the waste from the chemotherapy in your home.

Chemotherapy Drugs Are Hazardous

Chemotherapy drugs are hazardous. Equipment or items that come into contact with the medicines (such as syringes, needles) are considered contaminated. Regardless of how you take the medications, chemotherapy remains in your body for many hours and sometimes days after your treatment. Your body eliminates the chemotherapy in urine and stool. Traces of chemotherapy also may be present in vomit.

Disposal of Hazardous Drugs

Materials contaminated with chemotherapy must be disposed of in specially marked containers. You will be given a hard plastic container labeled "Chemotherapy Waste" or a similar warning. Place equipment and gloves that have been in contact with chemotherapy into this container after use. If the waste is too large to fit in the plastic container, place it in a separate plastic bag and seal it tightly with rubber bands. Place sharp objects in the hard plastic container. The company supplying your medicines and equipment will tell you who will remove the waste containers.

Body Wastes

You may use the toilet (septic tank or sewer) as usual. Flush twice with the lid closed for 48 hours after receiving chemotherapy. Wash your hands well with soap and water afterward, and wash your skin if urine or stool gets on it. Pregnant women should avoid direct contact with chemotherapy or contaminated waste.

Laundry

Wash your clothing or linen normally unless they become soiled with chemotherapy. If that happens, put on gloves and handle the laundry carefully to avoid getting drug on your hands. Immediately place the contaminated items in the washer and wash as usual. Do not wash other items with chemotherapy-soiled items. If you do not have a washer, place soiled items in a plastic bag until they can be washed.

Skin Care

Chemotherapy spilled on skin may cause irritation. If this happens, thoroughly wash the area with soap and water, then dry. If redness lasts more than one hour or if irritation occurs, call your doctor. To prevent chemotherapy from being absorbed through the skin, wear gloves when working with chemotherapy, equipment, or waste.

Eye Care

If any chemotherapy splashes into your eyes, flush them with water for 10–15 minutes and notify your doctor.

Questions and Answers

Is it safe for family members to have contact with me during my chemotherapy?
Yes. Eating together, enjoying favorite activities, hugging, and kissing are all safe.

Is it safe for my family to use the same toilet as I do?
Yes. As long as any chemotherapy waste is cleaned from the toilet, sharing is safe.

What should I do if I do not have control of my bladder or bowels?
Use a disposable, plastic-backed pad, diaper, or sheet to absorb urine or stool. Change immediately when soiled and wash skin with soap and water. If you have an ostomy, your caregiver should wear gloves when emptying or changing the bags. Discard disposable ostomy supplies in the chemotherapy waste container.

What if I use a bedpan, urinal, or commode?
Your caregiver should wear gloves when emptying body wastes. Rinse the container with water after each use, and wash it with soap and water at least once a day.

What if I vomit?
Your caregiver should wear gloves when emptying the basin. Rinse the container with water after each use, and wash it with soap and water at least once a day.

Is it safe to be sexually active during my treatment?
Ask your doctor or your nurse this question. It is possible that traces of chemotherapy may be present in vaginal fluid and semen for up to 48 hours after treatment. Special precautions may be necessary.

How should I store chemotherapy at home?
Store chemotherapy and equipment in a safe place, out of reach of children and pets. Do not store chemotherapy in the bathroom, as high humidity may damage the drugs. Check medicine labels to see if your chemotherapy should be kept in the refrigerator or away from light. Be sure all medicines are completely labeled.

(Continued on next page)

Appendix 3. Safe Management of Chemotherapy in the Home *(Continued)*

Is it safe to dispose of chemotherapy in the trash?
No. Chemotherapy waste is hazardous and should be handled separately. If you are receiving IV chemotherapy at home, you should have a special waste container for the chemotherapy and equipment. This includes used syringes, needles, tubing, bags, cassettes, and vials. This container should be hard plastic and labeled "Hazardous Waste" or "Chemotherapy."

Can I travel with my chemotherapy?
Yes. Usually, traveling is no problem. However, because some chemotherapy requires special storage (such as refrigeration), you may need to make special arrangements. Check with your nurse, doctor, or medicine supplier for further instructions. Regardless of your means of travel (airplane, car, or other), always seal your chemotherapy drugs in a plastic bag.

What should I do if I spill some chemotherapy?
You will have a spill kit if you are receiving IV chemotherapy at home. In the event of a chemotherapy spill, open the spill kit and put on two pairs of gloves, the mask, gown, and goggles. Absorb the spill with the disposable sponge. Clean the area with soap and water. Dispose of all the materials—including gloves, mask, gown, and goggles—in the chemotherapy waste container.

Note. Based on information from International Agency for Research on Cancer, 2004.

Appendix 4. Progression of Intravenous Extravasation

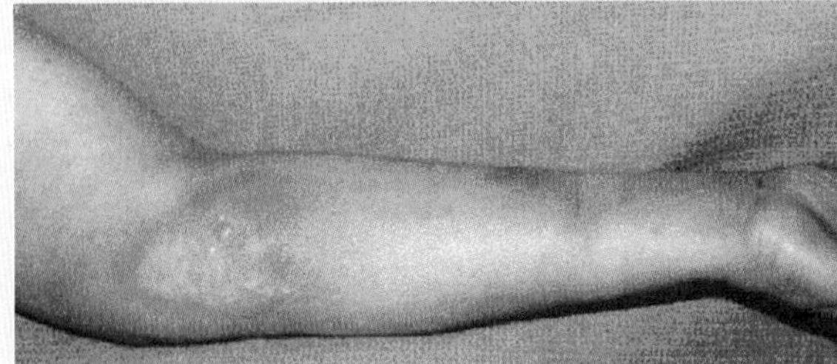

Photo 1. Erythema and Blistering

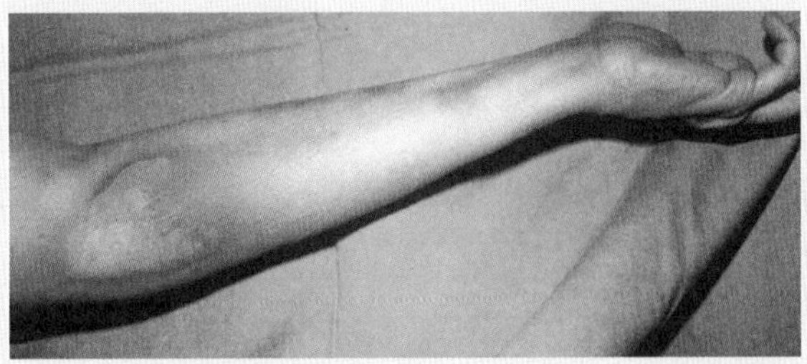

Photo 2. Painful Erythema and Beginning Tissue Necrosis

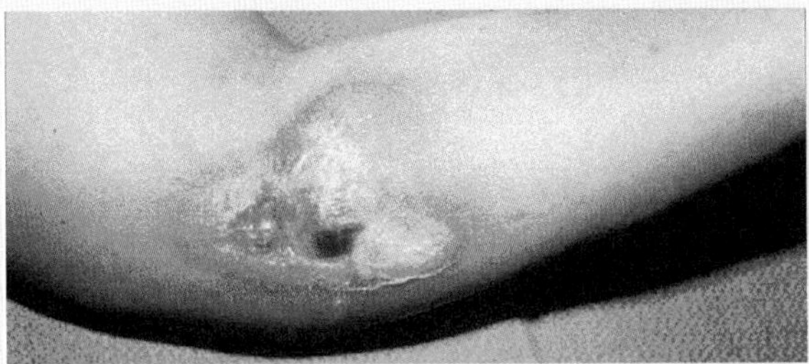

Photo 3. Progressive Necrosis and Ulceration

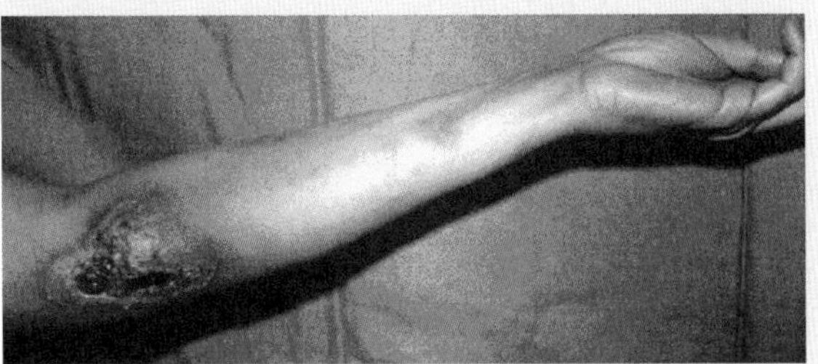

Photo 4. Surrounding Tissue Beginning to Heal

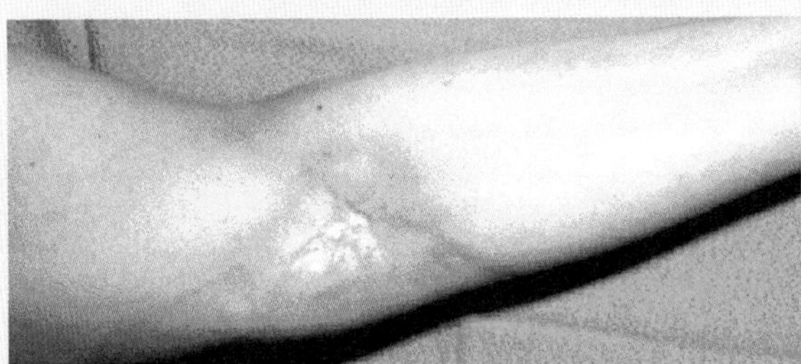

Photo 5. Healing Tissue With Resulting Tissue Defect

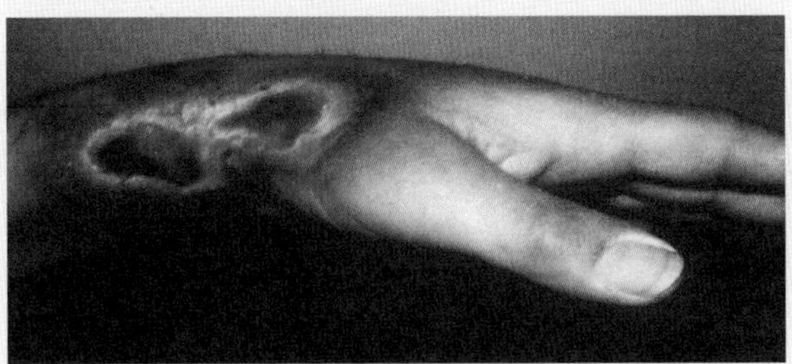

Photo 6. Severe Tissue Necrosis Secondary to Vesicant Extravasation

Note. Photos 1–5 are courtesy of Shirley Gullo, RN, MSN, OCN®, Cleveland Clinic Foundation; Photo 6 is courtesy of Rita Wickham, RN, PhD, AOCN®. Used with permission.

Appendix 5. Clinical Practicum Evaluation: Part I

Cancer Chemotherapy Administration Competency Record

Name ____

Chemotherapy-competent RN evaluators must validate competency on three occasions. Administer at least one vesicant under supervision.

RN Evaluators	Date	Drugs Administered

	Initials		
PRIOR TO ADMINISTRATION			
1. Coordinates time of administration with pharmacy and others as needed.			
2. Verifies that consent for treatment is signed.			
3. Checks that laboratory values are within acceptable parameters and reports results to MD/NP as needed.			
4. Verifies that original order is transcribed correctly.			
5. Recalculates BSA and drug doses.			
6. Checks chemotherapy order for drug, dose, schedule, and route.			
7. Verifies that patient education, premedication, prehydration, and other preparations are completed.			
ADMINISTRATION			
1. Compares original order to delivered drug (checks with RPH or RN).			
2. Verifies patient identification.			
3. Applies gloves and gown and uses safe-handling precautions.			
4. Verifies adequacy of venous access and appropriate IV-site selection.			
5. Checks IV patency and flushes line with 5–10 cc NS.			
6. Demonstrates safe administration:			
• Pushes through side arm, or at hub closest to patient; checks patency every 3–5 cc (or less if working with pediatric patients)			
• Ensures appropriate rate of administration			
• Flushes between drugs			
7. Demonstrates appropriate monitoring/observation for specific acute drug effects.			
8. Verbalizes appropriate action in the event of extravasation.			
9. Verbalizes appropriate action in the event of hypersensitivity reaction.			
AFTER ADMINISTRATION			
1. Flushes line with at least 5–10 cc NS.			
2. Appropriately removes device or flushes/maintains VAD.			
3. Disposes of chemotherapy waste according to procedure.			
4. Documents medications, education, and patient response.			
5. Communicates post-treatment considerations to patient, family members, and appropriate personnel.			

Appendix 6. Clinical Practicum Evaluation: Part II

Check the appropriate column to indicate whether the nurse performs the listed activities at a satisfactory level. If the nurse has not had the opportunity to carry out a particular activity, check the N/A (not applicable) column. Under Comments, provide examples of how the nurse met each objective or performed each activity.

	Yes	No	N/A
1. Participates in interdisciplinary care planning with physicians, nurses, and other healthcare professionals (e.g., home care or dietary workers). Comments:			
2. Anticipates complications of chemotherapy and takes action to prevent or minimize the complications. Comments:			
3. Involves the patient and family in care planning and attempts to establish interventions specific to the individual needs of the patient. Comments:			
4. Instructs the patient about hair and scalp care and takes measures to minimize hair loss and preserve body image. Comments:			
5. Reviews laboratory indices and gives a myelosuppressed patient correct information about conserving energy and taking precautions against infection and bleeding. Comments:			
6. Identifies patients at risk for stomatitis and instructs them about oral hygiene and preventive measures. Comments:			
7. Demonstrates knowledge of the use of drug therapy, relaxation, and diversional therapies in the prevention and management of nausea and vomiting. Comments:			
8. Instructs the patient about the prevention and management of gastrointestinal complications (e.g., constipation, diarrhea). Comments:			
9. Identifies and takes nursing action to prevent or manage potential or actual allergic reactions. Comments:			
10. Takes appropriate precautions in the preparation, handling, and disposal of chemotherapy. Comments:			
11. Demonstrates knowledge and skill in the assessment, management, and follow-up care of extravasation. Comments:			
12. Demonstrates skill in assessing the patient's need for a venous access device and knows the factors to be considered in selecting one type of device over another for a particular patient. Comments:			
13. Demonstrates knowledge of research trials by participating in data collection, drug administration, patient education, and follow-up. Comments:			

Index

The letter *t* after a page number indicates relevant content appears in a table; the letter *f,* in a figure.

C

D

E

F

G

H

N

O

T

U

V

W

Y

Z